Psychosomatic Classics

Psychosomatic Classics

Selected Papers from 'Psychosomatic Medicine', 1939–1958

Edited by a Committee from the Editorial Board
of 'Psychosomatic Medicine' consisting of
L. A. GOTTSCHALK, M.D., Davis, Calif.
P. H. KNAPP, M.D., Boston, Mass.
M. F. REISER, M. D., New Haven, Conn. (Editor-in-Chief, 'Psychosomatic Medicine')
J. D. SAPIRA, M. D., Pittsburgh, Pa.
A. P. SHAPIRO, M. D., Pittsburgh, Pa. (Chairman)

53 figures, 30 tables

19 72

S. Karger · Basel · München · Paris · London · New York · Sydney

S. Karger · Basel · München · Paris · London · New York · Sydney
Arnold-Böcklin-Strasse 25, CH-4000 Basel 11 (Switzerland)

Contents

Foreword

Psychosomatic medicine as a specific and sophisticated discipline is sufficiently youthful so that we can still, without too much difficulty and also without playing favorites, select a moderate number of examples of its best writings. The volume to which this is a foreword is composed of fourteen such contributions. They are all of American origin. This is not to imply that excellent work has not been done elsewhere. The present volume, however, was planned to contain papers written in this country and for the Journal *Psychosomatic Medicine*.

Since its beginning in 1939, to the present, our Journal has published 1,236 articles, plus two supplements. These had been culled from roughly twice the number submitted. In other words, a rigorous screening was exercised in their original selection. The present volume is composed of further selections chosen by a committee of experienced editors, who were charged with picking approximately fourteen articles, all of which ranked high in the minds of this committee.

A word should be said about the method of selection. The total number decided upon, namely, thirty-two, were judged on a scale of ten, and of these the ranking fourteen have been included in this volume. There were, of course, others of high merit, but in the opinion of the committee the final list here presented was a good one both from the point of view of interest and excellence of argument.

The first paper chosen was written by the late and greatly lamented Dr. FRANZ ALEXANDER, in 1939, as part of a symposium on Hypertension. This was printed in Vol. 1, No. 1, of *Psychosomatic Medicine*. In the same tissue he presented his tentative hypothesis of the Emotional Factors in this puzzling symptom complex, a theoretical formulation which by and large has withstood the test of time. The same issue contained his germinal article on the Psychological Aspects of Medicine, in which he distinguished between Conversion Hysteria, Organ Neurosis and Disturbances of Psychogenic Origin, thereby setting the stage for his subsequent psychosomatic studies and delimiting the field. I shall not attempt to outline all of the excellent work by Alexander and his collaborators which had its beginnings with our Journal and much of which appeared in its pages.

Skipping now the intervening decades, we come to two papers, one by LAWRENCE E. HINKLE, Jr. *et al.;* the other by J. W. MASON and his collaborators. These papers both appeared in Vol. 20 in the year 1958. They represent a sophisticated development in our field. The paper by HINKLE essays to correlate frequency of illness with certain biographical facts and is part of a larger study with the late HAROLD WOLFF of man's adaptation to his total environment. Mason and his collaborators demonstrated that the incidence of gastro-intestinal disease is significantly greater in a population of rhesus monkeys which had been subjected to chronic behavioral conditioning than in a control group of monkeys not so conditioned. Both papers introduce or emphasize important concepts in the field of psychosomatic medicine, the one based on statistical evidence, the other on experimental studies. They represent approaches not restricted to personal dynamics but inclusive of social factors as well.

I shall not attempt to comment specifically on the other contributions. They were selected with forethought and care, with an eye to being representative of some of the best work published in this Journal during the past twenty years.

I am honored to have been asked to write a foreword to this volume, representing as it does excellent work as judged by a committee of the authors' peers.

During the years of the Journal's existence, and as the discipline matured, psychosomatic medicine has undergone natural developmental changes. It began with a reformer's proselytizing zeal, striving to influence all of medicine and its ancillary sciences. Its chief aim then was to humanize medicine, which had become increasingly mechanized, to the detriment, it was thought, of patient care. The emphasis was on treating the patient as a whole person and striving always to find those emotional dynamic factors which might be held responsible for certain abnormal bodily processes. Great emphasis was placed on the notion of specificity.

As in all young sciences, new methods were needed. The descriptive ones which ushered in psychosomatic medicine soon proved wanting, although without them there could have been no beginning. Before long, new methods were introduced, borrowed from physiology, biochemistry, and dynamic psychiatry, and later from sociology, mathematics and statistics. Psychosomatic medicine thus became a congeries of basic sciences. Its continued growth and development will depend on our fundamental understanding of these sciences, and also of course on our ability to ask the right questions of nature.

This volume should be looked upon not as embodied evidence of pride or self-satisfaction, but as a milestone in our slow but we hope steady scientific enlightenment.

CARL A. L. BINGER, M. D.
Harvard University
Cambridge, Mass.

A Study of an Infant with a Gastric Fistula[1]

I. Behavior and the Rate of Total Hydrochloric Acid Secretion

G. L. ENGEL, F. REICHSMAN and H. L. SEGAL

Retrospective comment by Dr. I. A. Mirsky. Major new directions in the progress of science result from two distinct phenomena. One such turning point ensues from what may be best referred to as the 'intuitive leap' such as exhibited by EINSTEIN with his theory of relatively, by PAULING with the a helix, and by CRICK and WATSON with the concept that phylogeny is encoded in the sequence of nucleotides in the DNA that comprise the genes. Similar epochal developments ensue when the unusually intuitive, perspicacious observer meets a serendipitous event such as FLEMING's observations which led to the discovery of penicillin and BEAUMONT's observations on Alexis St. Martin which led to the modern era of gastroenterology. In both categories belong the studies by ENGEL and his colleagues on their now famous Monica. Their observations yielded new data, new approaches and new concepts on psychophysiologic integrations, the genesis of depression, the precipitation of various clinical disorders and other insights that mark the following as a classical contribution to physiology, psychology and sociology.

Since the classic investigations of BEAUMONT on Alexis St. Martin, a number of individuals with gastric fistula have been studied, mainly from a physiological point of view. WOLF and WOLFF's [1] classic study of Tom was the first systematic effort to relate manifest behavior, emotions, and gastric function in such a patient. MARGOLIN [2] subsequently psychoanalyzed such a patient and attempted to relate gastric activity and unconscious mental processes. Although a few observations of children [3] have been made, to our knowledge no detailed psychophysiologic investigation of an infant with a gastric fistula has been reported. This is a study of an infant girl with a congenital atresia of the esophagus on whom a gastric fistula was established in the fourth day of life. We began our research when the child was 15 months old and made detailed observations of behavior and gastric secretion until she reached the age of 22 months, when a substernal colonic anastomosis between esophagus and stomach was formed. During these 6 months we observed the child in 59 experiments and collected more than 600 specimens of gastric juice. This paper is a report on those data that have been analyzed to date. The literature will be discussed when all the material has been analyzed and prepared for publication.

History of the Infant

The infant girl, Monica, was born during July, 1952, in a small hospital about 90 miles from Rochester, New York. When it was discovered 2 days after her birth that she regurgitated all fluids, she was referred to the Pediatric Service of the Strong Memorial Hospital, where a diagnosis of congenital atresia of the esophagus was made.

[1] From the Departments of Psychiatry and Medicine of the University of Rochester School of Medicine and Dentistry and the Strong Memorial and Rochester Municipal Hospitals, Rochester, N.Y.

The next day a cervical esophageal fistula was established, and the day thereafter a gastric fistula. After a smooth postoperative course Monica was discharged, having been hospitalized for ten days. The mother was instructed to feed the baby through the gastrostomy on a four-hourly schedule. The parents were also told that when she was four to five months old, the child should receive an operation that would allow her to swallow normally.

At the time of Monica's birth her parents and her 20-month-old brother lived in the maternal grandmother's home. Our knowledge of this setting, particularly of the emotions and attitudes of the figures around Monica, is somewhat limited because of the guardedness of the parents in their communication with us and with others interested in the child. The mother was 19 years old when Monica was born. She appeared a child-like, timid woman, obviously dominated by her husband. She usually allowed him to do the talking and when faced directly with a question, often answered in a questioning tone through her husband. The father, 13 years older than the mother, was employed as a long distance truck driver. He spoke volubly and glibly and presented himself as a forthright, solid citizen. We know from other sources that he is considered unreliable and irresponsible. Both parents were brought up on farms, with restricted social background and limited education, but they seemed to have average intelligence.

Both parents were 'frightened' when the malformation was discovered, and particularly by the baby being taken to Rochester. At first they communicated with the doctors at the Strong Memorial Hospital by telephone only and had difficulty comprehending Monica's condition and what was being done for her. When Monica came home from the hospital, the mother was squeamish and anxious about the gastrostomy and the gastric tube. She could not reinsert the tube without 'feeling faint' and at times could not bring herself to do it at all. Furthermore, she was afraid to fondle and hug the child for fear of disturbing the gastric tube, which she regarded, with some justification, as the baby's lifeline.

For the first 5 months of her life, while she lived at the grandparents' house, Monica gained weight and to all observers seemed to be developing adequately. During this time the grandmother helped materially with the care of the malformed infant, picking her up when she cried and holding her on her lap for long periods. Toward the end of 1952 the relationship between the father and his inlaws, which apparently had been strained for some time, worsened. An open conflict erupted, particularly over the grandparents' handling of the children, and the parents decided to move. At about the same time, in December, two other events took place. The operation that Monica was to undergo about that time did not take place because, for some administrative reasons, the state aid to cover hospitalization costs did not materialize. Furthermore, the mother discovered that she was pregnant again. Throughout this unplanned and unwanted pregnancy she was afraid that this infant also might be defective.

In December, 1952, the family moved to an isolated farmhouse. During this winter they were snowed-in repeatedly for days at a time, on some occasions when the father was away on one of his trips. It was at this time that Monica started to go downhill. The mother said, 'She acted tired out, like a person who is discouraged.' Because the parents were quite reticent, we can only conjecture about the relationship between mother and child. We know the mother was a very dependent, immature woman who, in this situation, thrown on her own resources, was afraid to get too close to the child.

Monica's downhill course continued through the spring of 1953, while the parents made several moves in rapid succession (allegedly to avoid payment of rent). Her condition was further aggravated when she contracted chicken pox in May. She was described by the parents as 'cranky and irritable' and as 'crying all the time'. She began to refuse the sugar nipple that the mother had given her to suck before and during gastric feedings, in accordance with the doctor's instructions. The parents began, instead, to give her lollipops. Monica also would become quite excited during meal time and if sitting on a parent's lap would attempt to grab and devour any food she could reach. Swallowed food, of course, ran out through the esophageal fistula. She had failed to gain weight for some time and now began to lose weight. After a brief admission to a local hospital she was again referred to the Strong Memorial Hospital in June, 1953, where she arrived looking marasmic. The nurse described her as 'very neglected' and 'lethargic'. She was not studied by us on this admission.

During a hospitalization of one month Monica improved considerably, both physically and emotionally. She maintained this improvement at home for about one month, until the mother gave birth to a baby girl at the end of August. Following this event Monica's condition again declined sharply. She became very irritable and fretful and seemed particularly disturbed when the baby sister was held or fed. When the baby was held near her, Monica would push her away or claw at her. During this period she was particularly avid for food by mouth. When she heard her mother setting the table she cried to be fed by mouth, and when given juices by spoon, 'she couldn't get enough'. Within a few weeks she lost the weight she had gained during her hospitalization, and because of her increasing marasmus she was readmitted to the Pediatric Service on October 12, 1953; she was 15 months old and weighed 4,500 g. She was cachectic and the pediatric house officer described her as 'very depressed'. She was unable to sit up or even to turn over in bed.

During the first 2½ months in the hospital she gained only 1 kg. By the end of 5½ months she showed considerable improvement in strength and her weight had reached 7,500 g. During this time she became quite attached to one of the nurses and to one of the investigators, both of whom became quite attached to her.

During her 9 months in the hospital. Monica's parents visited only seven or eight times, three of these visits around the time of the operation. At times the social worker and public health nurse had to make extensive efforts to contact the parents. Because their visits were infrequent and unpredictable, we unfortunately have no direct observations of Monica's response to her parents. The nurses, however, reported that Monica always recognized them and responded with signs of pleasure. We do not know whether this response was immediate or delayed. The father was more active with her and she was reported to be more responsive in general to him than to the mother. The parents' visits were brief and they occasionally left her a small gift.

The nurses and doctors openly expressed their feeling that the parents were not sufficiently interested in Monica and that particularly the father seemed insincere in his display of affection and expression of interest. Some of them looked upon Monica as a deserted waif and were especially attentive to her for this reason. Throughout the prolonged period of hospitalization Monica became something of a celebrity and there was great interest in the outcome of her case. For some ward personnel she became 'the darling of the ward', a few resented the special attention she received. At the outset some of the hospital personnel identified the investigators with Monica's persecutors, but later most considered the interest of the investigators to exert a beneficial effect. At the end of 5½ months she was deemed physically fit for colonic substernal anastomosis between esophagus and stomach. After a somewhat stormy postoperative course, Monica regained her preoperative developmental level, and during the next 6 months she learned to feed herself, to stand, and to walk with help. She also developed some speech. Her subsequent development will be the subject of another paper.

The historical data are summarized below.

4   ENGEL/REICHSMAN/SEGAL

Summary of History

July 1952. Birth. Second day admitted to Strong Memorial Hospital, weight 2,700 g. 3rd day cervical esophostomy. 4th day gastrostomy. 10th day discharged home, weight 2,970 g.

Aug. 1952 to Dec. 1952. At maternal grandparents' home. Cared for by grandmother and mother. Gained weight.

Dec. 1952 to Jan. 1953. Friction between parents and grandparents. Monica and family move to isolated farm home. Mother pregnant – unplanned. Monica's operation postponed through administrative tangle.

Jan. 1953 to May 1953. Monica begins to go downhill. Tired, irritable, loss of weight. Mother frequently alone with children.

May 1953. Family moves several times. Chicken pox – rapid decline. Admission to Hornell Hospital.

June 1953. Admission to Strong Memorial Hospital, weight 4,830 g. Condition stabilized. Discharged in one month.

July 1953. Return to home weighing 5,180 g.

Aug. 1953 to Oct. 1953. Baby sister born. To grandmother's house for 5 days. Further decline until admission to Strong Memorial Hospital on October 12, 1953.

The Design of the Study

Basic to the design of this study is the concept that the experimenter is part of the experiment. An infant with a gastric fistula through which gastric juice is being aspirated manifests behavior in relation to the person withdrawing the gastric juice. The baby is behaving always in some way in relationship to the experimenter, the experimenter in some way to the baby, and the behavior of each is modified thereby. To this extent we are dealing with a transactional system which must itself be observed. We, therefore, regard the more or less naturally developing relationship between the baby and the experimenters as a behavioral variable, not to be controlled, but to be observed carefully and recorded by

one or more observers behind a one-way vision screen.

A second major premise of this study is that human behavior and associated physiological processes cannot be expected to follow the imposed time schedule of the experimenter. Since a variety of significant events, known and unknown, precede any period of observation, and since to a large degree baby and experimenter influence each other in unpredictable ways from the moment the two come in contact, we discard the concept that regards the initial period of observation of any experiment as a base line or control for what follows. Instead, we assume that we deal with analogical, that is, continuous, functions that are being observed simultaneously in different conceptual frameworks – physiologic, interpersonal, behavioral – and that from these can be derived categories or classes, any two or more of which can be compared. The methodologic problem is to set up categories that are clearly identifiable or measurable by any observer. In this study we measured by chemical techniques a variety of components of gastric juice and by observational techniques a variety of categories of behavior. For each specimen of gastric secretion there were corresponding observations of the behavior during the time that the gastric juice was being secreted and aspirated. The more than 600 specimens of gastric juice obtained provide ample material for statistical analysis.

Actual operation of the study was carried out as follows: During the 5 months there were 59 observation periods during which gastric juice was examined, 44 fasting and 15 after eating. Only the 44 fasting observations are reported in this paper. In nearly all experiments one of us (F.R.) was the experimenter, but on 13 occasions the experimenter was a relative stranger to the baby. The observation periods occurred 2–4 times per week and each lasted from 1–5 h, making a total of 161 h. Most of the studies took place in the laboratory, with the observers behind a one-way vision screen; some were in a cubicle on the infant

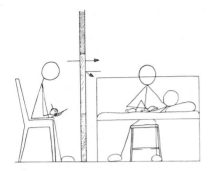

Fig. 1. The experimental set-up in the laboratory. The experimenter withdraws gastric juice and makes behavioral observations. The observer records behavior of baby and experimenter from behind a one-way vision screen.

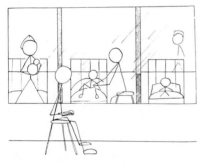

Fig. 2. The experimental set-up on the ward. The baby and experimenter were in a cubicle, while the observer was behind a glass partition. The observer was visible to the baby, as were nurses, doctors, attendants, and other babies concerned in ordinary infant ward routine.

ward with the observer behind a glass partition, visible to the baby. In the latter setting the usual activities of a busy infant ward were visible and audible to the baby, experimenter, and observer (fig. 1, 2). Additional sources of psychological data were:

Sources of Psychological Data
(1) Interview with parents. (2) Interview with public health nurse. (3) Daily diary of Miss D., pediatric nurse. (4) Spot observa-

tions of pediatric resident staff. (5) 1–3 hour observation periods on ward by Mr. CHIN-CHINIAN and Mr. WRIGHT. (6) Multiple daily visits by Dr. REICHSMAN. (7) Psychological testing by Dr. PARSONS. (8) 1–5 hour observation periods in ward or laboratory with simultaneous gastric analyses.

Both the experimenter and the observer(s) behind the screen made detailed minute-by-minute notes on the behavior of the baby (and of the experimenter) that was apparent to them. The experimenter either made brief notes or dictated his observations to a secretary who was out of the baby's view. Thus for each experiment there were two or more detailed behavioral protocols, which were subsequently analyzed into discrete categories. Clock time was meticulously recorded so that for the period of collection of each gastric juice specimen the corresponding behavioral data were available. (The criteria for the behavioral categories are presented later.)

Particular attention was paid to the development of object relationships between Monica and the various experimenters. F.R. quickly became the favored experimenter, and the relationship became highly invested on both sides. Within the framework of this relationship, Monica manifested her more advanced ego development. When new experimenters were introduced they were first experienced as strangers, from whom Monica withdrew, lapsing into a state that we have called the 'depression-withdrawal reaction'. This is discussed in more detail elsewhere [4]. With repeated contacts, this reaction became attenuated and Monica made efforts to establish contact with the new experimenter. The experimenter was not instructed specifically how he should respond to these overtures. The depression-withdrawal response was always alleviated promptly when the stranger left and F.R. returned. F.R.'s return invariably evoked unmistakable signs of pleasure. These characteristic responses to different experimenters offered a convenient method of studying the behavioral and gastric secretory responses to variations in object relationships. When pediatric care necessitated procedures such as catheterizations we obtained behavioral and secretory data characteristic of such periods of external stress.

Physiological Methods

Our physiological observations were purposely limited to studies of secretion. The small diameter of the gastric stoma would have necessitated interruption of aspiration for the study of mucosal color or of gastric motility; we thought it of greater importance to aspirate gastric secretion as completely as possible.

Gastric aspiration was performed by gentle manual suction on a 20 cm³ syringe attached by a metal adapter to a No. 18 rectal tube which fitted somewhat loosely into the small gastrostomy opening. By alternating the tube between the fundus and pylorus of the stomach secretions were aspirated as completely as possible. Both volume of secretion and the length of time it took to collect the specimen were accurately recorded. During the earlier experiments there were often pauses of 5–10 min between the individual gastric specimens, but later aspiration was carried on almost continuously. The volume of the individual specimen was determined by the necessity of obtaining at least 3–4 cm³ of secretion for the determination of pH, hydrochloric acid, and pepsin. Our physiologic measurements are as follows:

Gastric Analyses
(1) Gross appearance. (2) Volume of secretion in cm³/min. (3) pH. (4) Concentration of free and total HCl in mEq/cm³. (5) Rate of secretion of free and total HCl in mEq/min. (6) Concentration of pepsin in units per cm³. (7) Rate of secretion of pepsin in units per minute.

Of these we will deal in this paper only with the rate of secretion of total hydrochloric acid expressed in milliequivalents per minute. The concentration of total

hydrochloric acid was determined by titration with 0.1 N NaOH, using phenolphthalein as the indicator. The rates of secretion were calculated only when the stomach had been emptied of gastric juice immediately before the sample was collected and the exact time of collection and the exact volume of the sample were available. In most instances the interval between specimens did not exceed 3–4 min, and usually was one min. We arbitrarily excluded any specimen in which the preceding interval exceeded the duration of the specimen; in most instances the interval was much shorter.

In this paper we are reporting on 389 specimens of gastric juice in which the rates of total hydrochloric acid secretion in the fasting state were calculated.

Psychological Methods

In considering the psychological-behavioral observations, one should keep in mind that we were dealing with an infant with a chronological age of 15–21 months but who was much retarded physically and mentally. Monica was unable to sit up and she did not speak at all. Gesell rating at the age of 16 months was approximately 4–8 months; at 22 months it was 9–15 months[2]. Behavioral observations were therefore limited to recumbent bodily positions and movements, facial expressions, and a variety of inarticulate, but quite expressive, sounds. Although at first glance this may appear a serious limitation of the study, we believe that it was more than offset by the opportunity to observe a human being at a level of development at which emotions are expressed without any or with only slight disguise.

Our observations were recorded without preconceived ideas of what behavioral categories should be studied; only at the completion of the study were the various categories established. After criteria had been

[2] We are indebted to Dr. FRANCES PARSONS for these data.

established, the protocols of the observer and the experimenter were independently analyzed by two of us (G.E. and F.R.), without knowledge of or reference to the results of the gastric analyses. The independent judgments were then compared. With the rare exceptions noted below, there was agreement. The behavioral categories reported in this paper are as follows:

(a) Affects. (b) Object relations (OR). (c) Non-nutritional oral behavior (NNOB). (d) Sleep-waking status. (e) Non-nutritional feeding experiences (NNF).

We shall now discuss our criteria for identifying and classifying the different behavioral categories.

Affects

In this study we consider affects to be revealed by primary behavioral patterns that express the dynamic steady state of the organism and the deviations therefrom. We believe the basic behavioral pattern expressing the affect to be innate and essentially unlearned; it involves innervations of both the autonomic and voluntary nervous systems. Monica being in a preverbal stage no psychic representations of effect or manifestations of secondary process were observable. On the other hand, some affect, evoked by external or internal sources, was manifest during all observation periods except during sleep.

Our criteria for identifying affects were based on observations of posture, movements, facial expression, and vocalization that accompany the affects. The detailed descriptions by CHARLES DARWIN of the external manifestations of affects have been of great help to us [5]. Empathic responses of the observer were not unimportant in affect identification. Consistency of audience response to motion picture strips of the various affects has greatly enhanced our belief in the reliability of this method of classification.

In Monica we could identify 6 affects which we classify under two major headings:

Pleasure and *Unpleasure*. We distinguish two degrees of pleasure: *Contentment* and *Joy*; and 4 kinds of unpleasure: *Depression, Depression-Unpleasure, Irritation,* and *Rage,* the last two being different degrees of anger. These are illustrated in the accompanying photographs (fig. 3).

Contentment (fig. 3a)

This was a state of rather quiet relaxation. The posture was comfortable and uninhibited. It was appropriate for quiet play activity, self-stimulation, or repose. When she was flat on her back, her most usual position, her knees were usually flexed. Movements were generally slight and rather gentle, but occasionally more vigorous waving or reaching occurred. Movements included nodding and shaking the head; self-stimulatory scratching, rubbing, tickling, or oral manipulation; movements for manipulation of inanimate objects; movements toward a person, such as waving, touching with arms or legs, stroking, pinching, and reaching. The facial expression during contentment was placid, with not infrequent smiles, narrowing of palpebral fissures, and mimicking. Vocalization consisted of occasional cooing or gurgling.

Joy (fig. 3b)

This was a very active pleasure response. Movement overshadowed posture and usually was vigorous and almost continuous. It included waving, reaching, kicking with stretched legs, arching and turning of trunk. Facial expression was very active and mobile with much smiling and laughing. Vocalization consisted of almost continuous cooing, gurgling, or baby talk. Joy was marked by striking responsivity of the infant to the experimenter.

There was no sharp dividing line between these 2 degrees of pleasure. In general a period of observation was classified as joy either when the dominant behavior was as described above or when such behavior repeatedly broke through a background of contented behavior.

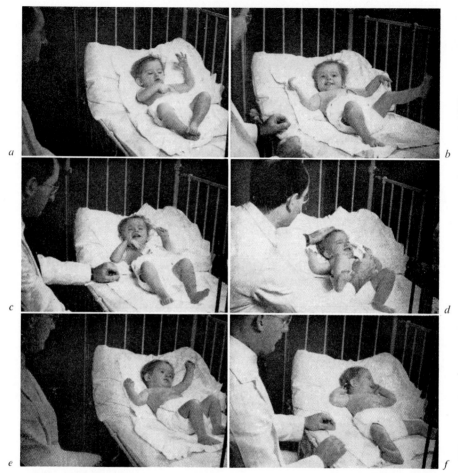

Fig. 3. Affects: (a) Contentment, (b) joy, (c) irritation, (d) rage, (e) depression, (f) depression-unpleasure. It is not possible to illustrate object relationship or non-nutritional oral behavior by photographs since evaluation of these categories depends on the sequence of behavior over a period of time. Motion pictures are the only effective means to do this. It is planned to make available soon a motion picture of the major behavioral data of this study.

Irritation (fig. 3c)

During this state Monica either had a relatively low tolerance to stimulation or was responding to disagreeable stimuli, as, for example, when intubation through the gastric stoma evoked pain or memory of pain. Under these conditions, stimuli that were ordinarily pleasurable often produced an unpleasurable effect. In this state her posture was relatively hypotonic; the legs often lay flat on the bed with the knees slightly bent. At the same time there was readiness for evasive movements, which were usually quick, slight, and jerky, with a tendency to turn away from the experimenter. Periods of muscular inactivity were interrupted by occasional self-stimulation. The facial expression was impassive, even to the usual pleasurable stimuli, or she responded with scowling or frowning. Vocalization consisted of whimpers, whines, or complaining grunts from time to time.

Rage (fig. 3d)

This was a vigorous and sometimes violent response to an excessive stimulus, be it pain or a threat, real or anticipated. Posture was stiff and vigilant at the same time. Movements were those of vigorous resistance and evasion: she arched her back, bounced her hips, and turned from side to side. She pushed, kicked, and hit with her extremities. At times the legs extended and interlocked scissor-like while she used her whole body as a lever. The facial expression was contorted, eyes were wide open or squeezed tightly shut. At times she covered her face with her arms. Her mouth was wide open, she cried, and her face was often reddened and moistened by tears. Loud crying, high-pitched wailing, screaming, and sobbing comprised her vocalizing.

As with joy and contentment, at times there was no sharp line dividing irritation and rage, and the observation period was classified under the predominant affect.

Depression[3] (fig. 3e)

The most striking feature of this state was the lack of movement and of any kind of activity. At the point of transition into depression, which always occurred in the presence of a stranger, movement ceased and the limbs tended to fall gravitationally. Posture remained hypotonic and flaccid; the arms were flexed along the head or body, and the legs also were in slight flexion. The extremities usually lay flat on the bed, although at times the knees were slightly elevated.

The trunk was either flat on the bed or slightly turned from the experimenter. The head was either turned away or straight ahead. Rarely she would look toward the

experimenter, sometimes without even turning her head. Either there were no bodily movements or, with less severe degree of depression, there were slight and slow movements, such as fingering inanimate objects, occasional scratching or tickling, or, rarely, turning the body and perhaps glancing at the experimenter. With severe degree of depression she closed her eyes and eventually fell asleep. When she was awake, her facial expression during this state was characteristic: the face sagged flabbily; the corners of the mouth were down; the inner parts of the eyebrows were elevated and the brow furrowed; all producing 'the omega of melancholy'. Although she was usually silent, there were occasional brief whimpers or wails.

Depression-Unpleasure (fig. 3f)

This reaction occurred during depression when the child could not entirely avoid external stimulation by withdrawing. Elements of the fight-flight pattern of the anxiety reaction were then superimposed upon the underlying depression. In contrast to depression, there was more tendency to flex the thighs on the abdomen and to turn away more actively from the experimenter, positions which were regarded as self-protective. Bodily movements were evasive and resistive and included turning, pushing, and arching the back. Such movements, however, were less vigorous and less well-integrated than similar ones during the rage response. Facial expression and vocalization included crying, wailing, whimpering, and sobbing, added to the underlying expression of depression; the brow became deeply furrowed, the face puckered, and the mouth opened in a square fashion. Occasionally there was flow of tears.

The question may be asked whether what we describe as depression might be an anxiety state in which the child became frozen with fear instead of showing the more usual hyperkinetic response of anxiety. We inves-

3 This term is used to denote the behavioral pattern of an affect which will be discussed later as the depression-withdrawal reaction [4].

tigated this possibility by recording electro-cardiographically on 4 occasions Monica's heart rate while she exhibited the withdrawal response in the presence of a stranger. Although marked tachycardia occurred during rage and depression-unpleasure, during depression, the heart rate either did not change or slowed slightly. Figure 4 illustrates one of these experiments. We consider this additional evidence that we are not dealing here with the anxiety reaction, in the sense of a preparation for flight or fight, but with some other reaction, which we chose to call depression-withdrawal, a matter discussed in more detail elsewhere [4]. We do recognize that free anxiety (anxiety reaction) is indeed present in the affects of irritation, rage, and depression-unpleasure.

Mixed Affect

When an affect changed during a specimen, this was designated as *mixed affect*. The usual change was from contentment to irritation or *vice versa*. The 25 mixed affect specimens have not been included in this report; they will be considered at a later time.

Comments

The identification from the protocols of the major affect categories – contentment and joy, irritation and rage, depression-unpleasure and depression – presented no difficulties. The investigators (G.E and F.R.), who independently categorized affects, always agreed on these major categories. There were occasional disagreements between contentment and joy and between irritation and rage. These disagreements were resolved by mutual discussion of the detailed recorded data. Audiences viewing motion pictures illustrating the various affects also found the affects readily distinguishable.

Object Relations (OR)

Monica's interest in things or persons in the environment, as expressed behaviorally,

was classified in different degrees of object relations (OR). We first established 5 such degrees but later reduced these to three when it became clear that the finer subdivisions, although easily distinguishable, did not differ materially in correspondence to the secretory data. Thus OR 2 and 3 were grouped together to become OR 2, and OR 4 and 5 became OR 3.

Object Relation 1

For the most part the child was motionless and relatively unresponsive. She did not look at the experimenter. Her eyes were often closed, and at most she glanced occasionally toward the observer. No activity could be interpreted as effort to contact the experimenter by either motor behavior or vocalization. Those activities that occurred were usually limited to small movements.

Object Relation 2

For the most part she was actively concerned with looking, examining, manipulating, dissecting, touching, or stroking such objects as a piece of gauze, a clamp, a piece of tubing, or parts of her body such as fingers, the stomal region, face, neck, feet. The motor patterns were appropriate for such activities and her attention was largely occupied by them. Occasionally she might look toward, smile at, or even touch the experimenter, while continuing the previous activity. More often she appeared oblivious of the experimenter.

Object Relation 3

In this category the child's visual, vocal, and motor behavior all were directed predominantly towards attracting, contacting, or maintaining contact with the experimenter. These included looking, calling, smiling, reaching, touching, grasping, stroking, hitting, pushing, and kicking the experimenter. Although they were infrequent, we regarded placing her fingers in the experimenter's mouth or bringing the experimenter's fingers to her mouth as patterns indicative of high OR.

Comment

Whenever mixtures of patterns occurred during the period corresponding to a specimen of gastric juice the evaluation was based on the pattern that predominated. The commonest mixture was OR 2 and 3. Much less common were occasions when OR 1 included short periods of OR 2, usually in the form of manipulation of some inanimate object; or mixtures of OR 1 and OR 3, when the activity of the experimenter evoked evasive movements or struggling. There were few disagreements between the two investigators in their judgments of degrees of object relation.

Non-nutritional Oral Behavior (NNOB)

Mouth activities not related to actual ingestion of food were classified in three categories:

NNOB 1. There was no (or only fleeting) oral behavior during the period of observation.

NNOB 2. The behavior during the observation period fell between NNOB 1 and NNOB 3.

NNOB 3. At least half the period was occupied with vigorous oral activity, or there was some kind of oral activity during the entire period.

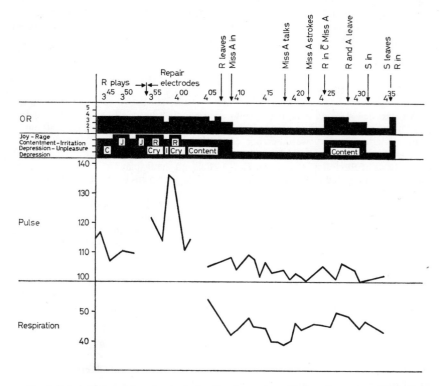

Fig. 4. Respiration and heart rate during the depression-withdrawal reaction. While there was a marked acceleration of heart rate during rage and irritation, both of which undoubtedly also included an element of fear, during depression there was no change or even a slight slowing. In this experiment 'Miss A' and 'S' were strangers, both of whom provoked the typical depression-withdrawal reaction.

Those classified as oral were activities in which the mouth and adjacent structures alone were involved, such as smacking, sucking, licking, protruding tongue, swallowing, and biting; activities involving fingers or hands and mouth, or objects and mouth, such as touching of lips, teeth, tongue or buccal mucosa, sucking, chewing, biting, and licking. In rare instances there was biting of the favored experimenter's finger, which was always classified as NNOB 3.

Comment
There were no disagreements between the identification of NNOB1 as compared to NNOB2 and NNOB3. Disagreements in t he judgment of NNOB2 and NNOB3 were few because the duration of oral activity was generally quite accurately recorded.

Sleep

We classified sleeping periods (1) depth and (2) the setting.

In the latter category we differentiated between *fatigue sleep* and *withdrawal sleep* on the basis of the following criteria. *Fatigue sleep* was preceded by yawning, stretching, scratching, seeking a comfortable position, and resisting any disturbance of this comfortable position. After the eyes had begun to close, they reopened only infrequently for an occasional glance. There was a gradual, fluctuating reduction of spontaneous activity preceding sleep, and the affects preceding it were those other than depression or depression-unpleasure.

A relative lack of yawning, stretching, and sleep positioning preceded *withdrawal sleep*. After the eyes had closed, they would reopen frequently to glance. During this period there was often a sustained, if quite low, level of activity. The preceding affect was depression or depression-unpleasure.

In classifying depth of sleep, we regarded arbitrarily as deep sleep all periods during which either no motor activity occurred or not more than one movement in 5 min. If

there was any more activity the period was classified as light sleep.

The first specimen obtained after falling asleep was not included under *sleep* unless Monica had been asleep for 10 min or longer.

Comment
There was no disagreement between the two investigators in their independent judgment of depth and kind of sleep.

Non-nutritional Feeding Experiences (NNF)

Two procedures were followed in observing the responses to feeding situations in which food did not reach the stomach.

Sham feeding. Lollipops and crackers were given by mouth, and the swallowed material was extruded through the esophageal fistula.

Bottle. The baby was shown or permitted to handle a bottle of her formula that was tightly stoppered so that no contents entered the mouth. Monica was accustomed to seeing her formula before receiving it through the fistula.

The specimens following non-nutritional feeding experiences were not included in the analysis of the behavioral categories in the fasting state.

Table I is a sample protocol of primary behavioral data and the corresponding analysis. We realize the inadequacy of providing such a small sample of our raw behavioral data. It is our intention to include all behavioral protocols when the completed study is published as a monograph.

Results

Some Typical Observations

From the total of 59 observation periods we present four as representative.

Observation No. 43 (fig. 5) illustrates spontaneous behavior in the laboratory

Table I. Sample protocol. Experiment No. 30, January 14, 1954

Spec. No.	Time	Observed behavior	Affect	OR	NNOB	Sleep
	10:16	On E4. M lying on back, knees drawn up. Right hand holding toy, left hand fingering neck. Watches us thru glass partition. Puts both hands to toy. Lies relatively motionless.				
	10:19	Doctors on rounds. M watches.				
	10:21	R arrives. M stretches legs out to him and smiles. She smiles at him. Exchange. Waves legs at R. R busy getting ready. Lowers bars. M reaches with arms and legs and smiles. R undressing M.				
	10:23	R takes off dressing. She whimpers a little. Watches him prepare tube. Finger at corner of mouth. Then beside head. R tries out glass electrode. M gives a little cry. R pleased and says it will work. M watches.				
	10:26	R inserts tube. Gives M paper. She picks up scissors and drops paper.				
1	10:26	Specimen. Playing with scissors. Miss D comes in view. M raises arms and legs to her. Miss D walks away. She looks after her. Tongue out. Moves restlessly. Pushes R's hands with foot. Crosses right leg on knee.				
	10:29	Holding scissors. Watching group behind glass. R takes her foot down and she kicks him. Holds scissors up. She smiles and coos. R coos. Smiles broadly. Bites on lower lip, M hears voices and looks behind her. Tongue out. Babies crying.	Content	3	2	—
	10:31	End specimen. Reaching. Tongue out. Finger in mouth. Both hands on mouth. Watching R who had taken scissors. R gives scissors back and after a few seconds takes them out.				
2	10:33	Specimen. M playing with scissors. Talking – smiles. Hears nurses and looks behind her. Holds scissors in right hand and touches syringe and tube with left. Holds scissors up with both hands. Holds right foot up. Tongue out. Miss D next cubicle. M smiles and reaches toward her. D turns back and M smiles and attends to scissors. D looks at her – they exchange smiles. Smiles at R. Tongue out. Smiles at D. Holds foot up.				
	10:37	Waves hand. Half smile. Wawawa. R answers. Smiles and laughs. R laughs. Miss D talks and she smiles. Handling scissors. Miss D looks and she grins and reaches. She puts scissors in mouth. Chews on them. Miss D reappears. M looks at her – back to her. Continues to chew on scissors. Raises foot toward D. D leaves without looking. She waves foot. Turns scissors around and puts handle in mouth. Smiles at R. He responds. Kicks at syringe. Holds it with left hand. Bites intermittently on scissors.	Joy	3	2	—

Table I. (Continued)

Spec. No.	Time	Observed behavior	Affect	OR	NNOB	Sleep
2	10:41	Puts it to side. Drops it. Tongue out. R gives her paper which she holds up. Leg up in air. Pulls at paper. Looks at R. Eh. R answers and she smiles. Awawawa. Pulls up kimono. Pulling at paper. Babies crying.	Joy	3	2	—
	10:43	End specimen.				
	11:15	In R-146. HS takes over. She looks wide-eyed.				
	11:16	In R-151. M looks wide-eyed. Eyebrows raised. Stares. S comes over. M begins to cry. Frowns. Omega. Hands up. Continues cry. S talks.				
	11:18	She cries vigorously. Tube in.				
5	11:19	Specimen. M quiet. Staring. Eyebrows raised. Hands beside head. Corners of mouth down. Looks to window. M looks up at S. Frowns. Eh. S answers. Whimper. Holding gauze. S makes noise and she startles. Tube out. Whimpers with tube in. Looks at S. Picks up metal, fingering it. Drops it. Picks up gauze. She whimpers. Red in face.	Depression-Unpleasure	2	1	—
	11:26	End specimen. Watches S. Playing with gauze. $3\frac{3}{4}$ cm^3 cloudy bile. S talking to us.				
7	11:47	Specimen. Looks to window. Looks back to S, stares at him. Looks to window. Staring with slight frown. Looks back. She sighs. Lying quietly. Looks toward S. Hands beside head, legs down. Arched brow. Stares at S. No movement, closing eyes. Eyes closed.	Depression	1	1	—
	11:53	Now is asleep. S says OK. End specimen. M awakens and looks at S. $4\frac{1}{2}$ cm^3 bile stained. Eh. Folds arms.				
8	11:54	Tube in. M whimpers and turns away from S. Cries as S manipulates. Lying on right with left arm over face. Staring toward window. Feet crossed. Lies motionless. Staring – eyes closed – open.	Depression	1	1	—
	11:57	Turns back toward S. Arms out. Closing eyes. Intermittent open and closed, but more closed.				
	11:59	Asleep.				
	12:05	Asleep – turns to right.				
	12:06	End specimen. S talks to us. She doesn't move, opens and closes eyes. Turns to left as S moves about. Puts crib side up and leaves. She looks toward door.				

with the favored experimenter. During the first $1\frac{1}{2}$ h the predominant affects were contentment and joy, object relation was mostly high, and there was intermittent non-nutritional oral behavior. During this period the rate of total hydrochloric acid secretion rose, and free acid appeared. Toward the end of this first period the baby became sleepy and then fell into a light sleep. With this the secretion of acid decreased markedly. During the 28-minute sleep the observer and experimenter disagreed as to how long to continue. The experimenter, who had a 1:00 p.m. appointment, wished to stop for lunch; the observer wished to secure data on the awakening period. The observer prevailed and the experimenter, somewhat disgruntled, resumed aspirating gastric juice. When the baby awakened, the experimenter was relatively uncommunicative, tended to be business-like and impersonal in collecting the specimen, and was relatively serious and unsmiling. As the baby responded with rage and irritation, secretion of acid increased sharply.

Observation No. 47 (fig. 6) illustrates the typical behavior with a stranger. Content

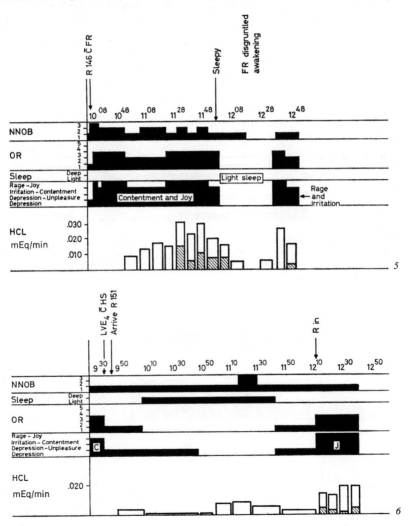

Fig. 5. Experiment No. 43: see text for description.
Fig. 6. Experiment No. 47: see text for description.

and outgoing for the first 10 minutes with the favored experimenter, she lapsed into the depression-withdrawal state when the strange experimenter arrived to take her to the laboratory. During the entire period with this experimenter she remained relatively motionless, turned away from the experimenter; her facial expression was sad. The affect was depression and the object relation was 1. There was no non-nutritional oral behavior. She closed her eyes; in about 30 min she was asleep and remained asleep

for 96 min. The secretion of acid was extremely low until the last 30 min of sleep, during which there was a slight rise; during this last 30 min of sleep there was active sucking. Upon awakening and finding the stranger still present, she remained in the depressed-withdrawn state and gastric secretion again fell to very low levels. With the return of the favored experimenter there was a joyful response and a prompt and sustained rise in the rate of acid secretion.

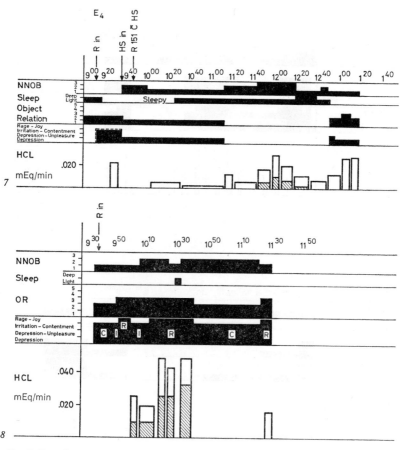

Fig. 7. Experiment No. 45: see text for description.
Fig. 8. Experiment No. 46: see text for description.

Observation No. 45 (fig. 7) also illustrates response to a stranger. It is of interest that the same response of depression-withdrawal was elicited and the rate of acid secretion was strikingly reduced; however, very active sucking behavior developed during the sleep period and acid secretion rose notably. Before her awakening the secretion of acid again diminished. After awakening the baby remained in the depressed state, but now made cautious overtures to the stranger. These consisted of slight rubbing and touching movements of her foot and hand. Although the experimenter did not respond, the secretion of acid increased.

Observation No. 46 (fig. 8) illustrates the high secretion of acid during a period of sustained irritation and rage. For reasons that were not clear, Monica had been fretful and irritable for two days. The skin around the stoma appeared somewhat reddened and may have been sensitive. The experimenter was firm in overcoming Monica's resistance to intubation. She responded with a vigorous rage reaction alternating with periods of irritation. When no aspiration was attempted, she was relatively content. The rate of hydrochloric acid secretion was high.

Affects

Figure 9 illustrates the range of rates of total hydrochloric acid secretion in mEq/min during the 6 affects. Each circle represents the rate of total hydrochloric acid secretion in one specimen of gastric juice collected during the period of the affect noted on the left. N refers to the total number of samples in each category. Mw is the mean secretory rate corrected for the mean collection time in each category.

While there is considerable spread within each affect, the data reveal that the secretion was lowest during depression (Mw $= 0.007 \pm 0.001$ mEq/min; N $= 31$) and highest during rage (Mw $= 0.027 \pm 0.003$; N $= 28$). Statistical analysis by t-test[4] shows

that the mean rate during depression was significantly less than during all other affects. These differences are significant at 0.01–0.001 levels, except for that with depression-unpleasure, which is significant only at the 0.02 level. The mean rate during rage was significantly higher than the mean rates during all other affects. The significance again is at the 0.01–0.001 levels except for the differences between irritation and rage which are significant only at the 0.02 level.

There were no statistically significant differences between rates of hydrochloric acid secretion during irritation, depression-unpleasure, contentment and joy.

Object Relations

These data are presented in figure 10. This reveals that the mean rate of total hydrochloric acid secretion during OR1 (Mw $= 0.006 \pm 0.001$; N $= 23$) is significantly less than during OR2 and OR3 (P <0.001). The mean rates for OR2 and OR3 were 0.018 ± 0.001 and 0.021 ± 0.001 mEq/min, respectively, a difference not statistically significant at the 5% level (t $= 1.82$; P $= 0.05$–0.1).

Sleep (fig. 11)

The rate of secretion of total hydrochloric acid was significantly less during sleep than during any wakeful state except during depression and object relation 1. There was no difference in secretion rates during light sleep and deep sleep. The secretion rate was less during sleep coming on during the depressed-withdrawal state (0.007 ± 0.001 mEq/min) than during sleep coming on as part of the pattern of fatigue (0.010 ± 0.001 mEq/min), but this difference is not statistically significant (P <0.1). Since

[4] We are grateful for advice on statistical methods to Dr. S. LEE CRUMP, Ass. Prof. of Radiation Biology and Chief of Section (Statistics), Atomic Energy Project, University of Rochester.

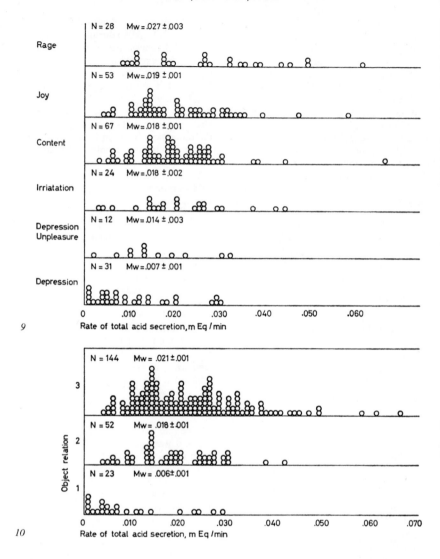

Fig. 9. Rates of total hydrochloric acid secretion in mEq/min during the various affects. Each circle respresents one specimen of gastric juice. N=the number of specimens. Mw=the mean weighted for the duration of the specimen. See text for significance of results.

Fig. 10. Rates of total HCl secretion in mEq/min and object relations (OR). See figure 9 and text for description of symbols and significance of results.

much higher rates of secretion generally preceded sleep-fatigue, in comparison with sleep-withdrawal, this difference may merely reflect a lag.

When we classified sleep specimens according to the amount of non-nutritional oral behavior during the sleep, we found a highly significant difference (P < 0.001) between hydrochloric acid secretion rates during periods of active sucking (sleep-NNOB 3 = 0.017 ± 0.001 mEq/min) in comparison with those with no sucking (sleep-NNOB 1 = 0.006 ± 0.001 mEq/min). This was already illustrated in figures 6 and 7.

In 2 experiments we were able to secure a continuous record of intragastric pH by placing within the stomach a glass electrode and a salt bridge extension of the calomel electrode. The pH was recorded on a photovolt pH meter. As illustrated in figure 12, when the baby fell asleep there was a fairly rapid rise in pH, after a lag of 10–20 min, corresponding to the affect preceding sleep.

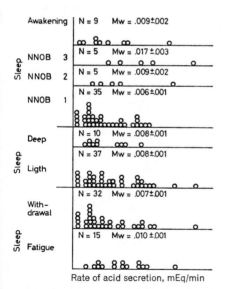

Fig. 11. Rates of total hydrochloric acid secretion during sleep. See text and figure 9 for description of symbols and for significance of results.

Then with sucking and other activity during sleep there were rapid decreases in pH, such fluctuations occurring until the baby awakened.

Histamine

Histamine diphosphate, in doses of 0.1 mg/10 kg body weight, was administered subcutaneously on nine different occasions. A striking correlation was found between the amount of acid secreted in response to this drug and the behavioral state of the infant. As illustrated in figure 13, when the baby was outgoing and relating actively to the experimenter, pleasurably or unpleasurably, the stomach secreted large amounts of hydrochloric acid in the 55 min after histamine administration, the total secretion ranging from 1.52–2.39 mEq. On the other hand, when she was depressed, withdrawn, or asleep, the same quantities of histamine were noted to have little or no effect. Total secretions were 0.16–0.68 mEq in 55 min, values which did not differ from those obtained in comparable behavioral states without histamine. The high rates, on the other hand, were considerably greater than those observed during comparable behavioral situations without histamine.

Range of Total Hydrochloric Acid Secretion Rates

Table II illustrates the mean fasting secretion rates of hydrochloric acid under the conditions so far analyzed. The highest mean rates occurred during sham feeding (0.035 ± 0.003 mEq/min) and feeding with the bottle of formula that she did not taste (0.039 ± 0.004 mEq/min).

It is noteworthy that individual specimens with higher secretion rates than those observed during sham feeding or feeding with the bottle occasionally occurred during rage, irritation, contentment, joy and OR 3. In these 4 affect categories there were 19 specimens (out of 172) in which secretion

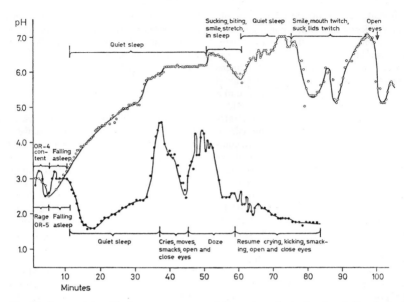

Fig. 12. Intragastric *p*H changes as measured by a glass electrode placed directly in the stomach. See text for description. It should be noted that *p*H is not charted on a semi-loga-rithmic scale and hence the fluctuations at the higher *p*H levels are relatively exaggerated.

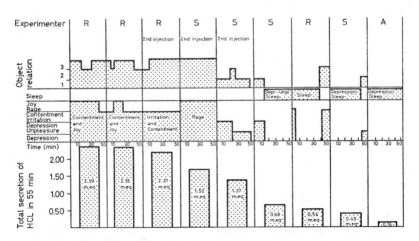

Fig. 13. Effect of histamine: Secretion is recorded as the output of total HCl in mEq in the 55 min after the histamine administration. When arranged in order of decreasing amounts, secretion is greatest in the outgoing states and least in the withdrawn states.

Table II. Total HCl-rates of secretion, mEq/min

Bottle	0.039 ± 0.003	Depression-unpleasure	0.014 ± 0.003
Sham feeding	0.035 ± 0.004	Sleep fatigue	0.010 ± 0.001
Rage	0.027 ± 0.003	Sleep-NNOB2	0.009 ± 0.002
Object relation 3	0.021 ± 0.001	Sleep-light	0.008 ± 0.001
Cry 2	0.021 ± 0.002	Sleep-deep	0.008 ± 0.001
Joy	0.019 ± 0.001	Depression	0.007 ± 0.001
Contentment	0.018 ± 0.001	Sleep-withdrawal	0.007 ± 0.001
Irritation	0.018 ± 0.002	Awakening	0.007 ± 0.002
Object relation 2	0.018 ± 0.001	Object relation 1	0.006 ± 0.001
Cry	0.017 ± 0.001	Sleep-NNOB1	0.006 ± 0.001
Sleep-NNOB3	0.017 ± 0.001	Depression-sleep	0.003 ± 0.001

rates ranged from 0.035 to 0.066 mEq/min. In OR3 there were 18 specimens out of 144 in which secretion rates were in excess of 0.035 mEq/min. In other words, the rates of secretion were consistently high in response to sham feeding and the bottle; however, sustained, active outgoing states were occasionally accompanied by secretion rates of a comparable order.

The lowest secretion rates occurred during the depressed, withdrawn state and during sleep. Rates of less than 0.001 mEq/min occurred occasionally during the sleep of the depression-withdrawal reaction, representing for all practical purposes a cessation of gastric secretion.

The table clearly indicates that when rates of gastric secretion are listed from the highest to the lowest, the corresponding behavioral processes fall from the most active and outgoing to the most withdrawn and inactive.

Discussion

We are aware that it is both tempting and hazardous to generalize from the study of a single infant. The detailed study of the single subject provides valuable information on the laws governing biological processes within that individual, but a different design is necessary to establish the range of variability of the same processes within a population. In this study we deal with a relatively unique individual, a baby born without continuity between mouth and stomach, who was fed for the first two years of her life through an opening in the abdominal wall. Food taken by mouth leaked out of an esophageal fistula in the neck. It is evident that this infant differs in a number of ways from infants without such a defect and that these differences in original endowment and in life experience resulting therefrom must be significant factors in her general development. In this sense she is a member of a population of infants who share the same defects and who may be studied as a group. On the other hand, she also shares many more qualities with infants not so afflicted and, therefore, can be viewed as part of the population of human infants. In discussing the findings of this investigation, the most reliable interpretations will be those that apply only to this one infant. Yet we will call attention to ways in which the data for this infant conform with, as well as differ from, data and concepts obtained from other sources, infant and adult. It remains for future study to establish their general validity.

Although many factors not investigated in this study undoubtedly influenced the rate of secretion of hydrochloric acid by the stomach in the fasting state (this is indicated by the wide spread of values in each behavioral category), it is nonetheless evident that gastric secretion was intimately integrated with the total behavioral activity of this infant. When the child withdrew and her activity was low, as during the depression-withdrawal state and sleep, there was marked reduction, at times almost cessation, of hydrochloric acid production. When she related actively to the experimenter, be it with pleasure or anger, the rate of hydrochloric acid secretion rose. The *highest* mean secretion rate occurred during rage, during which state she related most actively to the object in the environment and during which she appeared to have the least control over instinctual drives. Another situation that regularly evoked very active secretion was reunion with the favored experimenter after a period with a stranger. Under these circumstances hydrochloric acid secretion rates were sometimes as high as those during sham feeding. Even in sleep, during which the rate of acid secretion regularly diminished, sucking and other oral activity were accompanied by a highly significant increase in secretion. We interpret this behavior during sleep as expressing a returning contact with the outside world or its mental representations, that is, either awakening or dreaming.

These data suggest that in this infant, at the level of development at which she was studied, the processes whereby relationships with objects in the external world are established include a general intaking, assimilative organization in which the stomach participates as if the intention is also to take objects into it. In other words, along with other behavioral activities, such as reaching, touching, grasping, looking, hitting, pushing, kicking, all of which take very active cognizance of the object in the environment, the stomach also behaves as though preparing for food, as if that which is in external world is literally to be ingested and digested.

We also regard these findings as evidence that the oral phase of development in the infant, as postulated by FREUD, is indeed accompanied by corresponding physiologic activity of the stomach. Further, it would seem that such an oral phase represents not a behavioral organization that is necessarily dependent on the continuity of the connection between mouth and stomach, but rather a total assimilative pattern that includes activities in the service of feeding and the organs associated therewith. From this it appears that the genesis of early object relations includes an assimilative process, largely orally organized. The processes concerned in establishing mental representations of objects and their libidinal and/or aggressive cathexes involve an essentially oral, intaking model. In Monica the secretion rates of hydrochloric acid paralleled in a highly significant way the other behavioral expressions of object cathexes, libidinal or aggressive. Such a finding was predicted from the discoveries of psychoanalysis; whether this is a general phenomenon remains to be established from the study of a series of infants within the first year of life. Theoretically we would predict that this close correlation between gastric secretion and behavioral processes would diminish with further development of the mental apparatus. Whether regression to the oral phase in later life would also involve the corresponding physiological regression, a suggestion by ALEXANDER for the pathogenesis of peptic ulcer, remains to be demonstrated experimentally [6].

Whether the increased gastric secretion may be merely part of a general increase in the physiological activity of the body and not have the specific meaning we have proposed cannot be settled from a consideration of the data of this study. There is evidence, however, that vigorous muscular activity is usually associated with a decrease rather than an increase in acid secretion [7]. Further clarification may be obtained by studying gastric secretion at a later level of development and by studying other physiological systems not directly involved in intaking, assimilative processes.

The results indicate also that at the level of development of this infant affect may be regarded as the behavioral expression of instinct. In the relatively undeveloped ego one is able to see undisguised the attempts at discharge, e.g. instinct gratification. Here one might distinguish between attempts at tension reduction related to external objects and their mental representations (contentment, joy, irritation and rage), which are accompanied by patterned motor activity and augmented gastric secretion; and attempts at tension reduction of a narcissistic type (the depression-withdrawal reaction and sleep), in which muscular hypotonia, inactivity, and reduction of gastric secretion predominate. Other physiologic systems were not studied, but it was certainly established that the stomach participated in a major way in instinct expression, a phenomenon also predicted by psychoanalytic theory.

No less interesting than the data indicating that the oral phase has its physiological counterpart, is the indication of the existence of a relatively objectless, narcissistic phase in which secretory activity of the stomach largely ceases. In the depression-withdrawal reaction, as described above, there is a profound withdrawal of interest and activity in relation to the external world. This invariably occurred when the baby was confronted with a stranger. A more detailed consideration of the genetic dynamic background of this reaction will be published elsewhere [4]. Suffice it to say we believe that this reaction developed out of significant disturbances in the mother-child relationship in the first year of life, interfering seriously with the baby's capacity to tolerate object loss. As described in the history, she suffered two depressions in the first 15 months, variants of what SPITZ has called 'anaclitic depression' [8]. Both occurred in response to attenuations of the mother-child relationship and were alleviated by the establishment of more secure and satisfying object relationships in the hospital. Thereafter Monica responded, when confronted by a stranger, with the same mechanisms used in the earlier anaclitic depressions, withdrawing cathexes from the external world and from the systems concerned with it. The end result was a state of sleep, a narcissistic withdrawal with a reinstatement of the heightened stimulus barrier of the neonatal or fetal state. During this situation, as well as during natural sleep, secretion of acid by the stomach greatly diminished.

We interpret this to mean that when cathexes are withdrawn from the external world, when the child no longer seeks contact with persons in the environment and withdraws interest, not only does she abandon use of the motor system, as evidenced by the hypotonia and immobility, but also she behaves as if nothing is to be taken into the stomach. This is in contrast to the observation in the outgoing affective states described above. However, the last statement should not be interpreted to mean that the baby now decides nothing is to be taken into the stomach, an adultomorphic interpretation, but rather that a state of organismic organization exists, in which things are not taken into the stomach, a pre-oral organization. Such a state, of course, existed during fetal life, when nutrition was achieved passively through the umbilical circulation, and it perhaps is perpetuated to varying degrees in the biological withdrawals of sleep, even in the adult. GREENE has suggested the term 'umbilical stage' [9]. As one of us has developed elsewhere, biologic process and action precede the development of mental representations thereof, and therefore these data mainly point to the biologic anlage of processes that may later have psychologic expression [10].

Clinical and theoretical considerations have also led us to suggest that what we are calling the depression-withdrawal reaction represents an early developmental phase of depression, the anlage, so to speak, for depressive patterns of later life. Originating in a setting of helplessness unduly prolonged and accentuated by disturbances in the mother-child symbiosis, the reaction is reprovoked with exquisite regularity when the infant is threatened, through object loss, with a reactivation of the original shock state of helplessness. This fits well with the concepts of primal depression. The clinical manifestations are those concordant with the development of this child. Later libido and ego developments and the formation of superego add important features to adult depressions, not to be expected in infantile depression [4].

Finally, we wish to call attention to the remarkable reduction in the response to histamine in the depression-withdrawal reaction and in sleep. This suggests an alteration in physiological mechanisms and may provide an opportunity to elucidate some physiological processes in narcissistic states. This matter is now under investigation in our laboratory.

Summary and Conclusions

1. Gastric secretory, psychological, and behavioral observations were carried out in 59 experiments in an infant (with a gastric fistula) from the age of 15 to 20 months. Of a number of observed physiological variables, only the total hydrochloric acid secretion rate is considered in this paper.

2. The total hydrochloric acid secretion rate was intimately integrated with the total behavioral activity of the infant.

3. Outgoing affective states, be they libidinal or aggressive, were associated with rising rates of hydrochloric acid secretion.

4. During the depression-withdrawal reaction, characterized by sad facies, muscular flaccidity, inactivity, and withdrawal from the outside world, progressing into sleep in the more severe instances, there was a marked decrease in or even cessation of hydrochloric acid secretion.

5. The more active transactions with the environment were associated with rising hydrochloric acid secretion rates.

6. Histamine effect on gastric secretion during the depression-withdrawal state was slight or absent, whereas during outgoing states histamine proved to be a potent stimulant of hydrochloric acid secretion. This suggests the possibility of an altered organization at the cellular level under these two conditions.

7. These results support the psychoanalytic concept that, at this level of development, the establishment of object representations involves an oral, intaking model. Our study lends support to the concept of an oral stage of development: as the infant related outgoingly to an experimenter, be it aggressively or libidinally, her gastric glands reacted as if introjection of the cathected object was to take place. We want to emphasize that *our conclusions apply to this particular infant at this particular stage of development* and that generalizations should be made only with caution.

8. The depression-withdrawal reaction appeared to be a particular mode of the infant to object loss, the pattern for which had been established by her previous depressions as observed on two admissions to the hospital. The genetic dynamic background of this reaction, which may represent a regression to a preoral stage of development, will be considered extensively in a separate communication [4].

References

1. WOLF, S. and WOLFF, H. G.: Human gastric function (Oxford University Press, New York 1943).
2. MARGOLIN, S. G.: The behavior of the stomach during psychoanalysis. Psychoanal. Quart. *20:* 349 (1951).
3. WOLF, S. and WOLFF, H. G.: See references above.
4. ENGEL, G. L. and REICHSMAN, F.: Spontaneous and experimentally induced depressions in an infant with a gastric fistula: A contribution to the problem of depression. Amer. J. Psychoanal. *4:* (1956).
5. DARWIN, C.: The expression of emotions; in Man and animals. 1872 (New Edition, Philosophical Library, New York 1955).
6. ALEXANDER, F.: The influence of psychologic factors upon gastrointestinal disturbances: A symposium I. General principles, objectives, and preliminary results. Psychoanal. Quart. *3:* 501 (1934).
7. HAMMAR, S. and OBRINK, K. J.: The inhibitory effect of muscular exercise on gastric secretion. Acta physiol. scand. *28:* 152 (1953).
8. SPITZ, R.: Anaclitic depression. Psychoanal. Stud. Child *2:* 313 (1946).
9. GREENE, W. A., Jr.: Process in psychosomatic disorders. Psychosom. Med. *18:* 150 (1956).
10. ENGEL, G. L.: Homeostasis, behavioral adjustment and the concept of health and disease; in GRINKER Mid-century psychiatry (Thomas, Springfield 1953).

Etiology of Duodenal Ulcer[1]

I. Relation of Specific Psychological Characteristics to Rate of Gastric Secretion (Serum Pepsinogen)

H. WEINER, MARGARET THALER, M. F. REISER and I. A. MIRSKY

Retrospective comment by Dr. G. Engel. This study constitutes the first successful validation of ALEXANDER'S specificity concept, at least as applied to duodenal ulcer. Using psychological criteria derived from ALEXANDER'S original work, the investigators in a double blind fashion not only succeeded in correctly differentiating hypersecretors from hyposecretors on the basis of psychological data alone, but also were able to predict which hypersecretors would develop an active duodenal ulcer within the next 16 weeks. The study involved 2,073 army inductees from whom were selected 63 with serum pepsinogen levels in the upper and 57 in the lower 15 percentile. Without knowledge of the pepsinogen levels, the psychologist differentiated the two groups with remarkable success. The prediction of ulcer development was based mainly on the presence of intense needs to maintain relationships with others, a need likely to be frustrated during the period of army induction and basic training. Hyposecretors never developed ulcer while ulcer developed only among those hypersecretors for whom the military situation had been judged as capable of mobilizing the basic psychodynamic conflict. Hence, impressive support is provided for ALEXANDER'S hypothesis that a somatic predisposing factor (hypersecretion as measured by serum pepsinogen), a specific psychodynamic complex (as measured by the personality characteristics), and a precipitating situation that mobilizes the specific conflict (here induction into the military service) all are necessary for ulcer formation. Further elaboration of these concepts appears in subsequent papers.

More recently ADER has also been able to show that production of restraint induced gastric erosions in rats correlates not only with pepsinogen levels but also with whether or not the immobilization is carried out during a period in the animal's activity cycle when it would be maximally or minimally active; animals under the former circumstances proved more susceptible to gastric erosions. As with the human study, ADER's research demonstrates an interaction between somatic predisposing and behavioral factors and demonstrates that animal studies can be utilized to elaborate psychosomatic processes, e.g. genetic factors, which cannot readily be studied in humans.

The life history of a clinical syndrome and the various factors that contribute to the predisposition and precipitation of the syndrome in any particular person are usually inferred from data obtained after the clinical disorder has developed. Such inferences are frequently biased by the investigator's particular orientation. Thus, there are those who claim that the development of duodenal ulcer is determined solely by 'organic' factors [11] whereas others claim that 'psychic' factors are the sole determinants [8]. Such polar attitudes are inevitable when the data being considered is *post hoc* in nature. The ideal approach for evaluating the determinants responsible for precipitating any clinical disorder is to study the subject who is going to develop the disorder before he does so. This *propter hoc* approach requires criteria that will per-

[1] From the Division of Neuropsychiatry, Walter Reed Army Institute of Research, Washington, D.C., and the Department of Clinical Science, School of Medicine, University of Pittsburgh.

mit the selection of individuals who are susceptible to the development of the particular syndrome.

Previous studies have established that the concentration of pepsinogen in the blood is dependent upon the rate of pepsinogen production by the stomach [15]. In 87% of patients with duodenal ulcer, the pepsinogen concentration is greater than the mean of values found in subjects without duodenal or other gastrointestinal disturbances [16]. This observation is consistent with the general consensus that patients with duodenal ulcer tend to secrete more gastric juice, hydrochloric acid, and pepsin than do healthy subjects [10]. The fact that the high concentration of pepsinogen in the sera of such patients was found to persist even after the duodenal lesion was healed [16], as does also the increased rate of gastric secretion [13], suggested that gastric hypersecretion is an essential but not the sole determinant in the development of the lesion.

The concentration of pepsinogen in the blood of 14% of subjects without any gastrointestinal disturbance is greater than the mean of values found in patients with duodenal ulcer [16]. Presumably, the stomachs of such 'healthy' subjects are hypersecreting pepsinogen. If gastric hypersecretion is an essential determinant in the development of duodenal ulcer, it may be postulated that the high pepsinogen secretors represent that segment of the population with a maximal secretory capacity [9] that is most likely to develop duodenal ulcer when exposed to those circumstances responsible for precipitating the sequence of physiological events that result in the characteristic lesion. In accord with this hypothesis is the observation that apparently healthy subjects, without any previous history of gastrointestinal derangement, but with serum pepsinogen values in the range of those of patients with duodenal ulcer may go on to develop the lesion without any further significant increase in the concentration of pepsinogen in the blood [16, 17, 18].

The precise circumstances responsible for the precipitation of duodenal ulcer remain unknown. The consensus, however, is that psychic tension initiated by exposure to some environmental event is a prepotent factor. Although numerous studies have established that various manifestations of psychic tension can be related to a variety of gastrointestinal changes, no clue to the source of the tension became apparent until ALEXANDER and his colleagues applied psychoanalytical principles to the study of patients with peptic ulcer [1, 2]. Such studies by ALEXANDER and others [2, 12, 19] led to the generalization that patients with duodenal ulcer have in common a conflict related to the persistence of strong infantile wishes to be loved and cared for, on the one hand, and the repudiation of these wishes by the adult ego or by external circumstances, on the other hand. This psychic conflict is postulated to be responsible for initiating a sequence of physiological changes that result in the development of the duodenal lesion. Yet, as ALEXANDER [1] and others [12] have stressed, similar psychodynamic patterns can be demonstrated in subjects without any gastrointestinal disturbance or in subjects with some other derangement. Consequently, as ALEXANDER indicated, psychic conflict, specific or otherwise, cannot be the sole determinant in the precipitation of duodenal ulcer.

It is generally acknowledged that the response to some environmental event is a major factor in initiating the process responsible for the precipitation of peptic ulcer. Yet, there is nothing specific about the social situation that so frequently precedes the precipitation of duodenal ulcer [20]. The only inference that can be made is that the specific meaning of the environmental event to the particular individual determines whether or not the event is responded to as a noxious one.

From the preceding it would appear that there are 3 parameters which may contribute to the precipitation of duodenal ulcer a physiological parameter, which determines the susceptibility of the duodenum to ulceration; a psychological parameter, which determines the relatively specific psychic conflict that induces psychic tension; and a social parameter, which determines the environmental event that will prove noxious to the particular individual. Accordingly, a duodenal ulcer should develop when an individual with a sustained rate of gastric hypersecretion and the aforementioned psychic conflict is exposed to an environmental situation that mobilizes conflict and induces psychic tension.

This report deals with part of a study designed to evaluate the role of the three parameters in the precipitation of duodenal ulcer. The degree of gastric secretion gauged by the concentration of pepsinogen in the serum comprised the physiological parameter; subjects with serum pepsinogen values beyond one standard deviation of the mean were regarded as hypersecretors, and subjects with pepsinogen values below one standard deviation of the mean were regarded as hyposecretors. The selection of subjects representative of those with the highest and lowest concentrations of pepsinogen in the blood permitted one group to serve as a control for the other. The style of interpersonal interactions that could be inferred from projective and other psychological techniques comprised the psychological parameter. The exposure to 16 weeks of basic training comprised the environmental situation that might prove noxious to some and not to other subjects.

Method

A total of 2,073 draftees between the ages of 17.5 years and 29.2 years were chosen at random while being processed at induction at an army camp. Before entering service all had resided in the northeastern United States. Ten milliliter of blood was drawn from each man. The sample was identified by code number, refrigerated, and sent to one of us (IAM) for analysis. The concentration of pepsinogen in the serum was determined by a method described in an earlier paper [15]. The Cornell

Medical Index [5], the Saslow Screening Inventory [21], and a sociological rating scale[2] were administered to each man. Approximately 300 men were processed per week.

At the end of each week, the code numbers of 20 men were returned to the research group at the Induction Center without their levels of serum pepsinogen being revealed. These numbers identified men who were chosen for more detailed study because they were in the range of the highest and lowest values obtained in the group of men tested during the previous week. At the end of seven weeks, a total of 120 men had been selected for special study.

During the second week the 20 men who had been selected at the end of the first week were given a battery of psychological tests (Rorschach Test, Blacky Pictures, and Draw-A-Person Test). Each man was interviewed briefly by a psychiatrist and social worker, and each man was given a complete gastrointestinal roentgenological examination. The psychological tests were administered by a technician, and the test material was then sent to three of us (MT, HW, and MR) for evaluation.

After these studies were completed the men were sent to the basic training area. Subsequently, all but 13 men were again given the psychological tests and roentgenological examinations some time between the eighth and sixteenth week of the basic training period.

The Rorschach results were submitted both to a formal scoring[3] and to that devised by DeVos, which divides content into various categories and subcategories 'concerned with the symbolic expressions of affect' [6]. Each drawing from the Draw-A-person Test was classified as primitive, distorted, boyish, masculine, or adult. The Cornell Medical Index [5], Saslow [21] and Blacky [4] tests were scored as recommended by their originators. In addition, Card II of the Blacky Test was scored as to whether Blacky was seen as openly expressing anger or whether the expression of such affect was denied, rationalized, or ignored.

---

[2] Devised and evaluated by 1st Lt. SIDNEY CROOG, WRAIR, Walter Reed Army Medical Center, Washington 12, D.C.

Results

Figure 1 illustrates the normal distribution of the values for the concentration of pepsinogen in the sera of the population of 2,073 men who were screeend. The hypersecretor group selected for special study consisted of 63 of the 300 men who comprised those with the upper 15% of the serum pepsinogen values. The hyposecretor group selected for special study consisted of 57 of the 179 men who comprised those with the lowest 9% of the serum pepsinogen values.

The first roentgenological examination revealed evidences of a healed duodenal ulcer in 3, and of an active ulcer in 1 of the 63 men with gastric hypersecretion. Of these 4 men with evidence of duodenal lesions at the outset, one became a disci-

plinary problem and was confined to the stockade, one went absent without leave, one went through his basic training without incident, and the fourth man, who had the active duodenal lesion, was discharged from the service.

The second roentgenological examination at the eighth to 16th week revealed evidences of active duodenal ulcer in an additional five men who had no evidences of a gastrointestinal derangement at the outset of the study. All the subjects who had or developed evidences of duodenal ulcer were found among the 63 individuals with high blood pepsinogen values (fig. 1).

With no knowledge of the pepsinogen levels or roentgenological findings, we evaluated the psychological test material to test the hypothesis that the hypersecretor could be differentiated from the hypo-

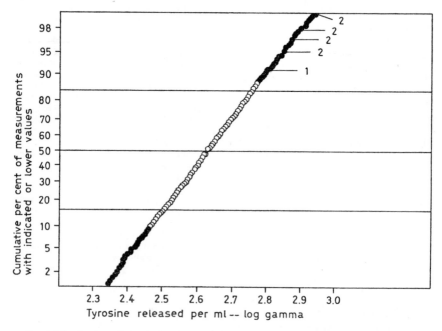

Fig. 1. Distribution of blood serum pepsinogen concentrations: the frequency distribution of the logarithm of the concentration of the pepsinogen in the serum plotted on a probit scale. The subjects selected for special study were among those designated with closed circles. The numerals refer to individuals with duodenal ulcer.

secretor and that men with or prone to duodenal ulcer could be identified. These hypotheses were based on clinical observations that suggested that the hypersecretor, like the patient with duodenal ulcer, would exhibit evidences of intense infantile oral dependent wishes, marked 'immaturity', tendencies to please and placate, and difficulties revolving particularly about the management of oral impulses and hostility [17, 18]. Similar clinical observations suggested that the hyposecretor, like the patient with pernicious anemia, would exhibit evidences of pseudomasculine defenses and paranoid trends [17]. Accordingly, in order to categorize those who might belong among the hypersecretor group, the psychological test material was examined specifically for the presence of strong direct references to the acts of feeding, of being fed and of incorporation. Indirect or inferred oral symbolism such as talking, smoking, kissing, blowing, etc., and responses referable to heat and cold (e.g., snow, people warming themselves, flowers growing in the snow) were also sought. It was anticipated that the hypersecretors would reveal diffuse anxiety in their answers, that many records might be characterized by depressive associations and that the drawings would be those of boys, or primitive and gross, or asexual.

To categorize those who might belong to the hyposecretor group, special attention was paid to indications of problems referable to activity and passivity, submissiveness and assertiveness, femininity and masculinity, as evidenced by responses suggesting conflict over sexual identification, passive sexual longing, and anal symbolism. It was postulated that the test material of the hyposecretors, in contrast to the hypersecretors, would show little or no oral, depressive, or anxiety content and a paucity of indications of a need to please and placate.

Using the above criteria, one psychologist and two psychiatrists independently rated the test records to determine whether the subject belonged to the hypersecretor or hyposecretor group. On the basis of a majority opinion, 61 % of the 120 men – 71 % of the hypersecretors and 51 % of the hyposecretors – were correctly designated on the basis of the postulated traits.

It had been anticipated that the psychological test material and social histories would permit the prediction of the way in which each individual would react to the social situation represented by the period of basic training. This anticipation, however, proved incorrect since no technique could be devised *post hoc* to permit the selection of individuals who would react to the situation as if it were a noxious one. Consequently, based on previous experience with test patterns from patients with duodenal ulcer [23] and on inferences derived from psychoanalytical and other clinical observations of such patients [1, 2, 7, 12, 14, 17, 19, 20, 22, 24] an attempt was made to predict which individual would develop a duodenal ulcer during the 16 weeks of basic training. It was postulated that the subject most likely to develop an ulcer during the period of basic training would show all the characteristics of the hypersecretor but with a much greater intensity than the individual who was not likely to develop the lesion. Accordingly, the psychological test material of the inductees was evaluated *before* the biochemical and roentgenological data became available.

Ten men were selected as those most likely to develop an ulcer because their test material not only suggested that they belong to the group of hypersecretors but also showed evidences of intense needs to maintain relationships with others. Their anxieties centered around a fear of expressing hostility lest there be a loss of supplies for their needs; they went out of their way to rationalize, deny, and displace such feelings. The need to please and placate authority figures as potential sources of affection was particularly striking. The predictions were accurate in seven out of the ten. Of the three who did not have or did not develop an ulcer, two were hypersecretors.

Post-hoc studies revealed that all of the nine men who had or developed a duodenal ulcer during the period of basic training had been classified correctly as belonging to the group with high serum pepsinogen values on the basis of the psychological criteria given above. Other than the intensity of their attempt to maintain relationships, no criterion was found to distinguish the hypersecretor who developed an ulcer from the hypersecretor who did not.

The attempt to differentiate the hypersecretors from the hyposecretors on the basis of clinical impressions of the available psychological test material indicated that the criteria used for such differentiation were inadequate. To develop a more accurate diagnostic tool, a variety of criteria from the test material of the hypersecretors and hyposecretors were analyzed statistically. Only those criteria that were significant at less than the 5 % level of confidence were used for a final classification. By means of a cluster of 20 such criteria it was possible to distinguish the two groups to the extent that 85 % of the 120 men could be assigned accurately to their group at a 0.001 level of confidence. Thus, of the 120 men, only 6 hypersecretors and 12 hyposecretors could not be correctly classified on the basis of the cluster of psychological test criteria.

The 20 criteria that permitted the relatively correct differentiation of the hypersecretor from the hyposecretor are listed in table I. No single criterion permitted the separation of the 2 groups with an accuracy exceeding 64.2 %, but all were significant at the 5 % level of confidence or better. The combinations of items, however, permitted the more accurate designation.

The overall impression of the psychological makeup of hypersecretors gained from the use of these scoring criteria was one of marked dependency in their relationships to others, of compliance, and of passiveness. Thus the affect of a greater number was childishly toned (criteria 1 and 2); they gave more texture responses (criterion 3), suggesting a greater awareness of,

or need for tactile contact with others. A greater incidence of responses symbolizing oral needs (criterion 4) and dependency on authority figures (criterion 2) were given by the hypersecretors. This group also displayed a greater incidence of immature body images on human drawings (crit. 5).

The majority of the hypersecretors gave responses symbolizing the expression, explicit or implicit, of anxiety (criterion 6), the source of which appeared to be hostile impulses (criterion 7) that they felt must not be revealed or directly expressed (criteria 8, 9, and 10). This was inferred from the resulting formal evidences of depression that were evident in the Rorschach scores (criteria 11 and 12). The hypersecretors had relatively few complaints about bodily symptoms, be they of discomfort, physical illness (criterion 13), or of the anxiety reaction (criterion 14). It is noteworthy, however, that the Rorschach associations of some individuals indicated both the presence of anxiety (criterion 6) in freely associated material, and a tendency not to complain of its physical concomitant and not to be aware of and/or acknowledge its presence on direct questioning (criteria 13 and 14). Thus, of the 27 individuals with high serum pepsinogen levels who gave anxiety associations (criterion 6), 12 denied that they felt anxious on the Saslow questionnaire. Yet anxiety associations (criterion 6) were given by 14 hyposecretors, 11 of whom admitted their anxiety openly (criterion 14).

Although the above features, so common to many of the hypersecretors, were also present in 12 of the hyposecretors, the incidence of such features was insignificant among the latter (criteria 1, 2, 4, and 5). The greater 'immaturity' of the hypersecretors, when compared with the hyposecretors, is also revealed in the fact that they consistently showed 2 of the 3 categories which best reveal juvenile traits (criteria 1, 2, and 5) when these criteria were combined to evaluate this feature.

Another distinction between the 2 groups was that the hyposecretors showed

Table I. Criteria distinguishing subjects with high and low concentration of pepsinogen in the blood

Criterion	Responses: Cut-off score	Serum pepsinogen concentration		No. correctly classified	% of total corr. classified	X^2	P Level
		High	Low				
1. Rorschach: Color-form	Present	31	17	71	59.2	4.684	<0.05
	Absent	32	40				
2. Rorschach: Childish and authority-dependency	Present	37	21	73	60.8	5.741	<0.02
	Absent	26	36				
3. Rorschach: Texture	Present	33	18	72	60.0	5.299	<0.05
	Absent	30	39				
4. Rorschach: Oral symbolism	31% or more	35	19	73	60.8	5.971	<0.02
	30% or less	28	38				
5. Draw-A-person: Boyish drawings	Present	24	8	73	60.8	7.67	<0.01
	Absent	39	49				
6. Rorschach: Openly symbolized hostility	3 or more	27	14	70	58.3	5.010	<0.05
	2 or less	36	43				
7. Rorschach: Per cent hostile responses	24% or less	50	30	77	64.2	9.624	<0.01
	25% or more	13	27				
8. Blacky test: Anger on Card II	Absent	32	18	71	59.2	4.546	<0.05
	Present	31	39				
9. Blacky test: Denial of aggression, Card IIIb	Present	29	16	70	48.3	4.119	<0.05
	Absent	34	41				
10. Saslow test: Anger expressed (N = 110)	No	36	22	66	60.0	4.296	<0.05
	Yes	22	30				
11. Rorschach: Per cent small details	8% or more	36	20	73	60.8	5.849	<0.02
	7% or less	27	37				
12. Rorschach: Poorly perceived responses	20% or less	31	14	74	61.7	7.755	<0.01
	21% or more	32	43				
13. Cornell medical index: No. of items	15 or less	46	26	75	62.5	9.153	<0.01
	16 or more	16	29				
14. Saslow test: Anxiety expressed (N=109)	No	30	14	67	61.5	6.64	=0.01
	Yes	28	37				
15. Rorschach: Hostile-sado-masochistic content	Absent	52	37	72	60.0	4.853	<0.05
	Present	11	20				
16. Rorschach: Feminine identification	Absent	52	37	72	60.0	4.853	<0.05
	Present	11	20				
17. Rorschach: Anxious face details	Absent	62	49	70	58.3	5.010	<0.05
	Present	1	8				
18. Rorschach: Hybrid combinations	1 or less	62	47	72	60.0	7.335	<0.01
	2 or more	1	10				
19. Rorschach: Per cent unpleasant content	39% or less	33	18	72	60.0	5.299	<0.05
	40% or more	30	39				
20. Rorschach: Per cent neutral content	35% or more	33	18	72	60.0	5.299	<0.05
	34% or less	30	39				
Total classification (20 Criteria)	10 or more	57	45	102	85.0		<0.001

Table II. Check list of 'disturbed' records

Sign	Responses: Cut-off score	Serum pepsinogen concentration		No. correctly classified	% of total (120) corr. classified	X^2	P Level
		High	Low				
1. Formal Rorschach N-33							
a) P %	12% or less	8	7				
	13% or more	6	12	20	60.0		N.S.
b) F minus % and i % combined	49% or more	9	9				
	48% or less	5	10	19	57.0		N.S.
c) W %	20% or less	9	8				
	21% or more	5	11	20	60.0		N.S.
d) Feminine on Card 3	Absent	14	12				
	Present	0	7	21	63.0	4.417	<0.05
e) Elaboration	Absent	14	10				
	Present	0	9	23	69.0	6.76	<0.01
2. DeVos scoring:							
f) Ahyb	1 or less	13	13				
	2 or more	1	6	19	57.0		N.S.
g) AA and Aa combined	2 or more	13	6				
	1 or less	1	13	26	78.0	9.874	<0.01
h) Oral	2 or more	10	6				
	1 or less	4	13	23	69.0	4.515	<0.05

high hostility scores (criterion 7) in which sadomasochistic associations figured prominently (criterion 15), or they openly expressed their anger (criteria 8 and 10).

To test the consistency with which the hypersecretor group appeared to avoid or evade the evidences of the expression of hostility, responses to criteria 7, 8, 9, 10, and 15 were combined. Using a simple majority tally as a cut-off score, the direct expression of hostility was found to be rarer among the hypersecretors than among the hyposecretors (P < 0.001).

Bodily preoccupation (criterion 13) and more complaints about bodily symptoms generally characterized individuals in the group with low serum pepsinogen concentrations. The hyposecretors gave a mean of 19 complaints, whereas the hypersecretors gave a mean of 12 complaints. Furthermore, using Brodman's criterion of 30 or more complaints as an indicator of potentially inadequate military performance [5] there were 4 hypersecretors and 15 hyposecretors who gave 30 or more of these answers; the difference is statistically significant (P<0.01).

Twenty of the 57 hyposecretors drew very masculine and adult figures on the Draw-A-Person Test, but 20 of these had an apparent difficulty in sexual identity, revealed by their identifying the figures on the third Rorschach card as women or by giving only female human content on the entire test.

That a small number of hyposecretors handle their anxiety by focusing on profile details on the Rorschach test is indicated by criterion 17. Other subjects gave two or more autistic and hybrid combinations of humans and animals (criterion 18).

In the overall group of 120 soldiers, there were 33 (14 hypersecretors and 19 hyposecretors) whose test records on in-

Table III. Overall clinical judgment of Rorschach record

DeVos index No. of responses	Hypersecretors		Hyposecretors	
	Not disturbed (49)	Disturbed (14)	Not disturbed (38)	Disturbed (19)
0	32	4	22	5
1	12	1	9	3
2 and more	5	9	7	11
	$X^2 = 8.75$ $p < 0.01$		$X^2 = 7.399$ $p < 0.01$	

spection indicated sufficient psychological difficulties to rate the protocols as 'disturbed' [6]. The contrast between 'disturbed' hyper- and hyposecretors was consistent with the inference drawn above for the entire group. In fact, the 'disturbed' records of hypersecretors revealed that their anxieties were the product of variants of primitive oral impulses in dependent relationships. The hyposecretors, in contrast, evidenced marked somatic preoccupation, predominantly projective defenses, and an elaborate form of thought disorder.

Discussion

In the present study, the criterion chosen as an index of the susceptibility to the development of duodenal ulcer was the concentration of pepsinogen in the serum. This criterion was selected because long-term studies still in progress have indicated that duodenal ulcer develops only in those with high serum pepsinogen concentrations [17, 18].

The data reported herein reveal a remarkable correlation between the concentration of pepsinogen in the serum and specific personality characteristics of a group of young men inducted into the army. The group of subjects with high serum pepsinogen concentrations show intense needs that are principally 'oral' in nature and which are exhibited in terms of wishing to be fed, to lean on others, and to seek close bodily contact with others. Satisfaction of these needs for external support and external sources for satiation is attempted by many means. When such attempts fail, the resultant frustration arouses anger that cannot be expressed lest there ensue a loss of supply for their needs. Consequently these subjects usually do not make complaints or express any feelings of anger.

In contrast to the above, the subjects with low concentrations of pepsinogen in the serum exhibit fewer problems about and less dependency on external sources of supply and support. They are more narcissistic and exhibit more problems relative to internal, bodily discomfort, and react to the sources of the discomfort with intense hostility which they express relatively freely. They show evidences of a disturbance in language style that is characterized by elaboration and pretentiousness. Some of the subjects show a hostile feminine identification which they defend themselves against by a masculine overcompensation. Projective defenses against anxiety are common.

In accord with the hypothesis stated at the outset, the men who had or developed a duodenal lesion were among those with high concentrations of pepsinogen in the circulation; that is, among the hypersecretors. Further the personality characteristics of those who did develop a duodenal ulcer are essentially the same as most of the subjects comprising the hypersecretor group. Although the prediction were accurate in seven of nine subjects who had or developed duodenal ulcer, it proved impossible in the present study to use the available data to determine why only some of the hypersecretors reacted as they did to the social situation or developed the duodenal lesion. In another study in which psychoanalytically oriented anamnestic interviews were conducted, however, it has been possible to predict the character of the social situation that would prove noxious to the specific individual, and subsequently to observe that when such exposure occurred, a duodenal ulcer ensued. These observations, as well as the mechanism whereby exposure to a social event that is noxious to the individual induces the development of a duodenal lesion, will be described in another communication.

The present study does not provide an explanation for the high correlation between the serum pepsinogen concentration and the relatively specific personality characteristics. Studies on siblings and twins reveal that the secretory capacity of the gastric mucosa as gauged by the serum pepsinogen concentrations is genetically determined [18]. Even at birth, the concentration of serum pepsinogen is distributed normally with some newborn infants having values that are beyond the mean of patients with duodenal ulcer. Consequently, it is improbable that the psychological characteristics described above are responsible for the physiological state of the stomach. Although the psychological development of the infant is largely dependent upon his human environment, the secretory capacity of the stomach with which the child is born may play a significant role in his relationship with that environment [17]. Studies on the manner in which the quantitative aspects of a physiological system influences the child-mother unit and thereby the child's psychological development are in progress and should provide data that may clarify the mechanisms involved.

Although it is possible to postulate that the inherited secretory capacity of the stomach plays a role in determining not only the psychological development of the infant but also his physiological predisposition, it does not account for the marked individual differences that characterize the manner in which the needs described above are handled. Study of these individual differences suggest that the vagaries of each person's life experiences determine the

manner in which impulses and wishes are mastered, whereas the hypersecretor's persistent wishes for support and succor from the external environment are determined by early childhood factors. The manner in which he handles these wishes is determined by all his life experiences, that is, by the factors that determine his integrative capacity.

Summary

1. Serum pepsinogen was determined for each of 2,073 army inductees. Sixty-three with values in the upper 15% and 57 with values in the lower 9% of the blood pepsinogen distribution were selected for special study. Each of these was given the Rorschach, Blacky, Draw-A-Person, Cornell Medical Index, and Saslow tests, and a complete upper gastrointestinal roentgenological examination before being sent to basic training.

2. One hundred and seven subjects were reexamined between the 8th and 16th week of basic training. The first roentgenological examination revealed healed duodenal ulcers in three subjects and an active ulcer in one. The second roentgenological examination revealed active duodenal ulcers in 5 additional men. All 9 subjects with peptic ulcer were in the upper 15% of the blood pepsinogen distribution, 8 of them being in the upper 5%. Thus, 15% of men in the top 5% developed peptic ulcer.

3. Independent evaluation of the psychological data revealed that subjects with peptic ulcer displayed evidence of major unresolved and persistent conflicts about dependency and oral gratification, the characteristics of which are described.

4. Classification of the selected test population into 2 groups on the basis of criteria derived from the psychological tests was found to correlate (85%) with the 2 groups (hyper- and hypo-pepsinogen secretors) derived from the physiological tests.

5. The study indicates that neither a high rate of gastric secretion nor a specific psychodynamic constellation is independently responsible for development of peptic ulcer. Together, however, these 2 parameters constitute the essential determinants in the precipitation of peptic ulcer on exposure to social situations noxious to the specific individual.

References

1. ALEXANDER, F.: The influence of psychologic factors upon gastrointestinal disturbances: General principles, objectives and preliminary results. Psychoanal. Quart. 3: 501 (1934).
2. ALEXANDER, F.: Psychosomatic medicine (Norton, New York 1950).
3. BECK, S. J.: Rorschach's test (Grune and Stratton, New York 1947).
4. BLUM, G. S.: Revised scoring system for research use of the Blacky pictures (Male form – 1951). Ann Arbor, Mich., Univ. of Mich., 1951.
5. BRODMAN, K.; ERDMANN, A. J., Jr.; LORGE, I.; DEUTSCHBERGER, J., and WOLFF, H. G.: The Cornell medical index. Health questionnaire VII: The prediction of psychosomatic and psychiatric disabilities in army training. Amer. J. Psychiat. 3: 37 (1954).
6. DEVOS, G.: A quantitative approach to affective symbolism in Rorschach responses. J. Proj. Techn. 16: 133 (1952).
7. GILDEA, E. G.: Special features of the personality which are common to certain psychosomatic disorders. Psychosom. Med. 11: 273 (1949).
8. GARMA, A.: Internalized mother as harmful food in peptic ulcer patients. Int. J. Psycho-Anal. 34: 102 (1953).
9. HUNT, J. N. and KAY, A. W.: The nature of gastric hypersecretion of acid in patients with duodenal ulcer. Brit. J. 2: 1444 (1954).
10. IVY, A. C.; GROSSMAN, M. I., and BACHRACH, W. H. Peptic ulcer (Blakiston, Philadelphia, 1950).
11. JONES, F. A.: The problem of peptic ulcer. Ann. Intern. Med. 44: 63 (1956).
12. KAPP, F. T.: ROSENBAUM, M., and ROMANO, J.: Psychological factors in men with peptic ulcer. Amer. J. Psychiat. 103: 700 (1947).
13. LEVIN, E.; KIRSNER, J. B., and PALMER, W. L.: Twelve-hour nocturnal gastric secretion in uncomplicated duodenal ulcer patients: Before and after healing. Proc. Soc. exp. Biol. N.Y. 69: 153 (1948).
14. MINSKI, L. and DESAI, M. M.: Aspects of personality in peptic ulcer patients. Brit. J. med. Psychol. 28: 113 (1955).
15. MIRSKY, I. A.; FUTTERMAN, P.; KAPLAN, S., and BROH-KAHN, R. H.: Blood plasma pepsinogen: I. The source, properties, and assay of the proteolytic activity of plasma at acid reactions. J. Lab. clin. Med. 40: 17 (1952).
16. MIRSKY, I. A.; FUTTERMAN, P., and KAPLAN, S.: Blood plasma pepsinogen: II. The activity of the plasma from 'normal' subjects, patients with duodenal ulcer, and patients with pernicious anemia. J. Lab. clin. Med. 40: 188 (1952).
17. MIRSKY, I. A.: Psychoanalysis and the biological sciences; in ALEXANDER and ROSS Twenty years of psychoanalysis (Norton, New York 1953).
18. MIRSKY, I. A.: In preparation.
19. RUESCH, J.: The infantile personality. Psychosom. Med. 10: 134 (1948).
20. RUESCH, J.; CHRISTIANSEN, C.; DEWEES, S.; HARRIS, R. E.; JACOBSON, A., and LOEB, M. B.: Duodenal ulcer, a sociopsychological study of naval enlisted personnel and civilians (University of California Press, Berkeley, Cal. 1948).
21. SASLOW, G.; COUNTS, R. M., and DUBOIS, P. H.: Evaluation of a new psychiatric screening test. Psychosom. Med. 13: 242 (1951).
22. STREITFELD, H. S.: Specificity of peptic ulcer to intense oral conflicts. Psychosom. Med. 16: 315 (1954).
23. THALER, M. B.; WEINER, H., and REISER, M. F.: An exploration of the doctor-patient relationship through projective techniques. Presented at lllth Annual Meeting, American Psychiatric Association, Atlantic City, N.J., May 12, 1955.
24. ZANE, M.: Psychosomatic considerations in peptic ulcer. Psychosom. Med. 2: 372 (1947).

Psychosomatic Disease and the 'Visceral Brain'[1]

Recent Developments Bearing on the Papez Theory of Emotion

P. D. MacLean

Retrospective comment by Dr. L. Kubie. In 1949, twelve years after the publication of PAPEZ's basic paper, 'A proposed mechanism of emotion', MACLEAN published a paper entitled 'Psychosomatic disease and the "visceral brain"' with the sub-title 'Recent developments bearing on the Papez theory of emotion'. This was MACLEAN's first step towards the reconciliation of experimental neurophysiology with modern dynamic psychology. Over the years he has pursued this goal in the work of C. JUDSON HERRICK, HUGHLINGS JACKSON, PENFIELD, KLÜVER, BUCY, BROWN, SCHAFER, SPIEGEL, MASSERMAN and many others. His earlier studies were of the neural centers and paths which activate the autonomic nervous system in affectively-charged processes. His later work considered the mechanisms involved in the subjective experiencing of feelings as feelings. Then he focused on a wide range of instinctual processes and their interdependence. With courageous and logical inevitability this brought him to a consideration of the relationship of all of this to certain psychoanalytic formulations concerning oral and oral-anal needs and drives, as well as respiratory needs, aggression and vigilance. This paper was the first of a long series of studies which moved from the study of the part to the study of the whole. Many have studied with precision and accuracy the parts of the central nervous system which are involved in affective processes and how they operate. There have been some who have studied how the whole machine works as a unit. PAUL MACLEAN is one of the few who has done both. This places him in the great tradition of WALTER CANNON, Sir CHARLES SHERRINGTON and STANLEY COBB. His philosophic sophistication made it unnecessary for him ever to deny the importance or the reality of either end of the spectrum. Consequently his studies of how the brain as a whole is organized and of the functions of its parts have built a bridge between modern dynamic psychophysiology and certain basic concepts of psychoanalysis. He has never had to use either in an attempt to destroy the other; and his interest in psychological implications has never warped his interpretation of his experimental data.

If those who work in the organic field would study more carefully his comments on the psychological significance of his organic findings, and if in turn the analyst and psychologist would study his organic contributions more carefully, we would not still be plagued by meaningless feuds between organo-phobic psychologists and psycho-phobic organicists. I have no doubt that in the end PAUL MACLEAN's beneficent and unifying influence will have the final word.

In most of those diseases where emotional states are thought to be etiologically related to focal or systemic lesions, it is generally assumed that the pathologic process is mediated by the autonomic nervous system and the humoral mechanisms under its control. There is considerable experimental and clinical evidence to support such an assumption. But little information has accumulated to indicate by what mechanism the emotions can so act on autonomic centers as to lead to diseases as diverse as essential hypertension, peptic ulcer, asthma, etc.

[1] From the Department of Neurology and Psychiatry of the Harvard Medical School and the Psychiatric Service of the Massachusetts General Hospital, Boston.

The first part of this paper will be devoted to a review of certain neuroanatomic and neurophysiologic evidence now at hand that contributes to the understanding of emotional mechanisms and points to a variety of ways by which the affective qualities of experience could act on autonomic centers. In the subsequent section it will be suggested how this evidence perhaps ties in with some of the current psychodynamic formulations regarding those psychosomatic diseases where lesions are present.

The problem pertaining to emotional mechanisms is basically one of communication in the central nervous system. It may be assumed that messages from both without and within the organism are relayed to the brain by nervous impulses traveling along nerve fibers and possibly by humoral agents carried in the blood stream. Ultimately, however, any correlation of these messages must be a function of a highly integrated body of neurones capable of sorting, selecting, and acting upon various patterns of bioelectrical activity. The indications are that both the experience and the expression of emotion are the resultant of the association and correlation of a wide variety of internal and external stimuli whose messages are transmitted as nervous impulses in cerebral analyzers. The manner in which these impulses can give rise to the subjective feeling of emotion remains a complete mystery. But in the light of what is known about the capacity of small electrical chargers to trip large scale mechanisms into action, it is more readily understood how nervous impulses set going the various phenomena associated with emotional expression.

The hypothalamus is considered to be the head ganglion of the autonomic nervous system [31]. On the basis of investigations showing the role of the hypothalamus in sham rage [6, 11] it has often been inferred in the literature on psychosomatic medicine that this nerve center is responsible both for the experiencing and expression of emotion. MASSERMAN, however, has amassed considerable evidence to show that whereas the hypothalamus is the main neural center for mediating the expression of emotion, it does not share in the experiencing of emotion [46]. Although the thalamus probably participates in a crude awareness of somesthetic sensations [38], the present evidence indicates that only the cerebral cortex is capable of appreciating all the various affective qualities of experience and combining them into such states of feeling as fear, anger, love, and hate [15, 46, 52, 69].

To emphasize the role of the cerebral cortex in the experiencing of emotion, however, is to require one to stress at the same time its connections with the hypothalamus, the effector mechanism of emotional expression. In the light of this it is an interesting and significant observation that the neopallium, despite its forming most of the cerebral mantle, has (as far as is known at the present time) comparatively little autonomic representation. If one accepts YAKOVLEV's interpretation that the orbitomesial surface of the frontal lobes belongs to the mesopallium [79, 80][2], there remains only a relatively small area of the neocortex – namely, the rostral part of the motor cortex – from which autonomic responses can be obtained by appropriate stimulation [31]. The anatomic pathways over which these responses are mediated have yet to be ascertained. There are known to be relay circuits from the frontal lobes to the hypothalamus by way of the septal nuclei and medial forebrain bundle (fig. 2), as well as through the dorsomedial nuclei of the thalamus and the periventricular system [70]; but the anatomic details of these fiber connections are still obscure. It is only within the last 2 years, as the result of further microanatomic studies [50] and physiologic neuronography [74], that there has been any clear indication of *direct* pathways to the hypothalamus.

The difficulty in demonstrating pathways between the neopallium and the hypothalamus is in marked contrast to the ease with

[2] Transitional cortex between 'old' brain and 'new' brain.

38   MACLEAN

which one can point to many and strong connections between the old brain (rhinencephalon) and the hypothalamus, some of which, such as the fornix, are almost the diameter of a pencil (fig. 1 and 2).

On the strength of this intimate relationship of the phylogenetically older cerebral structures with the hypothalamus, together with certain experimental and clinical considerations, PAPEZ in 1937 published a paper called 'A proposed mechanism of emotion' in which the theory was advanced 'that the hypothalamus, the anterior thalamic nuclei, the gyrus cinguli, the hippocampus and their connections consitute a harmonious mechanism which may elaborate the functions of central emotion, as well as participate in emotional expression' [52].

General Considerations of the PAPEZ *Theory*

The theory expressed in this paper has done much to revive interest in the rhinencephalon. As PAPEZ observed, many of the structures he listed as being involved in emotional experience have commonly been 'represented as dealing with some phase of the olfactory function'. He felt that there was 'no clinical or other evidence to support this view'.

To be sure, the doubt has long been expressed that the cingulate gyrus should be included as part of the rhinencephalon [19]. It has been noted that not only this gyrus, but also the hippocampal system, are present in such forms as the dolphin and the porpoise where the sense of smell is absent[3]. Furthermore, it is remarkable that in man where the olfactory bulbs are small compared with macrosmatic animals, the hippocampal formation and the cingulate gyrus reach their greatest development [9]. Recently BRODAL, in a review dealing with the hippocampus and related structures, has concluded that only a comparatively small part of the cerebral cortex usually assigned to the rhinencephalon is directly involved in olfaction [9]. On the basis of extensive

comparative studies, C. JUDSON HERRICK maintained that the rhinencephalon, in addition to mediating the sense of smell, served as a nonspecific activator for all cortical activities, influencing appropriately, in an excitatory or inhibitory capacity, such functions as memory, learning, and affective behaviour [30].

The mechanism of emotion proposed by PAPEZ will require further elaboration during the course of this paper. Briefly, the concept, as first presented in 1937, is formulated as follows (fig. 1): 'The central emotive process of cortical origin may ... be conceived as being built up in the hippocampal formation and as being transferred to the mammillary body and thence through the anterior thalamic nuclei to the cortex of the gyrus cinguli. The cortex of the cingular gyrus may be looked on as the receptive region for the experiencing of emotion ... Radiation of the emotive process from the gyrus cinguli to other regions in the cerebral cortex would add emotional colouring to psychic processes'.

In the light of subsequent experimental findings, PAPEZ's delimitation of this region in the experiencing of emotion strikes one today as a considerable *tour de force*. For, other than the known comparative and neuroanatomy of this region, there was little experimental data to support his thesis, and the clinical evidence was more suggestive than definitive. He emphasized that lesions directly involving or impinging on the anatomic circuit shown in figure 1 caused a variety of symptoms that were confined largely to the affective behaviour of the individual. Starting with the hippocampal formation (fig. 1, 2, and 4), PAPEZ noted that in rabies where the disease appears to have a predilection for the hippocampus and cerebellum, the patient is subject to anxiety, apprehensiveness, and paroxysms of rage or terror. I might add that both the 'dreamy state' and epileptic automatisms

---

[3] See 9, 19, 69 for review and further references.

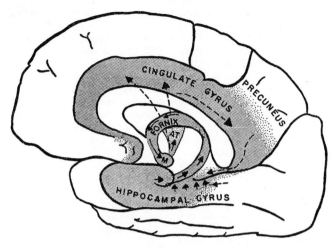

Fig. 1. The shaded area of cortex represents what was formerly known as the limbic lobe of Broca and subsequently termed the rhinencephalon by TURNER. It corresponds to what is arbitrarily referred to in this paper as the visceral brain. M, mammillary body. AT, anterior thalamic nucleus.

indicate that the hippocampal formation and associated structures are concerned in emotional experience. HUGHLINGS JACKSON who preferred the term 'dreamy state' to 'intellectual aura', described the condition as a kind of 'double consciousness' or 'mental diplopia' [32]. It was as though the individual had the sense of being in contact with reality, but at the same time had the *feeling* he was experiencing a dream or something that had happened before (déjà vu). JACKSON associated the dreamy state with 'discharges' or lesions in the uncinate region. In the experience of PENFIELD and ERICKSON the lesion responsible for the dreamy state has usually been situated deep within or underneath the temporal lobe [58]. They have stressed that the sense of reminiscence that occurs with discharges in this region is often '*only the feeling*[4] which normally accompanies the act of remembering'.

Patients subject to epileptic automatisms perform bizarre acts for which they have no memory. These seizures, as well as the dreamy state, are frequently associated with

a variety of visceral, emotional, and other sensory manifestations. There may be a visceral aura such as a sense of smell, taste, epigastric uneasiness, or asphyxia. Chewing and tasting movements, grinding the teeth, etc., may accompany the seizure. The author has seen one case where a feeling of hunger and frequency of urination and bowel movements persisted for a day or more following a seizure. Crude auditory sensations or peculiar visual impressions are sometimes present. A feeling of fear or terror may accompany the visceral aura, or may be the only premonitory symptom. As JACKSON noted, 'The occurrence of gastric and intestinal symptoms in some cases of uncinate fits with abnormal emotional states is obviously significant' [32]. Patients with automatisms are commonly afflicted by severe emotional and psychologic disturbances (nervousness, obsessive thinking, depression etc.,) between seizures. Since the introduction of electroencephalography it has been shown that in the type of epilepsy

[4] Italics mine.

under discussion there are abnormal electrical discharges arising in the region of one or both temporal lobes [27, 33]. The author, in association with Arellano, has demonstrated, by use of special leads at the base of the brain, that in a majority of the patients studied the origin of such discharges was nearer the electrodes in the vicinity of the basilar part of the rhinencephalon than those recording from the scalp [45a].

Papez cited a number of references to show that preservation of the nervous pathways from the mammillary bodies, through the anterior nuclei of the thalamus to the cingulate gyrus, are necessary to a state of vigilance and wakefulness in both man and animal. By inference, therefore, this circuit would be concerned in affective behaviour. The involvement of the mammillary bodies in Korsakoff's psychosis and Wernicke's syndrome also suggests the significance of this pathway in the elaboration of emotional experience [9]. In light of the bearing of emotional factors in essential hypertension, it is pertinent that stimulation in what appears to be the region of the mammillotegmental tract will produce in the cat a great rise in blood pressure [13].

In reference to the possible emotional function of the cingulate gyrus, Papez noted that tumors of the corpus callosum impinging on it are often associated with changes of the personality, loss of affect, and various degrees of somnolence and stupor. He also referred to one case where a softening of the left paracentral lobule and cingulate gyrus was accompanied by a marked disturbance in the emotional realm.

In view of the part played by smelling and mouthing in sexual activity, it is interesting that these various elements of experience may have the opportunity to be associated in the regions defined by Papez. The precuneus (fig. 1) which broadens out posteriorly from the cingulate gyrus is contiguous with the sacral representation in the paracentral lobule. Papez has 'noted that in the two sexes the precuneus shows a greater difference in size than any other portion of the cortex, being more highly developed in the male', and has suggested that representation of the sex organs may be localized there [52]. Further support for this speculation is suggested by the remarkable case of nymphomania reported by Erickson in 1945 [20]. The patient was a 55-year-old woman who for more than ten years complained of a persistent 'passionate feeling'. Later she developed convulsions. It is notable that perfume was thought to exaggerate her symptoms. At operation she was found to have a hemangioma of the right paracentral lobule which anatomically is just above the cingular gyrus and ahead of the precuneus. Penfield has described a patient with a lesion of the temporal lobe who exhibited sexual ideas as a component of his dreamy state [59].

Recent Developments in Neurophysiology Bearing on the Papez *Theory*

Since 1937 there have appeared a number of experimental reports which would lend support to Papez's thesis that the rhinencephalon plays a fundamental role in the affective sphere. Perhaps the most striking observations are those of Klüver and Bucy on a series of monkeys deprived of both temporal lobes [36]. It is important to stress that where only one lobe was removed or where bilateral lesions spared the rhinencephalon, the animals failed to show significant changes in their behaviour. The bilaterally lobectomized animals, on the other hand, presented a dramatic picture. Formerly wild and intractable, they became docile and showed neither signs of fear nor anger. They would not fight or retaliate when abused by other monkeys, and obviously would not have survived in a natural habitat. They displayed also what the authors refer to as 'psychic blindness', 'oral tendencies', and 'hypermetamorphosis', a kind of compulsive behaviour. It was as though they could no longer discriminate between objects that were either potentially dangerous or useful to them. The 'hissing tongue' of a snake or feces might be selected as readily for examination as a piece of food. Such an animal would go around its cage, and as if by compulsion smell and mouth everything – dirt, feces, nail, food – that captured its attention. Unless the object was edible, it would be immediately dropped. If presented with a nail a hundred times in succession, the animal would smell and mouth it in each instance as though he had not examined it before. Finally, these animals showed striking changes in their sexual behaviour. They appeared hypersexed, masturbated excessively, sought partnership with male or female indiscriminately, and manifested bizarre oral-sexual behaviour[5]. It is interesting that many of these phenomena described by KLÜVER and BUCY were noted sixty years ago by BROWN and SCHÄFER, who performed similar ablations, but their significance was not appreciated [10].

In 1940 SPIEGEL and co-workers reported a number of acute experiments in which they claimed that appropriate lesions in various parts of the rhinencephalon would produce in cats or dogs the picture of sham rage [70]. They emphasized that the lesions must be bilateral. Such lesions when confined to the olfactory tubercles, or the anterior portion of the amygdaloid complex, or to parts of the hippocampus and fornix (fig. 2), all led to manifestations of the rage reaction. These findings are reminiscent of those of FULTON and INGRAHAM, who in 1929 described rage reactions in cats following bilateral, prechiasmal lesions at the base of the brain [25]. These lesions probably involved rhinencephalic structures in the region of the olfactory tubercles. BARD and MOUNTCASTLE, in chronic preparations on cats, have confirmed the findings of SPIEGEL et al. in reference to the amygdala [7]. In contrast to the observations of KLÜVER and BUCY on the monkey, however, these investigators report that bilateral temporal lobectomy in the cat 'leads to savageness'[6]. 'They have noted that a removal of the entire neocortex results in a state of 'placidity' provided rhinencephalic structures are not significantly damaged. It is their

opinion that the amygdala acts as a 'funnel' through which inhibitory influences originating in the cingular gyrus, the neocortex, and the amygdala itself, exert a suppressing action on brain stem mechanisms.

As regards hypertension it is pertinent to note that stimulation of the anterior perforated space, which is posterior to the olfactory tubercle, will cause 'sharp rises' in the blood pressure of the monkey [65]. In the same animal stimulation in the region of the hippocampal gyrus produces vocalization and vagal-like vasomotor changes that last well beyond the cessation of the stimulus [67]. In one instance CHAPMAN et al. have had the opportunity to stimulate the region of the temporal pole in man and found there resulted a considerable rise of both the systolic and diastolic blood pressure [12].

Recently the cingulate gyrus has been subject to extensive experimental investigation. The results of experiments on the dog [37] and the monkey [69, 75] have been consistent and establish this part of the brain as an important autonomic center. In light of the bearing of emotion on asthma, it should be noted that the anterior part (area 24) of the cingular gyrus can exert a powerful vagal effect on respiration. A considerable rise of blood pressure can also be obtained by appropriate stimulation of this area. Besides its influence on visceral activity, area 24 can exert a profound effect on

---

[5] The temporal lobectomy as performed in these experiments spared part of the hippocampal formation posterior to the lesion. This should be kept in mind when the possible correlation of sexual and visceral sensations in this region receives further discussion. The indications are that these animals could still smell and taste; on an anatomic basis it is conceivable that some gustatory, olfactory, and other visceral sensations could have been transmitted from the septal nuclei and parolfactory area to the remaining dentate gyrus and hippocampus by fibers passing over the corpus callosum (fig. 2).

[6] Perhaps less of the hippocampal formation was removed in these experiments.

the electrical activity of the brain as well as the body musculature [5, 69, 75]: According to McCulloch, area 24 sends impulses by way of the caudate to the thalamus which block spontaneous thalamocortical activity and cause a suppression of electrical activity of the cortex [49]. And Ward has presented evidence to show that area 24 is able, through its connections with the reticular substance in the brain stem, to inhibit all motor activity [75]. These mechanisms suggest a possible explanation of how intense emotion could paralyze both thought and action. Finally, ablation of area 24 in the macaque is said to cause a loss of fear of man and other changes of affective behaviour peculiar to the monkey [68, 75].

It is now recognized that a great number of automatic responses can be obtained from the orbitomesial surface of the frontal lobes [4, 41]. Yakovlev maintains that this part of the brain is as much a part of the mesopallium as the cingulate gyrus, and along with the latter 'may be looked upon as part of the highest representation of visceral functions' [80]. Appropriate stimulation of this area will cause inhibition of respiration, rise of blood pressure, and

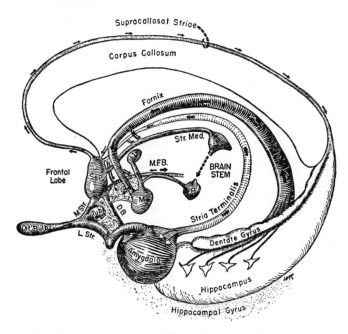

Fig. 2. A schematic representation of the relationship of the main subcortical structures and connections of the rhinencephalon, drawn as though all of them could be seen from the medial aspect of the right hemisphere, with the intervening tissue dissolved away. The composite was suggested by illustrations from W. J. S. Krieg's Functional neuroanatomy (The Blakiston Company, Philadelphia, 553 pp.), but for diagrammatic purposes some of the added or altered connections have been given an arbitrary course. Abbreviations: AT = anterior nucleus of thalamus; DB = diagonal band of Broca; H = habenula (a part of the epithalamus); IP = interpeduncular nucleus; L Str = lateral olfactory stria; M = mammillary body (a part of the posterior hypothalamus); MFB = medial forebrain bundle; M Str = medial olfactory stria; Olf Bulb = olfactory bulb; Sep = region of the septal nuclei; Str Med = stria medullaris; Tub = olfactory tubercle (head of the caudate immediately underneath).

decrease in tonus of the gastric musculature [4]. LIVINGSTON *et al.* have recorded a considerable rise of the blood pressure in man after stimulation at a critical frequency in this region [42]. Finally, it is highly significant that stimulation of this area (as well as the posterior hypothalamus and other points along the sympathetic chain to the kidney) will produce a blanching, and hence ischemia, of the renal cortex [16]. If emotion found chronic expression over these pathways, it is conceivable how the renin enzyme system could be so activated as to lead to persistent hypertension.

The island of Reil, which lies buried beneath the frontal and temporal lobes, is also intimately associated with the rhinencephalon. But all one can emphasize here is how little is known about the comparative neurology, neuroanatomy, and physiology of this region. PENFIELD has indicated in recent lectures that the insula is concerned with gastrointestinal sensation and function. Experiments are now under way at the Laboratory of Physiology at Yale which suggest that the orbitomesial surface of the frontal lobes, the anterior insula, the temporal pole, and the pyriformamygdaloid complex are mutually related in their bearing on autonomic activity and emotional behaviour [26, 35, 48].

Possible Anatomic, Physiologic, and Psychologic Correlates

The recognition that the cerebrum is an outgrowth of the olfactory brain is obtrusive evidence of the part played by the sense of smell in the evolutionary development of the vertebrate [29]. Smell not only has a fundamental role in obtaining food, but warns the animal of enemies; it participates in the sexual functions of mating and copulation [30]. In primitive forms where life seems to be a matter of incorporating or being incorporated, it is the medial olfactory tract leading to correlation centers for smell, taste, and sensations from the mouth and viscera that shows the greatest develop-

ment in size [3] (fig. 2). Smell therefore might be thought of as an oral sense, or more broadly as a visceral sense. In the course of phylogeny, as other senses exert a greater influence in directing the movements of the animal, the lateral olfactory tract leading to the 'olfacto-somatic'[7] correlation center in the pyriform lobe[8] becomes larger than the medial tract [3, 34]. Although, in the ascension to higher forms, the rhinencephalon yields more and more control over the animal's movements to the neocortex, its persistent, strong connections with lower autonomic centers suggests that it continues to dominate in the realm of visceral activity. Hence the rhinencephalon might be justifiably considered a visceral brain, and will be so referred to in the remainder of this paper to distinguish it from the neocortex which holds sway over the body musculature and subserves the functions of the intellect.

In primitive forms the visceral brain provides the highest correlation center for ordering the affective behaviour of the animal in such basic drives as obtaining and assimilating food, fleeing from or orally disposing of an enemy, reproducing, and so forth. From anatomic and physiologic considerations previously referred to as well as those about to be mentioned, it might be inferred that the visceral brain continues to subserve such functions in higher forms, including man. Some of the neuroanatomy of the visceral brain that may have to do with the correlation of feeding and sexual activities and their bearing on affective states will be dealt with presently in more detail. As a preliminary, it will serve to point up the problems discussed in this paper if it is first indicated how the primitive brain perhaps ties in with behaviour that has been so often described as primitive, or infantile, in patients with psychoso-

---

[7] A term used in comparative neurology. Somatic, in this instance, refers to the body exclusive of the viscera.

[8] Refers to the forward pear-shaped expansion of the hippocampal gyrus.

matic illness [40, 45, 64]. Psychiatrists have resorted to these adjectives probably because so much of the information obtained from these patients has to do with material which in a Freudian sense is assigned to the oral and oral-anal level, or, as one might say all inclusively, the visceral level. In practically all the psychosomatic diseases such as hypertension, peptic ulcer, asthma, ulcerative colitis, that have been subject to fairly extensive psychiatric investigation, great emphasis has been placed on the 'oral' needs, the 'oral' dependencies, the 'oral' drives, etc., of the patient [71, 76]. These oral factors have been related to rage, hostility, fear, insecurity, resentment, grief, and a variety of other emotional states. In certain circumstances, for example, eating food[9] may be the symbolic representation of psychologic phenomena as diverse as (1) the hostile desire to eradicate an inimical person, (2) the need for love, (3) fear of some deprivation or punishment, (4) the grief of separation, etc. It will be useful to refer subsequently to the *excessive* oral manifestations of hostility and anger, as 'visceral aggression'; of insecurity and fear, as 'visceral fear'; of a feeling of dependence, as 'visceral need', etc. It is to be noted that many of the seemingly paradoxical and ridiculous implications of the term 'oral' result from a situation, most clearly manifest in children or primitive peoples, where there is a failure or inability to discriminate between the internal and external perceptions that make up the affective qualities of experience [77]. Visceral feelings are blended or fused with what the individual sees, hears, or otherwise senses, in such a way that the outside world is often experienced and dealt with as though it were incorporated. Thus the child looking at a leaf may say, 'It tastes green' [77]. Or the primitive may attribute a feeling of anguish to a squirming animal in his stomach. On the basis of interview material it is claimed that the patient with psychosomatic illness deals with the affective qualities of experience very much as a child or a primitive. In regard to interpersonal relationships, for example, such a patient may give evidence of a symbolic sort that he either identifies with, or seeks to master, other individuals by a process of incorporation. Hence his emotional life often becomes a matter of 'inviscerating' or 'exviscerating'. It is as though such a person never 'learned to walk' emotionally. A few of the psychodynamic formulations relating to psychosomatic disease will be touched on in the concluding pages.

The best way to comprehend the anatomy of the visceral brain and to derive a relatively clear picture of its tangle of connections with the hypothalamus and lower centers (fig. 2), is to consider it from the standpoint of comparative neurology. Space does not permit, however, a tracing of its history from the stage in primitive vertebrates where it is so diffusely connected with the epithalamus and hypothalamus as to be indistinguishable, to the point of development in man where the exuberant growth of the neocortex relegates it backward and downward into the mesial and basal parts of the cerebrum [3]. Anatomic emphasis therefore will be given to such of its structures as may have a bearing on the correlation of emotional experience.

Bucy and Klüver have remarked that 'of all the areas of the cortex the temporal is anatomically the one to which the term 'association area' is most suited' [10]. But it is generally not recognized that such a statement applies particularly to the hippocampal formation[10] in the basal parts of the temporal lobes. Here, as we shall subsequently see, the possibility exists for correlating not only olfactory, gustatory, and other visceral sensations, but auditory, visual, somesthetic, and, perhaps sexual, sensations as well [57]. And once correlated in the hippocampal gyrus, the impressions can be discharged through the motor cortex

_____

[9] Or indulgence in drugs, alcohol, etc.

[10] The designation 'hippocampal formation' is used in this paper to include the hippocampal and dentate gyri, the hippocampus and the amygdala (fig. 4).

of the hippocampus, or the nuclei of the amygdala.

The motor cortex of the hippocampus is infolded longitudinally into the inferior horn of the lateral ventricle, presumably as the result of expanding cortex around it [3]. The dentate gyrus, which suggests a receptive type of cortex and which may serve as a visceral correlation center[11], lies along most of the medial side of the hippocampus and discharges its impressions into it. The hippocampal gyrus, which also has attributes of a sensory type of cortex is contiguous with the entire lateral aspect of the hippocampus, and projects to the motor cells of the latter through the transitional region known as the subiculum. Its anterior portion is intimately associated with the amygdala (fig. 2 and 4).

According to LORENTE DE NÓ, CAJAL was the first to note that in addition to the angular bundle from the olfactory area, the subiculum of the hippocampal gyrus receives two other large contributions – one from the cingulum and one from the supracallosal striae. I had the opportunity to see Dr. PAPEZ dissect out these and other association tracts of the rhinencephalon and the temporal lobes. In gross dissection the cingulum is a most impressive bundle. It is possible that fibers passing in it could interconnect the hippocampal formation with the whole length of the cingulate gyrus. If the PAPEZ theory is correct, the cingulum could carry sexual impressions, among others, to the hippocampal region. The supracallosal striae possibly convey visceral sensations from the primitive smell-taste-visceral nuclei in the septal region [3] (fig. 2 and 3).

Dr. PAPEZ indicated that there is ample opportunity for auditory and somesthetic sensations to pass by way of association fibers to the hippocampal gyrus. He also pointed out fibers coming by way of the lingual gyrus from the part of the visual cortex where the periphery of the retina is represented. He noted that it is objects that move in the periphery of our vision that most startle and alarm us[12].

The anatomic pathways by which olfactory impulses are carried to the hippocampal formation have been fairly well established [14, 23, 43, 44, 61, 62]. It is not at all clear, however, how the other visceral sensations, which patients with lesions involving the deep or under part of the temporal lobes experience, reach this area. RUCH and PATTON have claimed from experiments in the monkey that the para-insular cortex of the operculum has primacy as a taste center [63], but the possibility exists that taste, as well as smell and other visceral sensations, have multiple cortical representation. The comparative neurologists suggest that taste and other visceral sensations from the septal region could reach the hippocampal formation by way of the diagonal band of Broca and the amygdala, or the supracallosal striae [3, 34] (fig. 2). Dr. PAPEZ has evidence that area 38 on the tip of the temporal lobe may receive a visceral projection of vagal origin by way of the central medial and central nuclei of the thalamus, the inferior thalamic peduncle, and the amygdala [54, 55, 56].

Figure 3 is a highly schematic diagram to demonstrate the number of sensory systems streaming into this region. The hippocampus has been externalized in the form of the little sea horse, after which it

---

[11] The dentate gyrus is the only part of the hippocampal formation absent in anosmatic animals. Comparative neurology suggests that it is the first cortical association area for smell, taste, and sensations from the mouth and viscera. It receives afferents from the primitive smell-taste-visceral nuclei in the septal region by way of the longitudinal striae running over the corpus callosum (fig. 2 and 3), as well as afferents from the hippocampal gyrus.

[12] It is possible that here may be a partial neuroanatomic explanation for such psychologic phenomena as anxiety and delirium frequently occurring in the sick with the onset of darkness; the mental state of the paranoid who feels he is being attacked from the periphery; or more generally the fear and apprehension that is commonly associated with the unseen both in the present and the future?

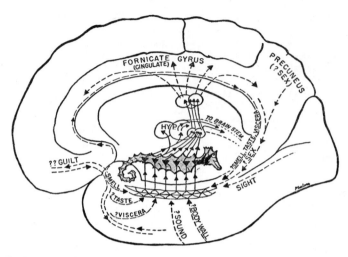

Fig. 3. Explanation in text. HYP, indicating the anterior, middle, and posterior divisions of the hypothalamus. Directly above are the three subdivisions of the right anterior nucleus of the thalamus.

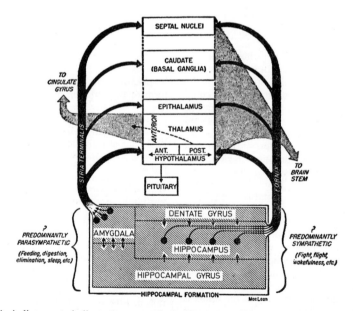

Fig. 4. A diagram to indicate the anatomical and possible functional relationships of various parts of the hippocampal formation. The latter designation is used in this paper to include the hippocampal and dentate gyri, the hippocampus and the amygdala.

got its name from ARANTIUS who first described it in 1587 [37]. The layer of large pyramid cells in the hippocampus suggests a keyboard on which the various elements of the sensorium can play. In the diagram the arch of the fornix has been straightened out to clarify the direction of impulses going to the hypothalamus, anterior nuclei of the thalamus, and the cingular gyrus. Most of the fibers in the fornix are said to terminate in the mammillary bodies [2]; but other parts of the hypothalamus and rhinencephalon, as well as the epithalamus and basal ganglia, also receive contributions (fig. 4). The diagram emphasizes that the hippocampal gyrus may serve as affectoceptor cortex and the hippocampus as affectomotor cortex, somewhat analogous to the somatic sensory and motor gyri of the neocortex. The lobulations on the hippocampus, which suggested the body segments of the sea horse to Arantius, conceivably might represent parcellations of different functions [57]. Perhaps some day an 'animunculus' will be drawn for this region.

It has not been possible to include the amygdala in the diagram in fig. 3. As previously stated, this structure is intimately associated with the anterior part of the hippocampal gyrus (fig. 2 and 4). It is often emphasized that the olfactory fibers, unlike those of other sensory systems, have no known primary projection to the thalamus. When one regards the amygdala from the standpoint of its phylogeny and anatomy [3, 14, 34, 72], however, it is evident that it is a thalamus-like relay station for olfactory stimuli (as well, probably, as other visceral impressions) to the archipallium. One therefore might as justifiably refer to it as an olfactory thalamus as to designate the conventionally known thalamus the optic thalamus. The efferent fibers from the nuclei of the amygdala project in large measure to the region of the septum and the anterior hypothalamus [22, 34, 72][13]. It is notable that these latter regions have been implicated in such highly coordinated viscerosomatic acts as defecation, urination, etc. Since the amygdala seems to project

predominantly to the parasympathetic centers of the hypothalamus, and the hippocampus to the symphathetic, is it possible that these respective parts of the visceral brain are mutually antagonistic? Might the sham rage associated with bilateral lesions of the amygdala result in part from the release of the hippocampus and the posterior hypothalamus to sympathetic discharge? The possibly antagonistic relationship between the amygdala and hippocampus has been indicated in figure 4.

It is important to stress that there is an overlapping of the three main fiber systems coming into the subiculum of the hippocampal gyrus [44]. There are also longitudinal fibers associating the hippocampal formation throughout its entire length. In the light of these observations, there is a possible neuroanatomic mechanism to explain some of the seemingly paradoxical overlapping (or synaesthesia) of the various qualities contributing to emotional experience. The overlapping of oral and sexual behaviour, for instance, must be more than a fortuitous circumstance. In this part of the brain it is possible to conceive how sexual incitations could stimulate a crude, diffuse feeling of visceral yearning that would make the individual seek to mouth and incorporate the object of its desire. According to intensity, the sex-hunger pattern might lead anywhere from gentle kissing to the deviate forms of oral-sexual behaviour, or to such bizarre psychotic manifestations as a woman eating her menses. Likewise, the hunger-rage pattern susceptible to sexual firing might express itself in all gradations from aggressive, sadistic behaviour to sex-murder and mutilation. In regard to the influence of other sensations, it is possible that disturbing impressions from the realm of vision, hearing, etc., could generate appropriately either visceral need, visceral fear, or visceral aggression. To use a crude analogy, it is as though the various elements of the sensorium were gathered together in the hippo-

[13] Especially the pre-optic nuclei.

campal gyrus and placed on a party line. The ringing of the bell for one party, particularly if persistent and intense, might bring one or more of the other parties to the phone. Much of the gossip going back and forth in this area is what we have commonly come to associate with the id, the beast, or sin in man (e.g. gluttony, lechery, etc.). In the light of this it is interesting that through the large uncinate fasciculus, the frontal lobes 'stand guard' over this region. Could it be that feelings of guilt are fomented here? It may have more than little significance that the uncinate fasciculus is apparently involved in lobotomy [51].

In the preceding discussion it has been implicitly assumed that the hippocampal formation provides the kind of analyzer that can derive universals from the particulars of experience and relate them symbolically in the experience of emotion. But in the light of current concepts of servomechanisms, it is pertinent to question whether or not the primitive structure of the hippocampal formation allows such an assumption. In his recent book on Cybernetics, Professor WIENER has indicated that a machine having to deal with the recognition and choice of forms may be served by a scanning mechanism in conjunction with a central clocking device [78]. McCULLOCH and PITTS have presented evidence to show that a structure exists in the auditory and visual cortex for scanning, and it was postulated that reverberating thalamocortical circuits provided the necessary clocking device or sweep mechanism [60]. Theirs is the first reasonable explanation of how the brain is able to recognize auditory and visual forms. One might further postulate that a sweep circuit exists between the pulvinar and the parietooccipital[14] cortex and between the dorsomedial nuclei and the frontal cortex, whereby the patterns of electrical activity built up in the sensory areas are carried along the association gyri, somewhat analogous to the moving letters across the light bulbs of a sign board [53].

But when one comes to consider the temporal lobes (exclusive of the auditory area) in the light of such a possible scanning mechanism, one finds a deficiency of the necessary neural apparatus. One of the anatomic enigmas is the apparent absence of projections from the thalamus to the temporal lobes save for the small acoustic area [48, 73]. This would indicate that no central clocking device was available to the greater part of the temporal region. As previously noted, however, the amygdala has a thalamus-like relationship with the archipallium. The large lateral nucleus of the amygdala deserves particular attention in regard to the present problem. It develops *pari passu* with association nuclei of the thalamus [57] and reaches its greatest size in man [17]. And like the pulvinar and dorsomedial nucleus of the thalamus it receives no projection from sensory systems [34, 72][15]. Since many of its fibers appear to run in the external capsule, it is possible they may be distributed to various parts of the temporal lobe, including the hippocampal formation. If this were true, there might exist a potential sweep mechanism for this cortex.

But regardless of any scanning and sweep mechanism that may exist, the cortical cytoarchitecture of the hippocampal formation indicates that it would have little efficiency as an analyzer compared with the neocortex. When LORENTE DE Nó undertook his studies of the cerebral cortex, he started with this region because, as he noted, it provides the simplest type of cortex [43]. In the regio entorhinalis of the mouse, for example, only 30 types of cells can be differentiated as compared with more than 60 in its most complicated cortical structure. Finally, it should be emphasized that the cortex of the hippocampal formation has a similar architecture throughout its entire length and presents the same general picture in all mammals from mouse to man

[14] Inclusive of a small area of temporal cortex.

[15] There is the possibility, however, that part of this nucleus may receive a visceral contribution by way of the inferior thalamic peduncle [54, 55, 56].

[44]. On the basis of these observations one might infer that the hippocampal system could hardly deal with information in more than a crude way, and was possibly too primitive a brain to analyze language. Yet it might have the capacity to participate in a nonverbal type of symbolism. This would have significant implications as far as symbolism affects the emotional life of the individual. One might imagine, for example, that though the visceral brain could never aspire to conceive of the colour red in terms of a three-letter word or as a specific wave length of light, it could associate the colour symbolically with such diverse things as blood, fainting, fighting, flowers, etc. Therefore if the visceral brain were the kind of brain that could tie up symbolically a number of unrelated phenomena, and at the same time lack the analyzing ability of the word brain to make a nice discrimination of their differences, it is possible to conceive how it might become foolishly involved in a variety of ridiculous correlations leading to phobias, obsessive-compulsive behaviour, etc. Lacking the help and control of the neocortex, its impressions would be discharged without modification into the hypothalamus and lower centers. Considered in the light of Freudian psychology, the visceral brain would have many of the attributes of the unconscious id. One might argue, however, *that the visceral brain is not at all unconscious (possibly not even in certain stages of sleep[16]), but rather eludes the grasp of the intellect because its animalistic and primitive structure makes it impossible to communicate in verbal terms.* Perhaps it were more proper to say, therefore, it was an animalistic and illiterate brain.

If the visceral brain functioned in the realm of emotion in the manner described, certain puzzling aspects of the psychologic status of patients with psychosomatic disease would be more readily understood. It strikes one as paradoxical, for example, that such patients often advance to superior attainments in the intellectual sphere, and at the same time, according to some psychiatrists, show evidence that their emo-tional life has been arrested at or near the oral level. This would suggest that more attention should be directed toward factors having to do with the emotional development of these individuals during infancy and childhood.

It has been stated that the first directed act the child performs on coming into the world is to smell and root its way to its mother's breast [1]. If hungry it cries, and it may be predicated in this instance that both hunger and crying are manifestations of insecurity in its new environment. If its hunger is unsatisfied, the instinctual patterns of response appear limited and stereotyped. It may scream in anger and bite the mother's breast, or if neglected for a long period lapse into a wailing type of cry. Once fed and satisfied, it becomes placid and goes to sleep. During the infantile stage, the majority of its preoccupations continue to be associated with obtaining food and being fed. It would not be unreasonable to suppose therefore that in its emotional development the act of being fed would symbolize for it being loved and cared for; whereas the contrary situation would be associated with feelings of insecurity, resentment and anger[17]. Once the child begins to sit up and to share in the

[16] The role of the rhinencephalon in sleep presents a fascinating problem when considered in the light of comparative zoology and neurophysiology. Animals without a neocortex appear to sleep at irregular intervals. The basal electroencephalogram in man (involving leads near the basilar rhinencephalon) recorded during early sleep has a different appearance from the tracing obtained in the region of the neocortex, resembling more the waking type of record (personal observation). It has been suggested that dreaming is a function of the temporal lobes [58].

[17] It may prove pertinent to the problem under discussion that, according to FLECHSIG, the process of myelination in the cerebrum commences in the eighth month of intrauterine life and involves first the afferent fibers passing to the somesthetic area in the postcentral gyrus and the afferent fibers to the hippocampal formation [28, p. 749].

activities of the home, its oral and visceral sensations must obviously fall into greater association with those of the eye, the ear, and the body wall. Stimuli from the genitalia would also be integrated with these other sensations. (Feelings from bladder and bowel, of course, fall into the visceral category). Although the child might live in an environment where all the requirements for food were satisfied, the harsh voice or look of rejection would have the opportunity in the hippocampal formation to be associated with the oral and visceral sense, and thereby serve as the stimulus to arouse visceral fear, visceral need, or visceral aggression. To cite examples of the great variety of ways anger, resentment, feelings of rejection, etc., reflect themselves in the eating habits of a child, and are therefore symbolically a function of the visceral brain, would not only be time-consuming, but also result in belaboring much that is well known. It should be stressed that the possibility exists for anger or fear to generate hunger as well as a paralysis of the desire to eat. Such a situation, as well as the symbolic content, is often more clearly evident in adults than in children. I might mention, for example, a hypertensive patient, who after a violent quarrel with her sister, proceeded to a restaurant and ate what she described as the biggest meal of her life. It is not unusual for persons with obesity to admit they constantly 'nibble' or eat excessively because they feel 'nervous', 'anxious', or 'frustrated'.

The question arises in reference to psychosomatic disease whether or not patterns of emotional behaviour leading to *excessive* visceral expression are repeated so often in childhood as to become permanently ingrained in the visceral brain, with the result that they are perpetuated in later life. The combined studies of neuroanatomists and neurophysiologists during the past 50 years have led to a fascinating concept of how transient memory is kept alive in the brain [18, 21, 43, 47, 60, 61, 78][18].

This in turn may have a bearing on permanent memory. Transient memory is

postulated to be a function of the self-re-exciting chains of neurones which exist at all levels of the nervous system [43] and which allow the electrical impulses transmitting information of a transitory sort to reverberate in a fixed pattern until they are dissipated in the discharge of an effector circuit. It is possible that if a certain electrical pattern of information were to reverberate for a prolonged period or at repeated intervals in a neuronal circuit, the nerve cells (perhaps, say, as the result of enzymatic catalysis in the dendritic processes at specific axone-dendritic junctions) would be permanently 'sensitized' to respond to this particular pattern at some future time. Such a mechanism would provide for one variety of enduring memory in a way that is remotely analogous to a wire recorder. These hypothetical considerations suggest how oft-repeated childhood emotional patterns could persist to exert themselves in adult life. They would also indicate the problems facing the psychiatrist in dealing with old memory patterns; to dissipate the impulses of an old memory reverberating in a circuit is not to affect the memory of the cell. But the possibility exists that new patterns of behaviour may be learned that could modify the old.

Only brief reference can be made to some of the psychodynamic formulations that have been made in regard to those psychosomatic diseases where lesions are present. In essential hypertension it has been postulated that the patient suffers 'chronic unexpressed rage' because of his inability either to satisfy his 'oral' demands (e.g., failure to elicit the love and protection of a dominating parental figure) or his ambitious independent strivings [66]. In patients with peptic ulcer unconscious 'oral', dependent needs (e.g. craving for continued maternal care) are said to stand in conflict with the conscious struggle to achieve independence and success [71, 76]. Similarly, the asthmatic patient is described as being in an emotional dilemma where lingering 'oral' dependence

[18] See [8] for a review.

on a parent makes it impossible to fulfill his strong desire for emancipation [24]. It has been suggested that asthmatic breathing is a form of wailing or crying which occurs whenever the patient is faced with the crisis of deciding to break the parental tie. The 'inclination' to primitive behaviour in patients with ulcerative colitis has been noted by LINDEMANN [40]. It might be generalized that these patients manifest the primitive psychologic state where other individuals are identified with, or mastered by, a process of incorporation. Unsatisfactory identification or unsuccessful mastery because of lingering resentment, anger, etc., may lead to a feeling of visceral turmoil, and defecation becomes the symbolic expression of the desire to extrude and rid from the body the incorporated figure. The part played by symbolic incorporation and defecation in grief reactions of patients with ulcerative colitis has received the attention of LINDEMANN and his co-workers. In a psychiatric and psychoanalytic study of patients with rheumatoid arthritis LUDWIG has observed that these individuals 'are unable to express their very strong emotions, but instead react to emotional crises with intense autonomic activity, in a manner which closely resembles the primitive and poorly organized techniques of mastery by destruction and ingestion described in the traumatic neuroses' [45].

It is not the purpose here to defend or criticize these formulations, but rather to indicate that a mechanism (possibly involving dominantly inherited neural patterns) may exist in the visceral brain to account for the phenomena described. It might be imagined that the 'rage' of the hypertensive patient, arising out of unsatisfied 'oral' demands, has a similar mechanism to the rage-producing hunger in the animal. In both instances the visceral brain might be postulated as participating in the release of the hypothalamus to sympathetic discharge (fig. 4). But in the hypertensive the conscious need for restraint would exert through the neocortex an inhibition of the somatic expression of rage

for which the autonomic responses are brought into play, and so interfere with the physiologic safety valve of muscular activity. On the other hand, the 'emotional hunger' of the patient with peptic ulcer might be considered as chronically activating that part of the visceral brain which is linked to the hypothalamic nuclei governing gastric function, with the result that the stomach is being constantly prepared for food (fig. 4). Similarly one might speculate about possible mechanisms for asthma, ulcerative colitis, and other diseases where the emotions are thought to contribute to the development of lesions.

Psychotherapeutic Considerations

Preliminary to a few comments on therapy, it should be remarked that one of the striking observations regarding the patient with psychosomatic illness[19] is his apparent intellectual inability to verbalize his emotional feelings. Anatomically it would appear that the intellect could obtain information from the visceral brain directly on the cerebral level by way of the long and short association fibers, or otherwise be left to determine at second hand from feed-back signals what messages the visceral brain had discharged autonomously to lower centers. In the psychosomatic patient it would almost seem there was little direct exchange between the visceral brain and the word brain, and that emotional feelings built up in the hippocampal formation, instead of being relayed to the intellect for evaluation, found immediate expression through autonomic centers. In other words, emotional feelings, instead of finding expression and discharge in the symbolic use of words and appropriate behaviour, might be conceived as being translated into a kind of 'organ language'. Such a concept would have a bearing on some of the differences

[19] Here again we have reference particularly to that variety of psychosomatic diseases where lesions are present. See introduction.

that have been noted between patients with psychoneuroses and those with psychosomatic illness. The former are claimed by the analysts to have an emotional disturbance involving more the genital, rather than the oral, stage of development. Furthermore, they are said to have a greater facility than psychosomatic patients in giving verbal expression to, and 'acting out' their emotional feelings. Perhaps this facility affords a reduction of traffic on the autonomic circuits and thereby helps to ward off the development of lesions.

If the psychosomatic patient is inarticulate about his emotional feelings, and if, as indicated, the visceral brain is an animalistic and illiterate brain, one would not expect at the beginning of psychotherapy to accomplish a great deal by verbal methods. Rather, at the onset of therapy, such a situation would suggest an emphasis on those activities of the doctor that have a 'disalarming' effect on the patient – such for example as the doctor's kindly manner, his interest, tone of voice, etc. In other words these activities would involve the kind of things that have been hypothesized as having meaning for the visceral brain, and which clinically are regarded as supportive measures. After a good patient-doctor relationship was once established, one might progress gradually to the verbal methods involved in insight therapy.

Summary

A notable deficiency attendant on psychosomatic theory at the present time is the inability to point to a mechanism of emotion that would account for the variety of ways the effective qualities of experience may act on automatic centers. The first part of this paper reviews certain neurophysiologic and neuroanatomic evidence now at hand that contributes to the understanding of emotional mechanisms. There are indications that the phylogenetically old brain (classically known as the rhinencephalon and arbitrarily referred to in this paper as the 'visceral brain') is largely concerned with visceral and emotional functions. This region of the brain appears to be

so strategically situated as to be able to correlate every form of internal and external perception. In other words, the possibility exists in this region for bringing into association not only oral (smell, taste, mouth) and visceral sensations, but also impressions from the sex organs, body wall, eye, and ear. And in contrast to the neopallium, the rhinencephalon has many and strong connections with the hypothalamus for discharging its impressions.

These relationships and alleged functions of the rhinencephalon have far-reaching implications for psychiatry. For they indicate that though our intellectual functions are carried on in the newest and most highly developed part of the brain, our affective behaviour continues to be dominated by a relatively crude and primitive system. This situation provides a clue to understanding the difference between what we 'feel' and what we 'know'.

In the remainder of the paper it is suggested how the mechanisms referred to may be related to 'oral' and visceral factors that are brought into play in the experience and expression of emotion by the patient with so-called psychosomatic disease.

In view of recent developments in electronics and cybernetics and the light these sciences have shed on neurophysiology, one can no longer be content to think of dynamic psychologic phenomena as existing apart from the restrictions of ordered neural mechanisms.

References

1. ALDRICH, C. A.: Ancient processes in scientific age. Feeding aspects. Amer. J. Dis. Child 64: 714–722 (1942).

2. ALLEN, W. F.: Degeneration in the dog's mammillary body and Ammon's horn following transection of the fornix. J. comp. Neurol. 80: 283–291 (1944).

3. ARIËNS KAPPERS, C. U.; HUBER, G. C., and CROSBY, E. C.: The comparative anatomy of the nervous system of vertebrates, including man (Macmillan Company, New York 1936) 2 vol., pp. 864, 865–1845.

4. BAILEY, P. and SWEET, W. H.: Effects on respiration, blood pressure and gastric motility of stimulation of orbital surface of frontal lobe. J. Neurophysiol. 3: 276–281 (1940).

5. BAILEY, P.; VON BONIN, G.; DAVIS, E. W.; GAROL, H. W.; McCULLOCH, W. S.; ROSEMAN, E., and SILVEIRA, A.: Functional organization of the medial aspect of the primate cortex. J. Neurophysiol. 7: 51–55 (1944).

6. BARD, P.: A diencephalic mechanism for the expression of rage with special reference to the sympathetic nervous system. Amer. J. Physiol. 84: 490–513 (1928).

7. BARD, P. and MOUNTCASTLE, V. B.: Some forebrain mechanisms involved in expression of rage with special reference to suppression of angry behavior. Res. Publ. Ass. nerv. ment. Dis. 27: 362–404 (1948).

8. BRAZIER, M. A. B.: Neural nets and integration of behaviour. To appear in: Perspectives in Neuropsychiatry (Lewis, Ltd., London 1949).

9. BRODAL, A.: The hippocampus and the sense of smell. A review. Brain 70: 179–222 (1947).

10. BUCY, P. C. and KLÜVER, H.: Anatomic changes secondary to temporal lobectomy. Arch. Neurol. Psychiat. 44: 1142–1146 (1940).

11. CANNON, W. B. and BRITTON, S. W.: Studies on the conditions of activity in endocrine glands. XV Pseudaffective medulliadrenal secretion. Amer. J. Physiol. 72: 283–294 (1925).

12. CHAPMAN, W. P.; LIVINGSTON, K. E., and POPPEN, J. L.: An observation of the effect on blood pressure of electrical stimulation of the tips of temporal lobe in man (to be published).

13. CHU, H. N. and LOO, Y. T.: On vasomotor centers in the forebrain and the midbrain. Chinese J. Physiol., Lond. 11: 295–300 (1937).

14. CLARK, W. E. L. and MEYER, M.: The terminal connexions of the olfactory tract in the rabbit. Brain 70: 304–328 (1947).

15. COBB, S.: Borderlands of psychiatry, p. 166 (Harvard University Press, Cambridge 1943).

16. CORT, J. H.: Personal communication. Res. Publ. Ass. nerv. ment. Dis. 27: 405–417 (1948).

17. CROSBY, E. C. and HUMPHREY, T.: Studies of the vertebrate telencephalon. II. The nuclear pattern of the anterior olfactory nucleus, tuberculum olfactorium and the amygdaloid complex in adult man. J. comp. Neurol. 74: 309–352 (1941).

18. DUSSER DE BARENNE, J. G. and McCULLOCH, W. S.: The direct functional interrelation of sensory cortex and optic thalamus. J. Neurophysiol. 1: 176–186 (1938).

19. EDINGER, L.: The anatomy of the central nervous system of man and of vertebrates in general (tr., W. S. HALL), p. 446 (Davis Company, Philadelphia 1899).

20. ERICKSON, T. C.: Erotomania (nymphomania) as an expression of cortical epileptiform discharge. Arch. Neurol., Chicago 53: 226–231 (1945).

21. FORBES, A.; COBB, S., and CATTELL, H.: Electrical studies in mammalian reflexes. III. Immediate changes in the flexion reflex after spinal transection. Amer. J. Physiol. 65: 30–44 (1923).

22. FOX, C. A.: The stria terminalis, longitudinal association bundle, and precommissural fornix fibers in the cat. J. comp. Neurol. 79: 277–295 (1943).

23. FOX, C. A.; McKINLEY, W. A., and MAGOUN, H. W.: An oscillographic study of olfactory system of cats. J. Neurophysiol. 7: 1–16 (1944).

24. FRENCH, T. M.; ALEXANDER, F. et al.: Psychogenic factors in bronchial asthma. Psychosom. Med. Monograph, No. 2, 1941.

25. FULTON, J. F. and INGRAHAM, F. D.: Emotional disturbances following experimental lesions of the base of the brain (pre-chiasmal). Amer. J. Physiol. 90: 353 (1929).

26. FULTON, J. F.; PRIBRAM, K. H.; STEVENSON, J. A. F., and WALL, P. D.: Interrelations between orbital gyrus, insula, temporal tip, and anterior cingulate. Trans. Amer. neurol. Ass. 74 (1949).

27. GIBBS, E. L.; GIBBS, F. A., and FUSTER, B.: Psychomotor epilepsy. Arch. Neurol., Chicago 60: 331–339 (1948).

28. GRAY, H.: in LEWIS Anatomy of the human body, p. 1428 (ed. 24) (Lea and Febiger, Philadelphia 1942).

29. HERRICK, C. J.: A sketch of the origin of the cerebral hemispheres. J. comp. Neurol. 32: 429; 454 (1921).

30. HERRICK, C. J.: The functions of the olfactory parts of the cerebral cortex. Proc. nat. Acad. Sci. 19: 7–14 (1933).

31. HOWELL's Textbook of physiology, p. 1304 (ed. 15). J. F. FULTON (ed.) (Saunders Company, Philadelphia 1946).

32. JACKSON, J. H. and STEWART, P.: Epileptic attacks with a warning of a crude sensa-

tion of smell and with the intellectual aura (dreamy state) in a patient who had symptoms pointing to gross organic disease of the right temporo-sphenoidal lobe. Brain 22: 534–549 (1899).

33. JASPER, H. and KERSHMAN, J.: Electroencephalographic classification of the epilepsies. Arch. Neurol., Chicago 45: 903–943 (1941).

34. JOHNSTON, J. B.: Further contributions to the study of the evolution of the forebrain. J. comp. Neurol. 35: 337–481 (1923).

35. KAADA, B. R.; PRIBRAM, K. H., and EPSTEIN, J. A.: Respiratory and vascular responses in monkeys from temporal pole, insula, orbital surface and cingulate gyrus. J. Neurophysiol. 12: 347–355 (1949).

36. KLÜVER, H. and BUCY, P. C.: Preliminary analysis of functions of the temporal lobes in monkeys. Arch. Neurol., Chicago 42: 979–1000 (1939).

37. KREMER, W. F.: Autonomic and somatic reactions induced by stimulation of the cingular gyrus in dogs. J. Neurophysiol. 10: 371–379 (1947).

38. LASHLEY, K. S.: The thalamus and emotion. Psychol. Rev. 45: 42–61 (1938).

39. LEWIS, F. T.: The significance of the term hippocampus. J. comp. Neurol. 35: 213–230 (1923–1924).

40. LINDEMANN, E.: Psychiatric problems in conservative treatment of ulcerative colitis. Arch. Neurol., Chicago 53: 322–324 (1945).

41. LIVINGSTON, R. B.; FULTON, J. F.; DELGADO, J. M. R.; SACHS, E.; BRENDLER, S. J., and DAVIS, G. D.: Stimulation and regional ablation of orbital surface of frontal lobe. Res. Publ. Ass. nerv. ment. Dis. 27: 405–420 (1948).

42. LIVINGSTON, R. B.; CHAPMAN, W. P.; LIVINGSTON, K. E., and KRAINTZ, L.: Stimulation of orbital surface of man prior to frontal lobotomy. Res. Publ. Ass. nerv. ment. Dis. 27: 421–432 (1948).

43. LORENTE DE NÓ, R.: Studies on the structure of the cerebral cortex: I. The area entorhinalis. J. Psychol. Neurol., Lpz. 45: 381–438 (1933).

44. LORENTE DE NÓ, R.: Studies on the structure of the cerebral cortex: II. Continuation of the study of the ammonic system. J. Psychol. Neurol., Lpz. 46: 113–177 (1934).

45. LUDWIG, A. O.: Psychiatric studies in patients with rheumatoid arthritis (to be published).

45a. MACLEAN, P. D. and ARELLANO, A. P.: Basal lead studies in epileptic automatisms. EEG clin. Neurophysiol. 2 (1950).

46. MASSERMAN, J. H.: Behavior and neurosis. An experimental psychoanalytic approach to psychobiologic principles, p. 269 (University of Chicago Press, Chicago 1943).

47. McCULLOCH, W. S. and PITTS, W.: A logical calculus of the ideas immanent in nervous activity. Bull. math. Biophys. 5: 115–133 (1943).

48. McCULLOCH, W. S.: The functional organization of the cerebral cortex. Physiol. Rev. 24: 390–407 (1944).

49. McCULLOCH, W. S.: Some connections of the frontal lobe established by physiological neuronography. Res. Publ. Ass. nerv. ment. Dis. 27: 95–105 (1948).

50. METTLER, F. A.: Extracortical connections of primate frontal cerebral cortex; corticofugal connections. J. comp. Neurol. 86: 119–166 (1947).

51. MEYER, A.; BECK, E., and McLARDY, T.: Prefrontal leucotomy: A neuro-anatomical report. Brain 70: 18–49 (1947).

52. PAPEZ, J. W.: A proposed mechanism of emotion. Arch. Neurol., Chicago 38: 725–743 (1937).

53. PAPEZ, J. W.: Structures and mechanisms underlying the cerebral functions. Amer. J. Psychol. 57: 291–316 (1944).

54. PAPEZ, J. W.: Fiber tracts of the amygdaloid region in the human brain, from a graphic reconstruction of fiber connections and nuclear masses. Anat. Rec. 91: 294 (1945).

55. PAPEZ, J. W.: Human growth and development, p. 164 (The Cornell Cooperative Society, Ithaca 1948).

56. PAPEZ, J. W.: Unpublished data.

57. PAPEZ, J. W.: Personal communication.

58. PENFIELD, W. and ERICKSON, T. C.: Epilepsy and cerebral localization, p. 623 (Thomas, Springfield 1941).

59. PENFIELD, W.: Discussion. Arch. Neurol., Chicago 53: 226–231 (1945).

60. PITTS, W. and McCULLOCH, W. S.: How we know universals. The perception of auditory and visual forms. Bull. math. Biophys. 9: 127–147 (1947).

61. RAMÓN Y CAJAL, S.: Studien über die Hirnrinde des Menschen, 5 Vol. (Barth, Leipzig 1900–1906).

62. RAMÓN Y CAJAL, S.: Histologie du système nerveux de l'homme et des vertébrés, 2 vol. pp. 799, 823 (Maloine, Paris 1909, 1911).

63. RUCH, T. and PATTON, H. D.: The relation

of the deep opercular cortex to taste. Fed. Proc. *5:* 89–90 (1946).

64. RUESCH, J.: The infantile personality; the core problem of psychosomatic medicine. Psychosom. Med. *10:* 134–144 (1948).

65. SACHS, E., Jr. and BRENDLER, S. J.: Some effects of stimulation of the orbital surface of the frontal lobe in the dog and monkey. Fed. Proc. *7:* 107 (1948).

66. SAUL, L. J.: Hostility in cases of essential hypertension. Psychosom. Med. *1:* 153–161 (1939).

67. SMITH, W. K.: The results of stimulation of the uncus and adjacent portions of the hyppocampal gyrus. Fed. Proc. *3:* 42 (1944).

68. SMITH, W. K.: The results of ablation of the cingular region of the cerebral cortex. Fed. Proc. *3:* 42–43 (1944).

69. SMITH, W. K.: The functional significance of the rostral cingular cortex as revealed by its response to electrical excitation. J. Neurophysiol. *8:* 241–255 (1945).

70. SPIEGEL, E. A.; MILLER, H. R., and OPPENHEIMER, M. J.: Forebrain and rage reactions. J. Neurophysiol. *3:* 538–548 (1940).

71. Studies in psychosomatic medicine, p. 568. ALEXANDER and FRENCH (eds.) (The Ronald Press Company, New York 1948).

72. VAN DER SPRENKEL, H. B.: Stria terminalis and amygdala in the brain of the opossum (Delphis virginiana). J. comp. Neurol. *42:* 211–254 (1926).

73. WALKER, A. E.: The primate thalamus, p. 321 (University of Chicago Press, Chicago 1938).

74. WARD, A. A., Jr. and McCULLOCH, W. S.: The projection of the frontal lobe on the hypothalamus. J. Neurophysiol. *10:* 309–314 (1947).

75. WARD, A. A., Jr.: The cingular gyrus: Area 24. J. Neurophysiol. *11:* 13–23 (1948).

76. WEISS, E. and ENGLISH, O. S.: Psychosomatic medicine, p. 687 (Saunders Company, Philadelphia 1943).

77. WERNER, H.: Comparative psychology of mental development, p. 510 (Harper and Brothers, New York 1940).

78. WIENER, N.: Cybernetics, or control and communication in the animal and the machine, p. 194 (Wiley and Sons, Inc., New York 1948).

79. YAKOVLEV, P. I.: Motility, behavior, and the brain. J. nerv. ment. Dis. *107:* 313–335 (1948).

80. YAKOVLEV, P. I.: Personal communication Res. Publ. Ass. nerv. ment. Dis. *27:* 405–417 (1948).

Psychologic Mechanisms in Malignant Hypertension[1]

M. F. REISER, M. ROSENBAUM and E. B. FERRIS

Retrospective comment by Dr. A. P. Shapiro. In 1951, clinicians appreciated that blood pressure was variable and subject to emotional influence, but few studies were available to define the magnitude of this factor. This paper was one of a series from the Cincinnati group which provided such systematic information. In a group of 12 patients with malignant hypertension, REISER *et al.* clearly showed that emotional events, specific to the patient, were important precipitating events. They demonstrated not only the physical continuity of malignant acceleration from previous benign hypertension but continuity of the psychological events in the individual's life which reached a traumatic climax coincidental with the onset of the malignant episode. They clearly pointed out that it seemed unlikely that the psychological events constituted a sole cause of hypertension, either benign or malignant, but represented a potent contributing factor to the complex of events, the 'mosaic' as Dr. IRVIN PAGE has put it, which leads to the disease. What was also striking in this study, was the fact that a number of the patients reverted to the benign phase during a moderate amount of supportive psychotherapy which was oriented towards an understanding of the individual psychodynamics of the patients. (It must be remembered that at the time of this study there were no effective pharmacologic means of treating hypertension and malignant hypertension was a universally fatal disease.) It is unfortunate that in the explosion of information about physiologic mechanisms and pharmacologic influences in hypertension which has accumulated in the past twenty years, this small paper remains a gem only appreciated by those internists who have sought for confirmation of their own clinical experiences in handling malignant hypertensives with a 'listening ear'. Those who have 'listened' have repeatedly confirmed REISER's observation that one can almost always find emotional conflict of considerable meaning to the patient when hypertension accelerates to the malignant phase, but because of the other more easily communicated facts about this disease, the importance of the emotional factors is not transmitted sufficiently well in current teaching. This is a paper which should be read by each generation of medical students to indicate not only a significant observation, but a technique for study of a scientific problem which uses primarily psychological and psychodynamic interpretation to understand a patient's physiologic changes.

Hypertensive cardiovascular disease is essentially a nonepisodic condition in which there is no clear-cut relationship between symptoms and structural change. For this reason, it is often quite difficult to establish, with any degree of certainty, the exact date of onset or to reconstruct satisfactorily the previous course. The transition from the benign to the malignant phase, however, represents a relatively well delineated episode and thus provides the clinical investigator with an excellent opportunity for the study of psychosomatic relationships and mechanisms in hypertension.

As part of a comprehensive study of this disease, we have investigated 12 patients who were in various stages of the transition from benign to malignant hypertension. In each of these patients, examination of the relationship between the life history and

[1] From the Departments of Psychiatry and Internal Medicine, University of Cincinnati, College of Medicine.

the medical course of the disease revealed that the precipitation of the malignant phase could be chronologically correlated with emotionally significant life situations or events. In 8, where the time of onset of benign hypertension seemed reasonable clear, similar correlations could be made. The primary emphasis of this project was centered upon a simultaneous study of the medical, psychiatric, and physiologic aspects of the transition from the benign to the malignant phase of hypertension in each patient. This report then represents an exploratory effort to arrive at some understanding of the interrelationships involved in this basic phase of the hypertensive problem. This group of patients represented routine hospital admissions and were selected only on the basis of their ability to communicate adequately.

Material and Methods

Figure 1 summarizes the medical findings. Each of the patients showed evidence of diffuse cerebral edema and had hypertensive retinopathy corresponding to the grade IV classification of WAGENER-KEITH [8]. On this basis we have classified them as having malignant hypertension. In 7, the clinical findings were those of hypertensive encephalopathy without uremia. Six of these 7 patients recovered from encephalopathy and are still alive, having been followed for periods of 2 months to three and one-half years (as indicated in the last column on the right). The seventh subsequently developed uremia and died, as did the remaining 5 patients who showed renal decompensation in addition to encephalopathy[2].

Coexistent renal disease, in addition to arteriolonephrosclerosis, was diagnosed in 6 of the 12 cases. The remaining 6 patients are regarded as free of coexistent renal disease and are classified as having essential hypertension.

In addition to the routine medical workup, physiologic and pharmacologic studies were carried out in an attempt to determine the lability and range of blood pressure [4, 5], and some indication of the relative roles of neural and humoral mechanisms in the maintenance of the elevated pressure [3, 6].

The psychiatric material was obtained primarily by a series of face-to-face one hour flexible 'semidirective' interviews. The data derived and recorded included factual information regarding personal history, dream content, undirected associations and sequences, early memories, and transference phenomena. In addition, observations of the patients' clinical and physiologic responses to current situations on the ward, in the experimental laboratory, and in the general life environment were also recorded.

The data for each patient were then examined in regard to possible relationships between the major emotionally charged conflictual areas of the patient's personality (for which a functionally adequate system of defenses had not been developed), and (1) the conflictual meaning of the life settings in which benign and later malignant hypertension developed, and (2) the conflictual meaning of current situations which were associated with the observed clinical and physiologic responses.

In 6 of the cases where more intensive and penetrating psychiatric study was possible, we were able to obtain material relating to early traumata, and the stage of psychosexual development at which they occurred. These traumatic factors were also examined for evidence of relationship to the conflictual areas and the precipitating events (past and current).

Results

In order to illustrate the type of data obtained and the manner in which it has been handled, three case studies will be described.

Case 1 (No. 1, fig. 1 and 9; fig. 2, 3, and 4) E.B., a 43-year-old Negro male laborer, was admitted to Cincinnati General Hospital in

---

[2] Thirteen months have elapsed since the original preparation of this manuscript. Since that time, 2 of the 6 patients (I. O'L. No. 9, and F. J. No. 10) who were reported alive have expired. Of the remaining 4, 3 are alive and still in the benign phase (L. K. No. 4, J. S. No. 7, and O. H. No. 11). Contact with the fourth (E. B. No. 1) was lost when he left the city six months ago. Up to that time, his improvement had been maintained.

Patient		Age	Sex	Color	Medical status		
					Etiologic classification	Optic fundi (grade)	Cardiac state
1	E. B.	43	M	C	Essential	IV	Normal size heart, bundle branch block
2	V. F.	23	F	W	Chronic pyelonephritis (autopsy)	IV	Within normal limits
3	C. U.	42	F	W	Chronic pyelonephritis (autopsy)	IV	Enlarged heart, congestive failure, angina pectoris, EKG-myocardial damage
4	L. K.	32	F	W	Essential	IV	Moderately enlarged heart, EKG-mild myocardial damage
5	S. B.	28	M	C	Chronic glomerulonephritis	IV	Enlarged heart, congestive failure, EKG-myocardial damage
6	W. B.	49	M	W	Essential (autopsy)	IV	Normal size heart
7	J. S.	27	M	W	Unilateral hydronephrosis (biopsy)	IV	Within normal limits
8	P. T.	37	F	W	Essential	IV	Within normal limits
9	I. O'L.	44	F	W	Essential	IV	Enlarged heart, congestive failure
10	F. J.	45	M	W	Chronic pyelonephritis Kimmelstiel-Wilson syndrome	IV	Enlarged heart, congestive failure, EKG-myocardial damage
11	O. H.	36	F	C	Essential	IV	Within normal limits
12	F. N.	52	F	W	Chronic pyelonephritis	IV	Enlarged heart, EKG-left ventricular strain, no congestive failure

Fig. 1. Clinical data on twelve patients with malignant hypertension and hypertensive encephalopathy. Survey of the 'cardiac' status included routine electrocardiography, roentgenography, and measurements of venous pressure and circulation time (Decholin). Survey of renal function included urinalysis, assa of blood urea nitrogen content, phenolsulphonphthalein excretion

July, 1946, with acute hypertensive encephalopathy of six days' duration. His blood pressure had first been found elevated 2 years prior to admission.

The *personal history* revealed that he was an only child, whose parents separated when he was 2 years old. At this time, he was sent away to be raised by the mother's older sister and her husband. The patient's earliest memory is of this long, frightening journey, and he has been told that upon arrival, he was a very disturbed child, who refused to eat or talk for almost a week. He was then raised by rigid, demanding and punitive foster parents, who expected exemplary behavior and superior performance in return for physical sustenance. When he was 7 years of age, his aunt severely punished and humiliated him because of a childhood sexual escapade and the uncle threatened to turn him out of the home completely. Under this influence he developed into a precocious, model lad, who was, however, somewhat uncomfortable in the role and developed a ready facility with his fists and

Renal function	Cerebrospinal fluid pressure	Previous duration of hyper-tension	Course (since onset of malignant hypertension)
Normal	Increased	2 years	Living (2 years, 10 months)
Azotemia	Increased	14 years	Died
Azotemia	Increased	12 years	Died
Normal	Increased	7 years	Living (3 years, 7 months)
Azotemia		13 years	Died
Azotemia	Increased	26 years	Died
Normal		10 years	Living (6 months)
Restricted, blood urea normal	Increased	8 years	Died
Restricted, blood urea normal	Increased	2 years	Living (2 years, 6 months)
Slightly restricted, blood urea normal		4 years	Living (5 months)
Normal	Increased	7 years	Living (2 months)
Azotemia	Increased	13 years	Died

test, 18-hour concentration test, intravenous and/or retrograde pyelography, and urine cultures where indicated. Thirteen months have elapsed since original preparation of this table. See foot-note 2, p. 57, for current revision of the data regarding course.

found occasional outlet in surreptitious fight-ing, while totally suppressing sexual curiosity and urges.

At the age of 16, following the death of his aunt, which disturbed him greatly, he was expelled from school because of a violent outburst of temper. He then worked as a bell-hop and began to indulge in alcohol and sexual promiscuity and to allow free vent to his anger.

At 21, he married a girl whose father was a prominent minister and the pressure to con-form was again present. His relationship to his wife resembled that which he had experienced with his aunt, and by the age of 36, he had discontinued promiscuous sexual behavior and alcohol and had forced himself to control his explosive temper. He once more became a conscientious church goer. In 1944 (age 41) while working in a war plant, he became quite prominent in union activities, which brought him into open conflict with the company officials on many occasions. One month after a particularly severe union crisis in which the patient was prominently involved, he was called in for a routine physical check-up. This he interpreted as a direct personal retaliation for his union activities. On this examination his blood pressure for the first time was found to be elevated. He consulted his family doctor, who found it at normal levels repeatedly, but on each occasion examination by the company physician a few hours later revealed it to be elevated, and the patient was finally obliged to accept transfer to a less desirable job. He remained asymptomatic until July, 1946. Following an unusually heavy work assignment which he resented but carried out without

protest, he went home and in an automatic manner indulged in compulsive and repetitive sexual activity. During this episode, his wife's attitude became rejecting and threatening. The acute episode of encephalopathy immediately followed. The encephalopathy subsided in response to supportive care in the hospital. A remission, which has lasted now for 3 years, has been associated with relief of pressure in the crucial areas. Following discussion of his problems, he resigned from his union position and directed energies into managing a bowling league and sponsoring a young prize figther.

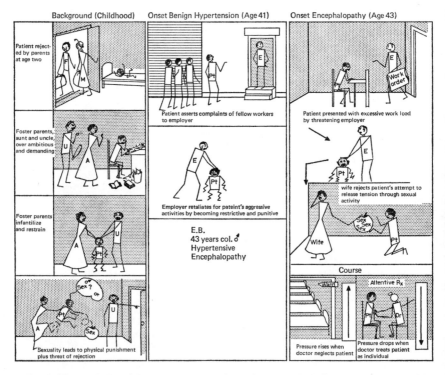

Fig. 2. Figures 2, 5, and 6 represent an experiment in the method of presenting case material of this sort. In them we have attempted through the use of a pictorial scheme to present a condensed visual summary of the correlations between early traumata and the psychodynamic content of important life events which were found to be associated with the medical phenomena studied. Note the resemblance between the dynamic emotional content and tone of the childhood traumatic events and the emotional content and tone of events which acted as the precipitating factors of clinical events in the course of hypertension in adult life. Figure 2 represents case 1 in the text.

Comment

This case, we feel, illustrates early pregenital trauma in the form of total parental rejection at the age of 2, followed by transfer to demanding foster parents, who were intolerant of any independent or aggressive display. Upon this was later superimposed severe physical punishment and threats of rejection at the time that first evidences of sexual curiosity emerged. It is felt that the major conflictual areas in this man's life were related to:

1. Intense hostility and dependence, with fear of rejection, in relation to demanding authoritative figures.

2. Guilt, fears of castration, and rejection for aggressive sexual behavior.

Early attempts at rebellion through unsocial behavior were relinquished in response to fears of rejection and retaliation. At the time of onset of hypertension, rebellious attitudes were being channelized through group identification in union activities. When this activity became personalized and punitive retaliation was threatened, the patient was forced to submit and hypertension developed.

Later, when again faced with intense hostility toward an employer because of demands for superior performance (similar to those made by the foster parents in childhood), the patient was unable to express this directly. At the same time, his wife was rejecting of his attempt to discharge energy in sexual activity. Thus, both phases of the early life trauma were combined and it was at this time that hypertensive encephalopathy appeared.

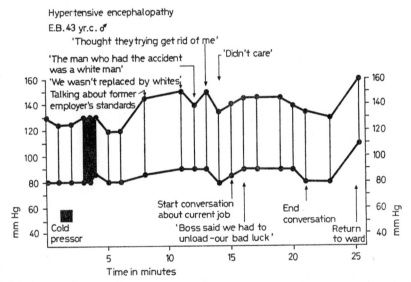

Fig. 3. Blood pressure readings in patient E.B. (case 1) during one experimental period in the laboratory. The patient's blood pressure at bed rest on the ward before coming to the laboratory was 175/105 mm Hg. After one-half-hour rest in the laboratory, it fell (45/25 mm Hg) to 130/80 mm Hg (first reading shown on the graph). Note that cold pressor test produced no significant rise in blood pressure over control levels (0/5 mm Hg). Interview topics noted in graph evoked pressor responses of 20/10 mm Hg. With discontinuance of interview, the blood pressure returned to the laboratory control level (125/80 mm Hg) but showed a prompt rise of 30/30 mm Hg upon the return of the patient to the ward. See text for interpretation.

Figures 3 and 4 illustrate the lability and range of the blood pressure in this patient. They illustrate also a certain specificity of the emotional pressor and depressor phenomena. An interview in which the precipitating events were discussed produced a greater rise in pressure than did the cold pressor test. The responses labeled 'environmental' in figure 4 illustrate the marked discrepancy between the low readings obtained in the laboratory as compared with the high ones obtained on the ward. This phenomenon is reminiscent of the discrepancy between the readings of the family physician and the company doctor at the time hypertension was first discovered. In the hospital, it appeared to be related to the fact that he

felt the investigator to be a reliable friend, who was intensely interested in helping him without making any demands upon him. On the contrary, he felt insecure and hostile in relation to the busy staff of the open thirty-bed ward. Thus, fluctuation in blood pressure was associated with a transference phenomenon, the content of which resembles that of the precipitating factors and relates to the same basic conflict; namely, that with authoritative parental figures. It has been our experience that the patient's unconscious response to a test situation may be of greater importance in determining his physiologic response than specific physiologic maneuvers or the conscious content of interview material.

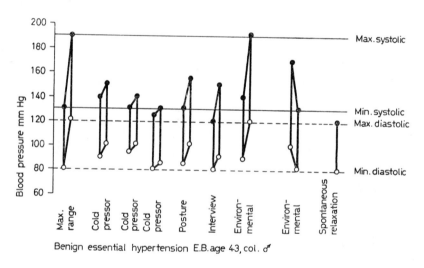

Benign essential hypertension E.B. age 43, col. ♂

Fig. 4. Summary of experimental blood pressure responses in case 1 (see text). Solid circles denote systolic pressure; open circles, diastolic pressure. Each parallelogram represents a single experimental blood pressure response; the left hand reading representing the starting (control) blood pressure and the right hand reading representing the end point blood pressures. The first parallelogram represents for purposes of comparison the maximum composite range of blood pressure obtained through the repeated pressor and depressor test maneuvers that were carried out over several weeks of study. Responses labeled environmental denote changes in blood pressure on transfer from the laboratory to the ward. The patient's blood pressure consistently fell upon transfer to the laboratory and rose on return to the ward. The magnitude of these changes was greater than those evoked by the other procedures used.

Case 2 (No. 2, fig. 1 and 9; fig. 5). V.F., a 23-year-old white, married female, was admitted to Cincinnati General Hospital on March 14, 1947, with a chief complaint of blindness and convulsions. Her blood pressure had first been found elevated 14 months previously, when she had begun to complain of listlessness and severe generalized throbbing headaches at the onset of her third pregnancy. This pregnancy was terminated at seven and one-half months (September, 1946) because of pre-eclamptic toxemia. She then felt better and was completely asymptomatic until 5 weeks prior to admission (February, 1947), at which time she began again to suffer from headaches, transient episodes of blurred vision, and nocturia. The day before admission, she had noticed headache and some blurring of vision, and on the morning of admission, she suddenly suffered a total loss of vision and entered the hospital with the findings of hypertensive encephalopathy.

At the time of the study, the patient was living at home in her own home, and had 2 children, boys, 6 and 3 years old. The child delivered 6 months previously had not lived and she had been sterilized at that time. Her husband was a steady working laborer.

Patient was born in Cincinnati, the fourth of 5 siblings, having 3 older brothers, 7, 6, and 3 years older, and a sister 4 years younger. She had no difficulty in pointing out that her father was not a good provider and because of his neglect of the family, mother was forced to work out of the home. He was described as being physically abusive to all the children and to the mother as well, when she attempted to protect the children. 'He didn't have no children and when he would come home he would be mean and hateful.' The patient idealized the mother and frequently emphasized what a horrible life she had had. As a child, the patient was cared for by grandmother or 'some other woman who was a relation'. The patient was married at the age of 16 to a man whom she had known all her life. She described her husband as an antisocial person who would drink sporadically, becoming mean and nasty when drunk, but aggressively hostile only if provoked. The patient was always afraid of provoking his anger at such times. The last pregnancy was not planned and patient felt discouraged when it occurred. She was able to give very little material regarding her psychosexual development. Mother had warned her against pregnancy and taught her the facts

of life at the age of 15. 'Mother was funny and wouldn't let the girls play with the boys.' She remembers mother spanking the boys for masturbating. She had no sexual experience before marriage. In association with this material, she said that she dreamed often about fighting with an unfamiliar figure and sometimes pushed her husband out of bed when she had these dreams.

She described with a good deal of confusion the sequence of events around the time of the onset of toxemia. She and her husband lost their apartment and had to move in with her mother. Shortly thereafter, her younger sister married a 'ne'er-do-well' navy deserter, who, the patient says, beat his fiancee even before marriage. The sister and her husband moved in with mother, forcing patient and her family to move out. Shortly after this, the sister's husband beat up the sister and the mother who was trying to protect her. In associating to this episode, the patient recalled an episode in which she had been shoved against a post by a cow, causing her abdomen to be 'squeezed'. As a result, she had bloody stools for several days thereafter. The next association was of an episode in which her husband kicked her 'in the belly' and mother had protected her. This, she said, was the only time that she could remember that he had ever abused her physically.

Her overt personality and behavior present an interesting picture. On her initial admission to the hospital, several clinicians spoke of her grim prognosis in her presence. Despite this, she remained in extremely good spirits, was always cheerful and denied symptoms. In relation to the doctors, she was always very defensive and would banter quick light conversation very skillfully. The only time that she lost composure in the interviews was when she was questioned about the most recent pregnancy.

She remained in the hospital on the first admission from March 14 until April 18, 1947. The blood urea nitrogen was moderately elevated but receded to normal. The cerebral manifestations subsided and vision improved, although the exudative retinopathy remained unchanged. Blood pressure remained high and patient left the hospital asymptomatic, having refused sympathectomy. She remained asymptomatic and managed her household until July 16, 1947, when she was readmitted with acute hypertensive encephalopathy. On this occasion, the blood urea nitrogen rapidly mounted to 140 mg% and she appeared moribund. After 10 days she began to improve spontaneously and for 2 weeks the blood pressure receded to levels of 150/90 to 119/78 mm Hg. Accompanying this period of remission, she showed evidence of a psychologic regression of psychotic proportions. She was discharged on September 27, 1947, with a blood urea nitrogen of 70 mg %, but without symptoms.

Three days later she was readmitted with acute encephalopathy and convulsions. The blood pressure was 250/190 mm Hg. On this occasion, the azotemia progressed and uremic pericarditis developed. Terminally, the blood urea nitrogen reached 230 mg % and creatinine 17 mg%. The patient died on October 13, 1947.

Comment

In this case, again, it is felt that there was early pregenital trauma in the form of oral deprivation due to the mother's having to work out of the home during patient's infancy. Upon this was superimposed further loss of the meager attention gained from mother when a younger sister was born. Sexual problems attendant to the witnessing of father's abuse of the masochistic mother led to an identification with the mother, with fear of and hostility to the father. The basic conflictual areas in this patient would appear to consist of: (1) Intense ambiva-

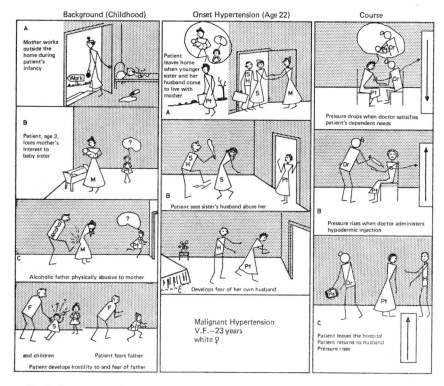

Fig. 5. See text, case 2.

lence to maternal figures stirred up by dependent frustration. (2) Hostility to sibling rivals. (3) Masochistic distortions, with fear of and hostility to men.

At the time of onset of hypertension (which apparently was of the malignant type from the start) all 3 of these conflictual areas were involved. First, patient was herself pregnant and hostile to the fetus. Secondly, she was rejected again by mother in favour of the younger sister. Third, the sister's experience with her husband replayed the old scene between mother and the abusive father.

The precise precipitating factors of the severe acute episodes of hypertensive encephalopathy with convulsions are not clear. However, such exacerbations occur-red regularly in relation to a patient's discharge from the hospital and return to her husband and sons.

In this patient, as in patient C.U. (case 3), temporary psychotic regression with loss of conflict and anxiety about dependent gratification was accompanied by a temporary remission of the malignant phase of the hypertension.

Laboratory procedures which evoked fear and hostility (probably related to sexual fantasies) regularly evoked pressor responses in this patient.

Case 3 (No. 3, fig. 1 and 9; fig. 6, 7, and 8). C.U., a 42-year-old recently separated housewife, had had benign hypertension for 12 years preceding the onset of the malignant phase.

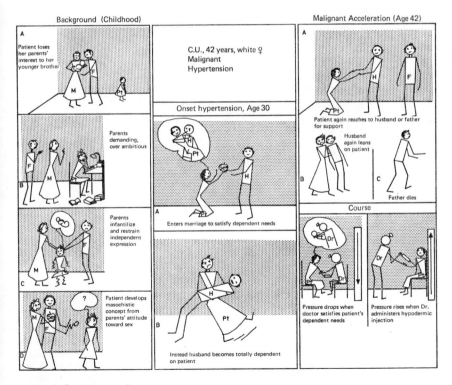

Fig. 6. See text, case 3.

Historical material indicated pregenital trauma in connection with the birth of 2 younger siblings by the time the patient was three and one-half years old. Genital problems appeared to be strongly colored by the unresolved oral conflict, since sexuality for this patient represented primarily an unpleasant but necessary means of gaining dependence. Benign hypertension developed shortly after marriage, when she realized that she would have to support her husband, who turned out to be an irresponsible alcoholic. Twelve years later, she separated from him but became so incapacitated by headaches that she decided to return for the meager support he might be able to offer in her illness. The frustration was more intense this time. Once again she had to go to work to support him. In addition, her father,

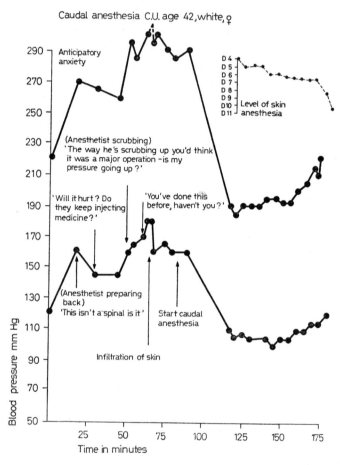

Fig. 7. Case 3: caudal anesthesia experiment. The patient's comments during preparatory phase of the experiment indicate clearly that her conception of the test was characterized by fear of pain and bodily damage. The mounting anxiety was accompanied by a steady rise in blood pressure which apparently was neurogenic in origin since the blood pressure promptly fell with paralysis of the autonomic fibers below the fourth thoracic segment. See text for discussion.

who was her only other possible source of help, died. Malignant hypertension developed in this setting.

Marked pressor responses were consistently noted in connection with procedures involving needles and may well reflect a response to masochistic interpretation of such a procedure. Figure 7 illustrates the pressor response evoked by preparation for caudal anesthesia.

The shaded area of figure 8 illustrates a temporary medical remission that occurred in connection with a transient psychotic episode in which the patient showed extreme infantile regressive behavior, which was characterized by an apathetic resignation and complete disappearance of conflict over frustrated de-

pendent needs. It is felt that the marked fall in blood pressure must represent a decrease in peripheral resistance since the blood urea fell concomitantly and there was regression of eyeground changes, disappearance of albuminuria and heart failure during this period. Thus, relief of dependent frustration was accompanied by temporary amelioration of the hypertension. It appears that with the temporary psychotic solution, the diffuse arteriolar spasm was relaxed and that circulatory dynamics reverted toward a more normal status. With emergence from the psychotic episode, evidence of emotional conflict and manifestations of malignant hypertension reappeared.

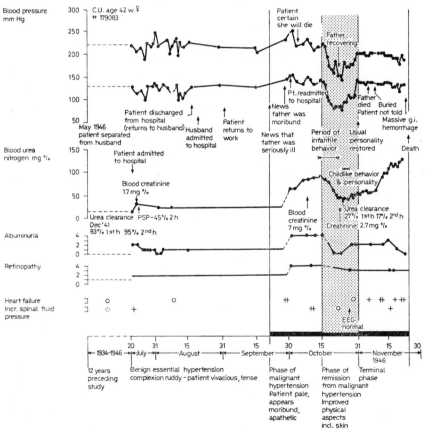

Fig. 8. Life chart (case 3) illustrating period of transient remission (shaded area) from malignant phase. See text for discussion.

Turning to a survey of the entire group of 12 patients, figure 9 lists the correlations within each individual case between basic conflictual areas and the emotional content of events associated with (1) the onset of benign hypertension, (2) the onset of malignant hypertension, and (3) the observed fluctuations in blood pressure and course.

A. Chronologic correlations between emotionally charged life events and clinical phenomena in the course of hypertension may be outlined as follows:

1. *Historical correlations. a) Precipitation of malignant hypertension.* Emotionally significant life events could be correlated with the onset of malignant hypertension in all cases; in 11 the life events were regarded as being of specific significance, in 1 it was felt to be of probable significance. *b) Precipitation of benign hypertension.* In 8 patients the date of onset of the benign phase was established with certainty. In 6 of these patients the onset could be correlated with specifically significant life events.

In the remaining 2, events of probable significance were noted. In one patient (V.F., case 2) the disease apparently was malignant from the onset.

2. *Current (observed) correlations.* During the course of observation and study, specific conflictual situations could be correlated with fluctuations of the blood pressure and the clinical course in 7 patients, and with fluctuations of the blood pressure alone in one additional patient.

B. Psychologic correlations. Ambivalence toward parental figures constituted the predominant central conflict for the group taken as a whole – such problems were encountered in 11 of the 12 patients, and were felt to be of primary importance in 11. Conflictual attitudes toward siblings were of importance in 8 instances, and sexual problems in 11. In all 6 patients in whom a history of early life trauma was obtained, there was evidence of problems having arisen in the pregenital phase of psychosexual development.

Fig. 9. A descriptive listing of the conflictual areas for each patient and the incidence of their occurrence as the central emotional content of the various precipitating life events. The summary for each case is recorded horizontally. The left hand column identifies the patient. The next column to the right designates whether or not a history of early genetic trauma was obtained, genital trauma being designated G, and pregenital PRE-G. The next (wide) middle column summarizes the data pertinent to the major conflictual areas of the personality structure. These have been grouped into three categories or 'areas': A = dependence and hostility to parents and parental figures; B = hostility to siblings or sibling figures; and C = sexual problems. For each area the conflictual dynamic forces are designated and the original childhood objects of ambivalent feelings are listed in upper case letters. Individuals involved in the current life constellation (as surrogates or objects of displaced or transferred conflictual feelings) are listed in lower case type. Those individuals actually involved in the precipitating events are underlined.

The next 4 columns to the right (enclosed by double lines) designate the correlations between conflictual areas and (reading from left to right) onset benign hypertension; onset malignant hypertension; observed fluctuations in blood pressure; and observed fluctuations in course.

Where a specific precipitating factor for onset of benign or malignant hypertension was found, this is designated by a + in the appropriate column. ? designates an episode of probable significance. Fluctuations in blood pressure are designated by appropriately directed arrows, and changes in course are identified by a descriptive word, such as *recovery*, *relapse*, etc. Beneath each designation indicating the presence of a precipitating factor, the basic conflictual area(s) touched upon by the episode is designated by the letter(s) (A, B, and/or C).

Thus, reading horizontally from left to right for each patient, there appears: (1) type of early trauma, (2) basic conflictual areas (with the involved past and current figures), (3) the correlations of these conflictual areas with the emotional content of events which precipitated benign, and/or malignant hypertension, and observed fluctuations in blood pressure and course.

It should be emphasized that case summaries are listed vertically for convenience only and do not indicate any specific similarities or correlations from one patient to another.

Within the individual patient, there was a striking consistency of the findings. In each instance, the emotional content of life situations associated (by history or observation) with clinical events was found to be related to the conflictual areas considered central for that particular individual. The course of the disease appeared to be affected when the individuals encountered life situations which evoked unresolved conflictual feelings which could not be adequately handled through normal channels

of expression or behavior. The precipitating events were considered specific for the individual patient in that they were related to specific areas of serious difficulty within his personality structure. Thus, each patient's central conflicts appeared as the common denominators of the various life events associated with the course of his hypertensive disease.

For example, patient E.B. (case 1) was able to act out or express hostile feelings except under specific circumstances, i.e.,

Part I

when they were directed toward an authoritative supporting figure from whom he would expect and fear either retaliating physical punishment or rejection (conflictual area A). He was unable to resolve such feelings because of the difficult childhood relationship with his foster parents. Benign hypertension appeared when this conflict was evoked in his relationship with his employers (who represented parental figures). The identical conflict situation was involved in the precipitation of the malignant phase; at this time there was engrafted additional tension because the feelings sought sexual outlet and were met with an attitude repetitious of the reception they had originally experienced in the strained childhood relationship with the foster parents (area C). Under study, it was repeatedly noted that situations which tended to arouse the conflict with authoritative figures (area A), e.g., the relationship to the ward physicians, were accompanied by a pressor response. A relationship which ameliorated this conflict – such as the experience of being the special patient of a doctor whom he had grown to trust – was productive of a depressor response. His recovery was related to relief of tension in both areas of difficulty (areas A and C) through supportive expressive psychotherapy and environmental manipulation.

Discussion

The events associated with the precipitation of malignant hypertension could in each patient be related to central or basic conflictual areas of the personality structure. Likewise, events associated with the precipitation of benign hypertension and situations related to current measurable changes in physiologic and clinical status involved the same set of basic conflicts. The observation that *current conflictual situations* (resembling those historically connected with the onset of benign and malignant hypertension) may be accompanied by *measurable* pressor responses and ob-

served fluctuations in the clinical course suggests that in each patient there is a close linkage between the hypertensive vascular mechanism and his specific central conflictual problems.

The differences between situations associated with clinical manifestations of differing severity appeared to be in large part quantitative – i.e., the basic constellations involved in the precipitation of the benign and the malignant phases in an individual were often the same, but the intensity of the conflict was greater (or difficulties in several areas seemed to be additive in their effects) at the time that the more severe manifestations appeared.

Of related interest is the finding that early in the malignant phase (before uremia has developed) reversion to the benign stage may frequently occur. This suggests a parallel or similar concept of the medical relationship of malignant to benign hypertension; namely, that it is a more intense form of the same basic disorder.

Specific correlations within the individual patient were found in the group with co-existent renal lesions, as well as in the group with essential hypertension. BINGER et al. have likewise reported finding similar psychologic data in hypertensive patients regardless of whether primary renal disease was or was not present [2]. Such findings are consistent with the 'multiple factor' concept of etiology – viz., that some physiologic predisposition toward involvement of a particular organ system must exist in order for it to be selected for involvement in the response to stress. Such organ vulnerability may be related to constitutional, hereditary, pathologic, or unknown factors. Of particular interest is the patient J.S. (No. 7, fig. 1 and 9) who had unilateral hydronephrosis. Hypertensive encephalopathy was here superimposed upon a ten-year pre-existent benign renal hypertension and its onset could be correlated with a highly charged life event. The encephalopathy began to subside in response to the support and protection provided by hospitalization alone, and the course reverted toward the pre-existent benign phase. Nephrectomy was then followed by return of the blood pressure to normal and complete disappearance of the retinopathy. His blood pressure has remained at a normal level for 16 months postnephrectomy, although he has returned to the same environmental problem. In this instance, the emotional and renal factors appear to have been combined in such a way that the renal hypertensive mechanism provided a physiologic pathway for the expression of specific conflictual energy. It seems probable that removal of the diseased kidney may have eliminated this patient's physiologic predisposition toward hypertension.

The selection of the hypertensive vascular mechanism in the group with 'essential hypertension' remains unexplained. It was found in the 6 more intensively studied cases of this series that significant problems had arisen in the first few years of life and there was evidence of severe insecurity in regard to the dependent relationship with parental figures. Evidence of genital-oedipal problems was also present and a marked masochistic orientation to femininity was prominent in each of the women. However, the genital problems seemed to be superimposed upon, and strongly colored by the earlier unresolved pregenital conflicts, since the heterosexual relationships were immature and seemed to be primarily oriented within a more infantile sphere. In the 6 remaining patients where historical data pertaining to early traumata is lacking, the general characteristics of the charged areas, with the marked emphasis on deep-going ambivalence in relation to parental figures, resemble those of the more thoroughly studied group, suggesting that the background may well be similar. These findings are consistent with the data reported in the psychoanalytic studies of ALEXANDER, SAUL, BINGER, and others [1, 2, 7]. This 'pregenital coloring' of the material may provide a speculative lead regarding the problem of the selection of the organ system in essential hypertension. The data suggest a linkage between pregenitally determined

conflicts and the hypertensive mechanism. It may be that the vascular phenomena characteristic of arterial hypertension represent an archaic physiologic concomitant of the stressful unconscious content of the precipitating life events. Such a response may at the age of the original trauma have constituted a usual and common physiologic mechanism involved in reaction to stress. Little is known about vegetative developmental patterns and vascular physiology in the early phases of life before verbal and controlled musculoskeletal pathways are available for the expression or discharge of energies induced by emotional stress. It seems possible that the physiologic response may be chronologically appropriate to the age at which the original unresolved conflict had its genesis. Any impression as to the role that early emotional trauma may play in determining a predisposition to hypertension must await more knowledge of vascular responsiveness in the first years of life.

Summary and Conclusions

In 12 representative patients with malignant hypertension in whom adequate study has been possible, we have found close chronologic correlations between the precipitation of malignant hypertension and the occurrence of emotionally charged life situations. It is felt that the data point toward the existence of a meaningful and understandable system of interrelated forces underlying these chronologic correlations. In the individual case, the precipitating events can be related to specific dynamic constellations in the patient's total personality. Further, these same constellations may in the individual patient be linked with the events associated with the onset of benign hypertension, fluctuations in blood pressure, and exacerbations of the clinical course. It should be emphasized that these correlations are specific within the individual patient. The data do not reveal any specificity of personality structure or conflict situations for the group as a whole and thus do not explain the selection of this organ system. The findings are consistent with the view that the specific choice of the hypertensive vascular mechanism may be related to an additional factor, or factors, such as the presence of a predisposing renal lesion in patients with coexistent renal disease, but as yet unknown in the patients with essential hypertension.

In 6 of 7 patients who had not yet developed renal failure, the course after hospitalization reverted without specific treatment to the benign phase, indicating that spontaneous remission may frequently occur in the early stage of malignant hypertension.

References

1. ALEXANDER, F.: Emotional factors in essential hypertension. Psychosom. Med. *1:* 175 (1939).
2. BINGER, C. A. L.; ACKERMAN, N. W.; COHN, A. E.; SCHROEDER, H. A., and STEELE, J. H.: Personality in arterial hypertension. Psychosomatic Medicine Monographs, NY, 1945.
3. FERRIS, E. B., Jr.; REISER, M. F.; STEAD, W. W., and BRUST, A.: Clinical and physiological observations of interrelated mech-
anisms in arterial hypertension. Trans. Ass. amer. Physicians *61:* 97 (1948).
4. GUBNER, R.; SILVERSTONE, F., and UNGERLEIDER, H. E.: Range of blood pressure in hypertension. J. amer. med. Ass. *130:* 325 (1946).
5. REISER, M. F. and FERRIS, E. B., Jr.: Clinical and experimental observations on the lability and range of blood pressure in essential hypertension, with special reference to physiologic mechanisms and significance of various pressor and depressor tests. (Abstract) J. clin. Invest. *26:* 1194 (1947).
6. REISER, M. F. and FERRIS, E. B., Jr.: The nature of the cold pressor test and its significance in relation to neurogenic and humoral mechanisms in hypertension. J. clin. Invest. *27:* 156 (1948).
7. SAUL, L.: Hostility in cases of essential hypertension. Psychosom. Med. *1:* 161 (1939).
8. WAGENER, H. P. and KEITH, W. M.: Diffuse arteriolar disease with hypertension and the associated retinal lesions. Medicine *18:* 317 (1939).

Studies of Syncope[1]

III. Differentiation Between Vasodepressor and Hysterical Fainting

J. ROMANO and G. L. ENGEL

Retrospective comment by Dr. D. T. Graham. This paper was one of a group of studies of fainting carried out by the authors. Its importance lies in its careful demonstration that not all faints called 'emotional' have the same mechanism, and in the encouragement it gave to efforts to delineate physiologically the processes involved in various responses that can too easily be dismissed as 'just psychological'. The logic of the distinction between hysterical conversions and vegetative neurotic symptoms, referred to in the paper as a 'complex problem', is unfortunately not much clearer today than it was in 1944. One continuing source of difficulty is the tendency to believe that there can be a non-physiological illness, and then to equate hysteria with this supposed lack of physiological process. Indeed, the authors say that the faint of their hysterical patient was 'not due to concomitant physiologic phenomena of an emotional experience'. Problems inherent in this conclusion do not, however, detract from the value of showing, as the authors did, that some faints are associated with changes in EEG, heart rate and blood pressure, while others are not.

In a recent communication, ALEXANDER clearly and succinctly outlined certain points of differentiation between hysterical conversion and vegetative neurotic symptoms [1]. It may be pertinent to quote directly his summary: 'While the similarities are rather superficial both conditions are psychogenic, that is to say, they are caused ultimately by a chronic repressed or at least unrelieved emotional tension. The mechanisms involved, however, are fundamentally different, both psychodynamically and physiologically. The hysterical conversion symptom is an attempt to relieve an emotional tension in a symbolic way; it is a symbolic expression of a definite emotional content. This mechanism is restricted to the voluntary neuromuscular or sensory perceptive systems whose function is to express and relieve emotions. A vegetative neurosis consists of a psychogenic dysfunction of a vegetative organ which is not under control of the voluntary neuromuscular system. The vegetative symptom is not a substitute expression of the emotion, but its normal physiological concomitant.'

We believe ALEXANDER's concept of this differentiation is valid and useful. We believe, too, that the concept does not constitute a fixed bipolar typology. Obviously there are many instances in which unrelieved emotional tension may be accompanied by normal physiologic processes, but at the same time, tension may be relieved through symbolic means. Perhaps it would help to consider the possible range of human expression as it relates to this differentiation as a wide spectrum, the extremes of which illustrate clearly the differences between hysterical and vegetative phenomena but the midzones may comprise features of both. One has but to consider hysterical skin lesions or involvement of certain areas of the gastrointestinal tract (cardiospasm) to illustrate the complexity of the problem.

In certain instances, it is possible to differentiate clearly between the two types. In the following, we wish to present certain physiologic and psychologic data which

[1] From the Department of Psychiatry, University of Cincinnati, College of Medicine and the Cincinnati General Hospital.

we believe demonstrate the distinction between hysterical conversion and vegetative neurotic mechanisms as it relates to the problem of fainting.

Fainting, that is, syncope is a common and somewhat terrifying human experience. It is well known that syncope may occur secondary to certain structural and physiological derangements which ultimately lead to reduction of blood flow to the brain, and in some instances, to local disturbance of cerebral circulation. These include such physiologic derangements as loss of blood volume, as in hemorrhage; relative increase of the vascular bed, as in high fever; derangements in the posture regulating mechanisms of the autonomic nervous system, as in true orthostatic hypotension; cardiac standstill, as in Stokes-Adams attacks or reflex asystole from carotid sinus and other vagal afferents; and local cerebral mechanisms, as in the cerebral type of carotid sinus syncope.

However, syncope occurs more commonly in individuals who have no previously demonstrable structural or physiological disturbance, but who develop syncope abruptly under conditions of phantasied, consciously anticipated or actually experienced emotional stress. This includes the large group of people who faint during venepuncture, minor surgical procedures or injuries, upon witnessing mutilation or accidents, upon hearing tragic news or facing situations of threatening nature, and occasionally with no obvious precipitating or provocative stimulus. That psychological factors play an important role in such fainting has been known since antiquity, but less well appreciated is the fact that two quite different mechanisms may be involved in the loss of consciousness that climaxes these reactions. When these patients are studied during spontaneous or provoked syncope, one finds that they may be classified into 2 groups. In one group the loss of consciousness is preceded by rather striking clinical manifestations, including pallor, sweating, sighing respiration, hypotension and sometimes bradycardia. In the second group, consciousness is lost without any demonstrable changes in circulation or respiration. The clinical characteristics of the first group are those of vasodepressor syncope. The clinical characteristics of the second group we believe to be those of hysterical fainting. By a more complete description of the psychological and physiological characteristics of these two types of syncope as illustrated by detailed data on one representative case of each type, we hope to demonstrate the validity of the concept formulated by ALEXANDER as it relates to fainting.

Vasodepressor Syncope

In previous communications, we have described the clinical and physiological characteristics of vasodepressor syncope [3, 5]. Briefly, it was found that the reaction could be initiated by a great variety of noxious stimuli, such as venepuncture, injury to deep structures, distention of hollow organs, viewing mutilation, facing threatening situations, etc., but once initiated, the subsequent course of the reaction was unrelated to the nature of the provoking stimulus. Vasodepressor syncope is common upon initial exposure to a new and threatening situation. Nurses and medical students frequently faint anticipating or witnessing the first dissection, the first autopsy, or the first surgical operation. With repetitive experiences, these individuals have less and eventually no trouble. Clinically, the first symptoms and signs of vasodepressor syncope are weakness, followed quickly by sighing respiration, nausea, pallor, sweating, falling blood pressure, changes in cardiac rate and rhythm (tachycardia, bradycardia, and varying degrees of heart block), and finally, unconsciousness within 1–5 min if the subject remains in the erect position. The complete picture, culminating in unconsciousness, is likely to occur in the erect position and most symptoms are relieved promptly upon returning to the recumbent position, although they may recur within a few minutes if the patient stands up too soon. The primary physiological change probably is an abrupt disturbance in the distribution of blood in the vascular bed. It is not known whether this is related to a decrease in venous or arteriolar tone, to a decrease in skeletal muscle tone, or to a shunting mechanism leading to pooling in splanchnic or other areas. In any case, the effect of gravity in the standing position greatly accentuates this disturbance, probably by impeding return of blood to the heart from dependent areas. The pallor and sighing respiration represent compensatory mechanisms designed to shunt blood from non-essential regions (skin and abdominal viscera) to aid filling of the heart. These signs, plus the sweating, nausea, air hunger, etc., are associated symptoms that occur during the phase of falling blood pressure. Unconsciousness does not result until arterial blood pressure or pulse pressure has fallen to extremely low levels, and then is accompanied by striking slowing of the brain waves. Recovery of consciousness and return of brain waves to normal occurs promptly upon resuming the recumbent position. Should the patient remain erect, the loss of consciousness is often followed within 10–20 sec by clonic convulsive movements. Recovery of consciousness usually occurs within 20–40 sec, with or without convulsive movements, even if the patient is maintained in the erect position.

The following case of typical vasodepressor syncope illustrates the concomitance of certain emotional experiences with these physiological changes.

The patient, J. B., 40-year-old twice-married Kentucky farmer and unskilled laborer, who had been employed in a Cincinnati war material factory, came to the Out-Patient Clinic of the Cincinnati General Hospital in October, 1943, because of increasing disability due to pain in the chest, diffuse weakness and 'spells' in which he lost consciousness. He remarked further that the symptoms, which had begun 4 to 5 months before, had prevented his return to work.

He was born on a small farm in Kentucky and had experienced little security in his relationships with parents or siblings, but found the kindness and interest of his maternal grandfather to be his chief support. This old gentleman, a preacher, taught him what he knew and impressed upon him the need for high ethical and social standards. During adolescence the patient broke away from his grandfather and from the religious beliefs, but was reconverted at the age of 19. He became deeply religious and succeeded in converting his entire family. The patient married shortly thereafter only to find his wife irreligious and irresponsible. She bore him a number of children. Although her slovenly and neglectful attitudes toward the home and children as well as her disrespectful attitude toward the church distressed him, he had no significant symptoms, somatic or otherwise, and had a fairly satisfactory work record. He remained deeply religious, was closely identified with his grandfather, the preacher, and, from time to time, assumed ministerial duties in the church. In spite of all this turmoil, he remained outwardly, at least, a fairly equable and easygoing person, who never was able to express his anger at anything or anybody.

Seven years before this report, his grandfather, while preaching a sermon, was suddenly seized with a severe chest pain, collapsed, and in a few minutes, died in the patient's presence. After this, the patient would occasionally complain of chest pain and weakness although neither symptom assumed any significant proportion. He usually experienced them during or after quarrels. Four years later, he divorced his wife, but the children, with the exception of the eldest son, remained in the wife's custody. Eight months later, he remarried and came to Cincinnati. He contracted gonorrhea soon after this marriage and concluded that his wife had been previously infected. She had borne no children and miscarried on one occasion. He worried constantly about his children, and insisted on visiting them frequently in spite of his former wife's objections. The visits often culminated in threats. In June, 1943, she brandished a gun and threatened his life if he returned. He had not been back since.

Another source of concern at that time was that his eldest son entered military service and suffered an injury to his leg which necessitated operative intervention. A third factor consisted of an altercation which the patient

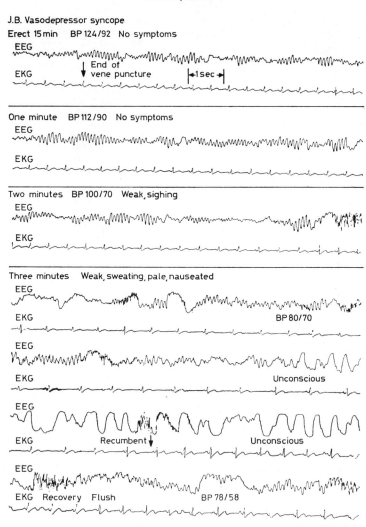

Fig. 1. The typical electroencephalographic and electrocardiographic changes in vasodepressor syncope. Weakness, sighing, sweating, nausea and pallor occur during the phase of falling arterial blood pressure. No change in the electroencephalogram occurs until consciousness is lost and then the EEG is characterized by high voltage waves of 2–3 per sec frequency. With the return to the recumbent position and recovery of consciousness, the electroencephalogram returns promptly to normal.

had with a guard at the factory. The patient stated he had been asked to show his badge of identification 6 times within an hour. He felt he was being discriminated against, became resentful and angry but was unable to express it. Immediately after this he felt faint and experienced pain in his chest. This was his first fainting sensation. Following this, the symptoms of weakness, faintness and chest pain increased in frequency and severity. He fainted following the extraction of a tooth which took place under local anesthesia. He became restless, diffusely anxious and exhibited startle patterns to sudden noises. His dreams became repetitive and consisted of two major themes; one, of life in the good old days before he married the first time; the second, of frightening content, such as someone breaking into his room, airplanes bombing him, animals, such as bears or hippopotami chasing him. Usually he would be awakened, panicky, just before he was about to be injured or destroyed. Occasionally, he would dream of funerals and on one occasion, the dream consisted of his grandfather's funeral in which in the middle of the ceremony the old gentleman arose hale and hearty from his coffin. He became extremely suspicious of his wife and believed that men were following her. He was distressed at her working in the same factory, and eventually insisted upon her quitting because she was forced to wear slacks.

During the initial physical examination, he became weak, pale and fainted while his blood pressure was determined. Following this, he fainted on two more occasions associated with venepuncture and attempt at dental nerve block.

The physical, neurologic and laboratory examinations revealed no significant abnormal findings. The following experiment was carried out:

The patient was brought to the laboratory, placed on a tilt table, and electroencephalographic and electrocardiographic electrodes applied. He was given little or no reassurance as to the objectives and possible hazards of this procedure. During 15 min resting quietly in the recumbent position, blood pressure ranged from 120/76 to 126/80 mm Hg; pulse, between 80–96/min, while the electroencephalogram (left and right fronto-occipital tracings) revealed a quite regular 9–10/sec alpha rhythm. The electrocardiogram (2nd lead) was normal. The patient was asked to hyperventilate vigorously for three minutes. Subjectively, he experienced heaviness in the chest, dizziness, and tingling of the hands and feet. The blood pressure dropped to 110/60 but then returned to its control value while the pulse rose to 144/min. During the last 20 sec the electroencephalogram showed a considerable amount of high voltage 3–5/sec activity, and the patient had diminished awareness as evidenced by amnesia for certain test phrases administered during this period. Subjectively, this did not resemble the patient's spontaneous symptoms and constituted, in our experience, a normal reaction to 3 min hyperventilation. After resting 10 min, the patient was tilted erect (75°). After 8 min in this position, the blood pressure was 112/82, pulse 114, the patient was slightly anxious and was experiencing slight pain over the left nipple. The electroencephalogram was unchanged. Stimulation of first the left and then the right carotid sinus produced no change in pulse or blood pressure and only some local pain. At the end od 15 min in the erect position, blood pressure was 120/86, pulse 114. He was questioned about the incident with the plant guard with no effect other than acceleration of pulse to 122/min. The patient was then told that he was to have a venepuncture. Within a minute after venepuncture the blood pressure began to fall and the patient experienced the progressive symptoms of weakness, sighing, sweating, pallor, and nausea, culminating within 3 min in unconsciousness and the appearance of high voltage slow waves on the electroencephalogram. Before collapse, blood pressure had fallen to 80/70 and bradycardia developed. The patient recovered consciousness and the electroencephalogram returned to normal promptly after being tilted back to the recumbent position, although relative hypotension (100/70) and bradycardia (66/min) persisted for 2 to 3 min.

The physiological data on this patient confirm in every detail those obtained in the previously reported patients with vasodepressor syncope [3, 5] as well as in other patients studied since then. In all instances, the reaction was characterized by progressive weakness, pallor, sighing, nausea, and finally falling blood pressure, culminating in unconsciousness if the patient remained erect. The loss of consciousness was always accompanied by a striking alteration in the electrical activity of the brain, with the development of high voltage 2–3/sec waves. If the patient were restored to the recumbent position before a critical fall in blood pressure had occurred, unconsciousness did not supervene and the electroencephalogram showed no significant changes. In short, the eventual loss of consciousness was the end result of a profound and acute alteration in circulatory dynamics.

The patient's personality structure, life experiences and behavior under experimental conditions lead to the conclusion that his fainting was determined principally by emotional factors. While we are unable to present in detail many important facets of his early life experiences, it appears that with the exception of a short-lived adolescent revolt, he identified with his grandfather, the patriarch preacher, and utilized successfully in his setting of multiple domestic discord, the defenses of passivity, submission and religious interests. These psychologic defenses remained more or less intact even after he witnessed the sudden death of his grandfather. However, the patient became aware of occasional chest pain and weakness which usually occurred following quarrels with his wife. Following the divorce and his second marriage, he began to experience chest symptoms more often. A number of factors probably contributed to his distress. These included (1) guilt over the second marriage, the veneral infection and the conflict with his religious beliefs; (2) grief resulting from the family separation, and (3) insecurity caused by the sudden transition from the small town to the big city. His anxiety

neurosis reached formidable proportions after his wife threatened to shoot him, after he received news of his son's military disability and more particularly, after the incident with the plant guard in which he experienced impotent rage with great anxiety. In addition to the rather characteristic anxiety neurosis symptoms, he reacted to stimuli, even remotely interpretable as threatening or mutilating, with vasodepressor syncope, (blood pressure cuff, dental injection, venepuncture). The interpretations we offer for this behavior is that the vasodepressor syncope in this patient was the physiologic concomitant of the emotions of fear and anxiety, particularly in situations which mobilized his aggressive phantasies, which assumed proportions beyond which his ego could form no defenses other than flight.

Parenthetically, this flight reaction suggests that it might be possible to relate the human experience of vasodepressor syncope, particularly as it concerns muscular relaxation, to the sham death of defenseless animals.

Hysterical Syncope

In the second group of fainters, consciousness seems to be lost without any associated changes in general or cerebral circulation or in respiration. It is this group that we have called hysterical fainters.

Clinically, hysterical fainting differs from vasodepressor syncope in a number of respects. It tends to occur more frequently among women, although not exclusively so. The patients often exhibit other hysterical manifestations and often manifest little concern about their frequent faints ('la belle indifférence'). Fainting is more likely to occur in the presence of others. The loss of consciousness is usually abrupt and dramatic and is not preceded by the premonitory symptoms so characteristic of vasodepressor syncope. Although the patient falls or slumps to the ground, injury is infrequent. In contrast to vasodepressor syncope, pallor, sweating and changes in pulse and blood pressure do not occur, and consciousness is not regained upon attaining the recumbent position. The patient may remain unconscious for an indefinite period, ranging from a few seconds to hours. During the period of unconsciousness there are no changes in vital signs although there may be varying degrees of anesthesia and occasional random or tic-like movements. Recovery of consciousness may be subtle, but is complete.

The following case is reported in detail. Clinical and electroencephalographic studies on 4 additional cases will be included in a later report.

The second patient, C.S., a 25-year-old single woman was admitted to the hospital for study because of fainting spells which were occurring as often as 4 to 5 times daily. She had begun to experience these fainting spells 3 years before. At that time, she had struck her head on a table and is said to have lost consciousness. Initially, her spells would occur infrequently, usually once monthly during her menses, but they had increased in frequency, and at times she would remain unconscious for as long as 90 min. Usually in the presence of others, she would suddenly fall to the floor and, although there appeared to be no significant changes in pulse, blood pressure or color as observed by physicians, she remained limp and unresponsive. One was struck by her indifferent, exhibitionistic and childish attitude. She was characteristically vague as to the details of the onset, character and course of the disabling attacks. However, it was learned that she lived with her parents in a rural home, that she had worked for a period of time in a clinic and hospital, but at present remained home to nurse her invalid father. She reported in detail an incident in which her father became annoyed and struck her, causing her to faint. In recounting some of her symptoms associated with her faints she spoke of having frequent repetitive dreams of rather violent sexual experiences or in which she was in labor. This led to a description of her severe menstrual cramps which she had often thought to be as severe as labor pains. She had had a period of a-menorrhea, nausea and abdominal distention at the time her sister-in-law was pregnant. She spoke constantly of pregnant women, of her love for babies, and when she worked in the hospital would take every opportunity to witness childbirth, Cesarian sections and surgical operations.

The usual physical and laboratory examinations elicited no significant findings. However, during the examination of the heart and lungs when the breasts were exposed, the patient became limp and unresponsive. When asked to stand at the bedside her legs were exposed in the move from the bed and with this she fell out of bed to the floor in a faint.

The following experiment was carried out. The patient was examined in the recumbent position on the tilt table. Blood pressure ranged from 108/80 to 110/76, and the pulse was 84. The electroencephalogram showed chiefly a low voltage fast pattern with only a small amount of alpha (8–12/sec) activity and some 14–16/sec activity. Electrocardiogram was normal. The patient was tilted to the erect position (75°). There was an abrupt increase in heart rate to 138/min and blood pressure rose slightly (118/84). After 10 min of standing, blood pressure was 100/90 and pulse 138. She had no symptoms. The left carotid sinus was massaged. In 10 sec the patient's head fell forward, and she did not respond. There was no change in pulse, blood pressure or color, and there was no sweating. The patient was unresponsive for 30 sec, but there was no detectable change in the brain wave pattern. Upon recovery, she described the faint as identical with those which led her to seek medical attention.

One minute later the left trapezius muscle was vigorously massaged. In 8 sec the patient's head fell forward and she failed to respond to any stimulus for 55 sec. Blood pressure during the syncope was 108/88 and pulse 144. Two minutes later the patient was asked to hyperventilate for 3 min. This resulted first in an increase in alpha activity and then in a moderate amount of higher voltage 4–7/sec activity but only slight tingling and light headedness. Thirty seconds after hyperventilation had been

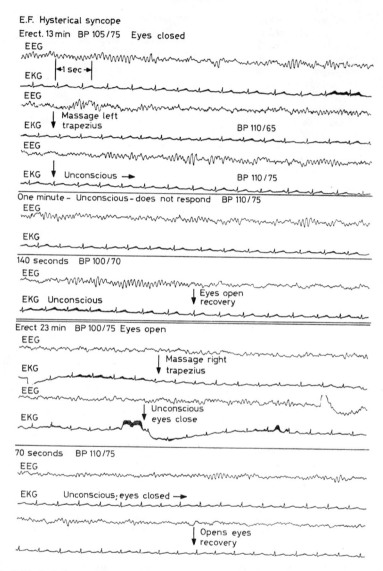

Fig. 2. Typical electroencephalographic and electrocardiographic data in hysterical syncope. With loss of consciousness following massage of the trapezius muscle, there were no changes in the electroencephalogram, electrocardiogram, pulses or blood pressure. Upon recovery of consciousness, the eyes were opened and alpha rhythm dropped out. The procedure was repeated with the patient's eyes open; with loss of consciousness the patient closed her eyes, and normal alpha rhythm appeared. With recovery of consciousness, eyes were opened and alpha rhythm again lost. The EEG actually became more 'normal' during the period of unconsciousness.

discontinued and the electroencephalographic pattern was returning to its original status, the patient again experienced syncope. She was unconscious for 80 sec, during which time the electroencephalogram returned to and maintained its control pattern of dominant low voltage fast activity. Blood pressure was 108/92 and pulse was 138. Three minutes later, as the experiment was about to be discontinued, the patient spontaneously experienced syncope, lasting 2 min. The electroencephalogram again showed no changes during this period. Physiologically, although this patient exhibited mild postural maladaptation, the syncope was marked by the absence of any significant changes in pulse, blood pressure, color, sweating, etc. In spite of prolonged unconsciousness, the electroencephalogram showed no abnormalities and, in fact, on the occasion following hyperventilation became more normal. Similar absence of change in pulse, blood pressure, color, respiration, sweating, and in the electroencephalogram during varying periods of unconsciousness was noted in 4 additional patients with hysterical syncope and will be cited in detail in a later report. This is in striking contrast to the findings in all other forms of syncope in which unconsciousness is complete and lasts for more than a few seconds [5].

Aside from the characteristic presumptive and traditional clinical hysterical behavior of this young woman as well as the negative physiologic data, it may be of interest to consider her fainting from the points of view of 'choice of neurotic symptom' and psychologic gains. Here again, because of our brief contact with the patient, we remain ignorant of many determinants. We are impressed, however, with the tenacity and intensity of her phantasies. Her dreams, directly or in disguised forms, were constituted of rape and violation, of pregnancy, labor, Cesarian births, and anesthesia. At the time of her sister-in-law's pregnancy, the patient's symptoms of nausea, amenorrhea and abdominal distention were undoubtedly identifications. Consciously the patient expressed constant interest in the welfare of pregnant women, in the care of infants, and during her hospital work as a technician arranged to witness surgical operations, childbirths and particularly Cesarian births. Her menstrual periods often were accompanied by cramps, severe enough for her to describe them as labor pains. Finally, she commented that frequently before fainting and at other times following recovery from the faint, she would remember details of dream fragments most of which were of a sexual nature. The total constellation of phantasies and consciously directed behavior of this patient are reminiscent of adolescent girls whose phantasies are full of pregnancy and birth ideas and of tendencies to identify themselves with pregnant women. As HELENE DEUTSCH [2] has pointed out, if these phantasies are to a considerable extent accompanied by feelings of hatred and by aggressive impulses they result in morbid symptoms and fear of death. Further, she states that fainting during puberty expresses the girl's flight from dangers or her passive abandonment of herself to them. With our patient the role of the invalid father whom she nursed but who punished and struck her seems particularly significant. It seemed to us that the fainting experiences of this young woman were hysterical in nature. The fainting, itself, appeared to be the attempt at relief of sexual excitation. Her rape dreams, associated pseudocyesis and conscious interests in surgery, Cesarian birth and anesthesia comprise evidence that sexuality to her meant passive acceptance of violent mutilating attack. The fainting then appeared to serve as a substitutive or symbolic expression of the repressed sexuality. However, the fainting also served to reject the repressed emotion. Because of her fainting, she not only avoided sexual experience but she remained at home more or less a child, unable or unwilling to meet the demands of adult life.

In other words, this patient's fainting, an hysterical conversion symptom, existed as a substitutive expression – an abreaction – of the emotional tension of sexual excitation which could not find adequate outlet through full fledged motor behavior. As FREUD, ALEXANDER and others have pointed out, these substitutive and symbolic innervations never bring full relief. The symptoms express at the same time both the repressed emotion and its rejection. It appears that our patient was able, through the repetitive hysterical syncope, to relieve partially the emotional tension of sexual excitation.

Discussion

It is the principal purpose of this preliminary report to illustrate certain points of differentiation between hysterical conversion and vegetative neurotic symptoms as they relate to fainting. We believe that the fainting experienced by the first patient was vasodepressor syncope. In that instance, the emotional experiences were accompanied by certain changes in the circulatory system which led eventually to loss of consciousness. These physiologic changes were clearly demonstrable in the form of pallor, sweating, changes in respiration and pulse, and in falling blood pressure leading finally to cerebral anemia and marked distortion of the electrical activity of the brain. The physiologic mechanism suggests flight. The concomitant emotional experience appears to be that of anxiety overwhelming the ego and preventing other compromise compensatory defenses.

The fainting of the second patient as well as of the other hysterical patients, may be contrasted by the notable lack of change in respiration, circulatory dynamics and electrical activity of the brain during periods of unconsciousness. In our experience, unconsciousness related to changes in cortical metabolism is always accompanied by alterations in the electroencephalogram if the unconsciousness lasts longer than 1 to 2 sec. This includes the cerebral type of carotid sinus syncope. FORSTER, ROSEMAN and GIBBS [4] have reported on negative

electroencephalographic data in patients stated to have a cerebral type of carotid sinus syncope. Our experience with 10 cases has been that slow EEG waves always accompany unconsciousness of more than 1 to 2 sec duration. In another report [2], we have criticized their data because of lack of control as to (a) duration of unconsciousness (b) position of patient during syncope, and (c) lack of proof that syncope could not be provoked from other sites. It will be noted in our second patient, as well as in the 4 other hysterical patients who were studied, that syncope was provoked not only from pressure on the carotid sinus, but from many other areas of the body. Obviously, if the specificity of the carotid sinus as the sensitive zone is not controlled, cases of hysterical syncope may easily be confused with the cerebral type of carotid sinus syncope.

The absence of any alteration of the electrical activity of the brain in these patients clearly distinguished the hysterical faint from fainting resulting from cerebral anemia due to general or local changes in blood flow to the brain. Essentially then, the fainting of the second patient was not due to concomitant physiologic phenomena of an emotional experience. Rather, from what we know of the patient's phantasy and the specific hysterical structure of the neurosis, the fainting appeared to be an attempt to express the repressed sexuality in a symbolic manner.

We do not intend to engage in polemics over the term 'consciousness'. Admittedly, it has a great number of meanings. Essentially, both patients, through contrasting mechanisms completely lost contact with reality, lost motor function, and fell to the ground.

Nor do we intend in this report to outline definitely the configurational personality structure or more specific conflict situation in vasodepressor and hysterical fainting. However, certain observations relevant to vasodepressor syncope may be made at this time. Vasodepressor syncope frequently occurs as a 'first-time' phenomenon. The incidence appears to be dependent upon many variables, the nature of the person, the setting, the preparation for the noxious stimulus, the capacity to diffuse individual anxiety through identification with a group, the specific nature of the ego defenses used previously and the acuity and intensity of the noxious stimulus. Most first-time fainters learn or adapt in one manner or another so that repetitive experiences find them free from trouble. Recently we were able to demonstrate this fact more quantitatively during a study of vasodepressor syncope provoked during high altitude (35,000 to 38,000 ft) exposures in a decompression chamber made by 78 male university students. During the course of 7 exposures the group incidence of syncopal reaction fell from 18% to 2% in spite of a sustained incidence of decompression sickness [3].

It is our clinical impression that vasodepressor syncope is more common in men and further that the men who have repetitive or neurotically determined syncope are characterized by considerable narcissistic consideration of their bodies. Any cut, bruise, injury, however trivial it may be, appears to mobilize an exaggerated degree of castration anxiety. Usually there has been considerable attention to the body, and pride in muscle mass and athletic endeavor. Perhaps the folklore opinion which is so familiar to all of us 'that the bigger they are, the harder they fall' has some validity.

Our clinical studies are as yet not extensive enough for us to know whether it would be possible for a patient to experience both hysterical and vasodepressor syncope. From a theoretical consideration it would appear that the principal determinants would be the nature of the personality

structure and the nature of the noxious stimulus.

In conclusion, then, we wish to point out that the material presented leads us to believe that vasodepressor syncope is a vegetative neurotic symptom in which certain disturbances in circulatory dynamics occur concomitantly with emotions of fear and anxiety which overwhelm the ego and lead to a flight marked by weakness, falling, and loss of consciousness. In contrast, hysterical fainting appears to be the substitutive or symbolic expression of an emotion – an attempt at a partial relief of the chronic unrelieved emotional tension in which loss of consciousness is not related to any demonstrable disturbance in circulation or metabolism of the brain.

References

1. ALEXANDER, F.: Fundamental concepts of psychosomatic research: psychogenesis, conversion, specificity. Psychosom. Med. 5: 205 (1943).
2. DEUTSCH, H.: Psychology of women, vol. 1 (Grune & Stratton, New York 1944).
3. ENGEL, G. L.; ROMANO, J., and McLIN, T.: Vasodepressor and carotid sinus syncope: clinical, electroencephalographic and electrocardiographic observations. Arch. intern. Med. 74: 100 (1944).
4. FORSTER, F. M.; ROSEMAN, E., and GIBBS, F. A.: The electroencephalogram accompanying carotid sinus reflex and orthostatic syncope. Arch. Neurol. Psychiat. 48: 957 (1942).
5. ROMANO, J.; ENGEL, G. L.; WEBB, J. P.; FERRIS, E. B.; RYDER, H. W., and BLANKENHORN, M. A.: Syncopal reactions during simulated exposures to high altitude in decompression chamber. War Medicine 4: 475 (1943).

The Correlations Between Ovarian Activity and Psychodynamic Processes

I. The Ovulative Phase[1]

THERESE BENEDEK and B. B. RUBENSTEIN

Retrospective comment by Dr. R. Grinker. The first issue of the new Psychosomatic Journal published in 1939, contained a number of general articles defining the subject matter of Psychosomatic Medicine, a few reviews and some pious hopes for the future. Only one paper represented a prototype of psychosomatic research oriented toward establishing specific relationships between the 'psychic apparatus' and physiological processes – that by BENEDEK and RUBENSTEIN. Looking back to those early days it is amazing that the methods used included a double blind setting, in that neither collaborator knew the other's results until the final correlation, that the best endocrine techniques available at the time were employed, that the psychological data with few exceptions were derived from daily sessions using the manifest content of dreams divulged in a psychoanalytic situation and that repeated menstrual cycles of the same patients were studied. The results indicated a close correlation between psychological trends and phases of the female gonadal cycle even verified by blind predictions.

From this beginning, BENEDEK has continued her studies of female sexuality to produce exciting speculations about maternal–child transactions, and menopausal processes. Her work still stands as a model of psychosomatic specificity among the ruins of most other research applied to other systems. Praising these contributions is however associated with concern and surprise that no one has repeated the research except for feeble incomplete attempts that masquerade as research. The psychological side does not require psychoanalytic techniques which are difficult and lengthy and for the physiological side, there are more improved modern systems of measurement available. Yet even without adequate replication, BENEDEK's research should be hailed as a great advance in developing a conceptual framework for psychosomatic unity.

The existence of relations between gonadal function and emotional states had been inferred before the dawn of history and can be traced in the folklore of nearly all people. The emotional changes associated with puberty and menopause in both sexes are well known.

The ebb and flow of emotion in the adult woman has also been associated in a vague way with the cycle of sex function. Premenstrual nervousness, apathy and depression have often been described in the clinical literature. Less well known, but recognized, are the sudden changes of mood associated with 'Mittelschmerz' and other midperiod symptoms, which have recently been related to ovulation. For a review of pertinent literature see SEWARD [22]. Proof of such correlations has, however, been strikingly absent due to ignorance concerning the precise details of the cycle in women on both the physiological and psychological sides. The recently described day-by-day study of vaginal smears and basal body temperatures [19–21] offers an approach to the problem on the physiological side. The psychoanalytic method offers a powerful tool for investigation on the psychological side.

[1] From the Institute for Psychoanalysis, Chicago, Illinois, and the Laboratory of Anatomy and Associated Foundations, Western Reserve University.

The cycle of sex function in the adult woman centers about ovulation. The process of ovulation is merely the rupture of a mature follicle and expulsion of its ovum. It implies preliminary phases of follicular maturation, and subsequent phases of corpus luteum formation. During this entire period, the ovary is the source not only of the ovum but also of hormones which exhibit their chracteristics throughout the body, preparing it for pregnancy. If the mature ovum is not fertilized, pregnancy does not occur. The uterine mucosa which hormonal stimulation had prepared for nidation of an ovum breaks down upon cessation of the hormonal stimulus and menstruation occurs. It is usual to think of the cycle from one menstrual period to the next. The present description will follow this scheme (fig. 1).

Usually, by the end of menstrual flow, the ovary shows first evidence of follicle development. Follicle maturation usually continues for about ten days during which time there is an increasing production of oestrone (the follicular or female sex hormone) which stimulates uterine proliferation. At about the time of maturity, but

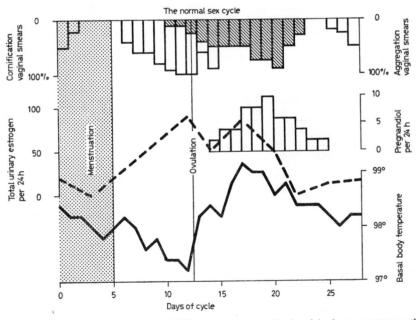

Fig. 1. The normal sex cycle: the solid curve represents the basal body temperatures; the broken curve presents the excretion of oestrogenic substances (female sex hormone); the clear blocks of the center are the excretion of pregnandiol sodium glucuronidate (metabolite of progesterone, the corpus luteum hormone); the uppermost set of blocks presents the vaginal smears, the clear blocks indicating cornification, the shaded blocks aggregation. The broken curve is a composite from the data of GUSTAVSON *et al.*, PEDERSEN-BJERGAARD, and PALMER. The pregnandiol excretion is after the data of VENNING and BROWNE. The temperature and smear representation is from my own data.

before rupture of the follicle, lutein cells appear in its lining (granulosa) and begin production of progesterone which stimulates the secretory activity of the uterus. Normally, follicular rupture, ovulation, occurs a few hours later, but is occasionally delayed for some days. After ovulation the former follicle space is invaded by more lutein cells from its lining (theca luteinization) and these produce both progesterone and an oestrogen (estriol?), which maintain the uterus in a state suitable for reception of the fertilized ovum. Upon atresia of the corpus luteum, progesterone production diminished, the uterine mucosa breaks down, and menstruation follows.

The existence of a hormonal cycle which is reflected in the vaginal smears and basal body temperature has been established. It was, therefore, interesting to see whether the psychological material could be correlated with the hormonal cycle. Our first question was whether the phases of the

ovarian function are reflected in the psychic processes as observed during the psychoanalytic procedure. Patients who were under treatment for various neurotic disturbances at the Institute for Psychoanalysis of Chicago were selected for this purpose. They were instructed to make their vaginal smears and take rectal temperatures daily. The smears and temperatures were sent to Dr. BORIS B. RUBENSTEIN of Western Reserve University, Cleveland, Ohio, for study. The psychoanalytic records were studied by Dr. THERESE BENEDEK at Chicago. After ten months had elapsed the two investigators met to compare for the first time the data of their independent investigations. Both sets of records had been summarized in tabular calendar form. The calendars were superimposed. We were pleased and surprised to find an exact correspondence of the ovulative dates as independently determined by the two methods. Table I represents such a procedure.

Table I

Case I. G.S.	Prediction on the basis of psychoanalytic material		Physiological findings
Cycle IV Aug. 28 to Sept. 23	Sept. 2:	Heterosexual tension starts	Sept. 2: Smear full of masculine secretion
	Sept. 4:	Preovulative tension	
	Sept. 7:	Preovulative	Sept. 3: Very beginning of cornification
26 days	Sept. 8:	*Postovulative* material	Sept. 4: Increasing cornification
	Sept. 14:	First premenstrual evidence	Sept. 8: *Ovulation*
	Sept. 23:	Menstrual flow	Sept. 14: First premenstrual evidence
			Sept. 23: Menstrual flow
Cycle V Sept. 23 to Oct. 19	Oct. 1:	Preovulative tension	Ovulation could occur from Sept. 28 to Oct. 7.
	Oct. 3–4:	Ovulation (?)	
	Oct. 4–5:	Ovulation (?)	There is evidence that it occurred before the 6th; assume Oct. 3rd
28 days	Oct. 9:	First premenstrual evidence	Oct. 10: First premenstrual evidence
	Oct. 18:	Increased premenstrual tension	Oct. 18: Cornification
	Oct. 20:	*Menstrual flow*	Oct. 20: Menstrual flow
Cycle VI Oct. 20 to Nov. 14	Oct. 23:	Heterosexual tension	Oct. 24: Minimal cornification
	Oct. 27:	Preovulative	Oct. 27: Increasing cornification
	Oct. 31– Nov. 1:	*Ovulation*	Oct. 31: Complete cornification Ovulative
25 days	Nov. 5:	First premenstrual evidence	Nov. 1: Postovulative
	Nov. 14:	Menstrual flow	Nov. 5: First premenstrual evidence
			Nov. 14: Menstrual flow

It might be assumed that the psychological structure of the patient whose records we first studied facilitated the location of the ovulative dates. We made the same comparative study of three other cases with various symptoms and different psychodynamic structures, with the same results. In those cycles in which hormonal and psychoanalytical material were available for the ovulative period, the date of ovulation was predicted. We missed complete coincidence only in those cycles in which either the patient failed to take the smears or when there were no psychoanalytic sessions.

After our first encouraging results our task was to find those characteristics of the psychoanalytical material which enabled us to distinguish the various phases of the cycle.

We therefore reviewed the same material day by day. We studied one case during ten cycles, a second case during eight cycles and the third and fourth cases during 5 cycles each and found that the psychoanalytic material in the normal cycle shows typical changes which are described briefly in the following paragraphs.

During the follicle ripening phase the psychological material is dominated by heterosexual interest. The libidinous tendencies are concentrated on the male. The heterosexual desire becomes increasingly strong during the ripening phase. With normal sexual adjustment the increasingly strong heterosexual desire finds normal gratification. Without sexual gratification, the heterosexual tension can be dammed up so that increasing hormone production causes an increased tension.

In neurotic persons we observe that this increasing oestrone production activates the psychological conflicts and thus the neurotic symptoms are intensified. The great psychic tension is suddenly relieved (but only for a short time) when ovulation occurs. The libidinous interest is withdrawn from the outer world and centered on her self. She is self-satisfied, wants to be loved and to be taken care of. She is content to be a woman. The period of postovulative relaxation is necessarily of short duration. Hormone production increases rapidly after ovulation. Although both hormones are produced during the luteal phase progesterone now dominates the hormone picture. The psychological material corresponding to this phase of the cycle shows the tendency to be passive and receptive. The tendency to be impregnated, the tendency to be pregnant, the tendency to care for a child and the various reactions to all these are reflected in the psychological material. After this phase of the cycle reaches its peak the corpus luteum starts to regress and with it the production of progesterone diminishes. After regression of the corpus luteum many new follicles begin their development. Ordinarily none of these follicles is destined to mature. However, they do produce oestrone in small quantities. This is immediately reflected in the psychological material by the reappearance of heterosexual interest.

The heterosexual desire of the premenstrual phase is similar to that of the preovulative phase. In the late premenstrual state this heterosexual tension is complicated by the expectation of menstruation. This expectation of the menstruation is in turn reflected in the psychological material.

Normally the follicles regress by the end of the cycle. Occasionally one of the immature follicles may be luteinized and therefore will complicate the hormone picture by producing minimal amounts of progesterone. This will also complicate the psychological material.

It should be noted that Dr. THOMAS M. FRENCH studied one case in which the vaginal smears were taken by the same technique and established the various phases of the cycle on the basis of the psychological material. This case is not included in the present paper.

As an example of our day to day study and the correspondences it demonstrated, we have presented table II, one cycle of patient R. E.

Table II. Case R.E.[1]

Date	Psychoanalytic Material	Prediction	Physiological findings
Oct. 19–24			Menstrual flow; no smears
Oct. 25	Cheerful; no dream		No smear
Oct. 26	Heterosexual dream content and associations	Starting oestrone tension	Beginning cornification. Extreme leukocytic invasion. Definitely preovulative
Oct. 27	Heterosexual desire and feminine exhibitionistic tendencies	Increasing oestrone tension	
Oct. 28	Cheerful. Dream material: admiration of brother – associations: fear of brother and of incest	Increasing oestrone tension	Increasing cornification
Oct. 29	Castration wishes – heterosexual material – impregnation wish – lutein; Mittelschmerz	Preovulative tension	Lowest point of temperature curve. Minimal folding of completely cornified smear – late preovulative
Oct. 30	No analytic material		Cornification 75 % (slight regression)
Oct. 31	Dream: Strongly heterosexual – fear of impregnation	Preovulative	Cornification 90 %. Minimal folding
Nov. 1	Dream: Heterosexual material. 1° Masochistic and identification with brother. 2° Identification with mother. Impregnation material	Preovulative	Cornification 100 %. Slightly more folding and aggregation
Nov. 2	Dream: Heterosexual wishes and fear of being attacked. During hour fear of pregnancy, increased fear and suffocation	Ovulative	Cornification 100 % with more luteal activity – Ovulative
Nov. 3	Cheerful, rushing: Analytic association superficial hypomanic	Postovulative	Leuk. influx – clearly postovulative
Nov. 4	No dream; excited, happy, eager, animated. Associations are resistive	Postovulative	Definitely postovulative

[1] The ovulative phase of this cycle, Oct. 30–Nov. 4 is presented in detail in the text of this paper, pp. 98/99.

Table II (continued)

Date	Psychoanalytic Material	Prediction	Physiological findings
Nov. 5	No dream. Feels full and bloated. Associations deal with fear of identification with mother. Fear of pregnancy	Lutein phase	Definitely postovulative
Nov. 6	No analytic hour		Clear lutein state
Nov. 7	No analytic hour		Occasional cornified cell. First premenstrual evidence
Nov. 8	Dream: heterosexual wish and aggression toward brother	Premenstrual	Premenstrual; low oestrone level
Nov. 9	Fear. Great need for protection. Great dependency		Premenstrual with low oestrone
Nov. 10	Craving for sweets. Dream shows castration wish toward a boy. Boy's bleeding – menstruation – castration	Premenstrual	Premenstrual
Nov. 11	Fear of identification with mother on sexual level; fear of insanity	Premenstrual with increased oestrone and minimal progesterone	Late premenstrual
Nov. 12	Tension increases. Pain in stomach. Fear of sexual attack. Relaxed during analytic hour	Increased premenstrual oestrone	Increased oestrone output. Premenstrual
Nov. 13	Aggravation of symptoms, especially fear, diarrhoea. Analytic material: Fear of sexual attack	Increased premenstrual oestrone material	No smear
Nov. 14	Heterosexual material	No relaxation of oestrone tension	Menstrual flow starts. Cornification 90%

On the basis of our preliminary study we set ourselves the following hypotheses: (1) Increasing heterosexual tendency is correlated with increasing estrone production. (2) Relaxation and contentment are correlated with ovulation. (3) The passive and receptive tendencies, the tendencies toward pregnancy and toward nursing are correlated with progesterone production. (4) The reappearance of heterosexual tendencies marks the onset of the premenstrual phase which results from new oestrone production.

Further studies were carried out in the light of these hypotheses. This report is based on our study of seventy-five cycles of which twenty-three were ovulative. It is of interest to note the frequency of anovulatory cycles in our neurotic patients although the patients were of child-bearing age. Even in the anovulatory cycles there was sufficient fluctuation of hormone production to define the characteristics of the cycle. The psychological material reflected these daily changes and naturally failed to show the psychological relaxation characteristic of ovulations.

Method

Physiological. For our evaluation of gonad function, we employed the vaginal smear-basal body temperature technique recently described by one of us [19–21] with certain modifications. Since the patients were in Chicago and the laboratory work was done in Cleveland, slides of the vaginal smears had to be shipped and, therefore, dried. To compensate for loss in cytological detail consequent on drying, we advised the patients to take the smears with a stiff wire loop inserted into the posterior fornix of the vagina; we thus obtained comparable smears from day to day. The smears were stained according to the method of PAPANICOLAOU [16] and evaluated without reference to either the temperature or the psychological data. In general, they were adequate for a decision concerning the phases of the cycle represented. It should be noted that since much of the material was pathological, we followed a scheme for evaluation of slides as follows.

Slides were examined and a rough quantitative estimate made of the proportions of various squamous epithelial cell types as follows: (1) Normal cells with vesicular nuclei. (2) Cells with granular cytoplasm and pyknotic nuclei. (3) Cells with keratinized cytoplasm and pyknotic nuclei. (4) Cells with keratinized cytoplasm and fragmented nuclei. (5) Cells with 'moth-eaten' edges, folded over. (6) Cells folded and aggregated into masses.

The presence of marked desquamation of epithelial cells in the absence of sperm and red blood cells was given careful consideration. The presence or absence of leukocytes, red blood cells, thick tenacious mucous and of spermatozoa was noted.

Since, under the influence of oestrone, whether produced by the maturing follicle or injected, all mucous membranes [14] and in particular the vaginal mucous membrane proliferates [4, 13], the superficial cells grow away from their blood supply and begin to undergo the degenerative processes called cornification (types 2 to 3 to 4). We assume, therefore, that in an untreated woman the progressive change in smears from type 1 through to type 4 is indicative of a progressively maturing follicle. Luteal cells appear in the granulosa of the follicle just before ovulation and frequently even when the follicle is doomed to atresia [6,15–17][2].

Minimal evidence of progesterone activity associated with a high oestrone level is therefore the criterion of the ovulative phase: in the vaginal smear it is recognized by either increased desquamation of type 4 cells or by the appearance of type 5 and 6 cells together with type 4. In the post-ovulative phase the increasing level of progesterone neutralizes the effect of oestrone on the mucosa [13, 24]. There is progressive desquamation and degeneration of the proliferated, cornified epithelium and therefore the preponderance in vaginal smears of type 5 and 6 cells, together with the appearance of occasional cells from deeper layers, i.e. non-squamous epithelium. Upon atresia of the corpus luteum, new follicles develop under stimulation by the uninhibited anterior pituitary, even before menstruation. Therefore, there is usually a recurrence of oestrone activity – of cornifica-

[2] Since preparing this paper 2 more publications have appeared which demonstrate that initial leuteinization occurs just before ovulation.

tion in the vagina in the premenstrual-menstrual phase. The smear evidence indicates that menstruation occurs despite the presence of a low or even moderate oestrone concentration.

The temperature data are interpreted independently. Recent studies [20, 21] confirmed by ZUCK [26] demonstrate the existence of a temperature curve in the normal, adult woman. There is a rise of temperature in the mid-month period correlated with ovulation as determined by smears [19], electrical disturbance [5, 18], and by pregnancy due to single coitus [26]. The temperature rises after ovulation to its zenith, about one week premenstrually, and is related to maximum corpus luteum function. The temperature then falls gradually during the next two to three weeks presumably under the influence of the gradually increasing oestrone level [20, 21, 23] which inhibit the pituitary progressively until several hours before ovulation when the temperature reaches its nadir (i.e. maximum oestrone, no progesterone production). As soon as leuteinization of the mature follicle begins, the temperature again starts to rise signalling impending ovulation. The patients selected for this research were given instructions by a woman physician as to how to take the vaginal smears and the rectal temperatures. They received also the necessary material and other instructions regarding the handling of the slides from a laboratory technician, to whom they gave the smears and temperatures every 2 or 4 weeks. This whole technical procedure was managed so that the analyst working with the case was not involved.

Psychological. One of the cases was studied for the period of 15 menstrual cycles, 2 cases for 12 cycles, one for 11 cycles and the others for a period of 4 to 6 cycles. Seventy-five cycles of 9 patients were studied; which means about 2,000 day-by-day diagnoses of their psychodynamics[3]. Besides this, the author (T.B.) studied and made similar diagnostic interpretations of the same cases during those periods of their psychoanalytic treatment when vaginal smear tests were not made. Of these nine cases, 2 were analyzed by the author (T.B.); 7 by other psychoanalysts in connection with the Chicago Institute for Psychoanalysis.

These investigations based on psychodynamic changes occurring every day and related to the day, would not have been possible except on the basis of daily recorded material.

We do not have mechanical records and therefore no verbatim record of any analytical session. In spite of this, a 'good record' conveys the content of the psychoanalytical session to another psychoanalyst. It contains the patient's recent important experiences, the emotional state, and the various topics of the session in the sequence of the associations. Even when the record is not verbatim it should cite the patient's own expressions. The patient's verbalisation reflects her feelings and enables the person studying the record to get in touch with the recorded emotional state. The most important parts of the records are the dreams. The dream is the most sensitive instrument for the registration of psychic changes. In these investigations the dreams were used as the 'objective' material of the psychoanalysis[4]. It is necessary, as far as possible, to record the dreams in the patient's own words and the flow of the associations. If the record does not contain the course of the analytical session at least partially expressed in the patient's own words, it offers a great source of error in interpretation. Records which contain mainly the summaries of the hour in psychoanalytic terminology permit only a review of the interpretations of the analyst. No matter how correct the interpretation may have been, psychoanalytic interpretation by another investigator is possible only with great tolerance for error.

Of course it is impossible to go into detail about the technique of interpretation of the

[3] A comparative evaluation of the daily findings by both methods – which offered practically complete correspondence – will be published later.

[4] THOMAS M. FRENCH in his recent dream studies, emphasizes that the manifest content of the dream is an 'index of the quantitative balance between repressed and repressing forces' [7]. And in another [8] paper 'Reality and the unconscious', he explains: 'I am using the chronological order of appearance of the manifest dream elements in order to trace the shifts of emphasis that bring into focus one after another during the act of dreaming different parts of the latent dream thoughts. These shifts of emphasis I regard as quantitative indicators of the balance between conflicting tendencies just as conscious thoughts and actions during waking life are indicators of the quantitative balance between the motives that activate them.'

recorded psychoanalytic material. Every kind of psychological material available was utilized. We had to evaluate the conscious emotional and physical condition of the patient, her actions and experiences. The symptoms of the patient belong partly to conscious material, and partly to unconscious material. Psychogenic symptoms are results of conflicting psychodynamic tendencies and can be analyzed in relation to the hormonal state. The most important materials for this investigation were the dreams, associations, and the transference[5]. The interpretation of all this material differs from the usual interpretation technique of any experienced analyst in but one respect – all the recent determinations and also overdeterminations are not emphasized as it would be necessary in the actual course of a psychoanalysis. The material is reduced to a few underlying determinants – to the instinctual biological tendencies.

The tentative conclusions utilized for the predictions of the hormonal state were also checked in another way. One of us studied the vaginal smears of unanalyzed cases. Those cases gave a day-by-day report of their conscious emotional state and report their dreams on a questionnaire. The material was submitted for psychological study and it was possible to determine in which phase of the cycle the dream occurred.

The aim of our investigations was to describe the emotional states as they are correlated with the hormonal states. The results show that the emotional states, as expressions of the underlying instinctual tendencies, easily coordinate with the conception of the instinct theory of psychoanalysis. Hence in these investigations which offer the first laboratory results to support the theoretical concepts of psychoanalysis, the terminology of the instinct theory is introduced. The meaning of the terms will be apparent from the context, but it may be useful to give a few definitions at once.

Libido is the psychic energy supplied by sexual drive.

Active-passive designates the direction of the drive. If its goal is achieved by action, it is called active. When the goal is achieved by experiencing activity of another person, it is called passive.

Object libido is the instinctual tendency directed toward another individual for its gratification.

Heterosexual object libido expresses a desire toward an individual of the opposite sex.

Narcissism is the psychic condition in which the sexual energy is concentrated on one's self.

Auto eroticism is the process of gratification of the narcissism.

Genital phase of libido organization designates the capacity of normal adults to experience full sexual gratification (orgasm) by normal heterosexual intercourse. The genital phase is characterised by the full acceptance of, and by the desire for, the genital organ of a person of the other sex, as the object of gratification of one's own genital drives.

The Libido Theory differentiates several phases of the instinctual development previous to the genital phase; for instance, oral.

'*Oral*' connects the so circumscribed subject with a sensation experienced on the mouth: oral gratification, oral aggression.

Oral receptivity is the term of the passive need of being fed. In the passive state of early infancy this need is experienced together with the passive need of being sheltered and taken care of. We refer to this attitude with the term *oral dependency.*

Anal eroticism refers to erotic pleasure derived from the anal region.

Data and Discussion

Follicle ripening phase. Oesterone is the hormone produced by the ripening follicle; it makes the animal ready for and desirous of copulation. The conscious and even more the unconscious psychological material during the phase of follicle development deals with the heterosexual tendencies of the woman. It is impossible to give a full account of all the ways in which heterosexual tendencies can appear in psychological material. Our comparative material shows clearly how complicated it may appear in the emotional state of women.

[5] Transference is the repetition of emotional experiences, which during the analytic procedure becomes manifest in relation to the analyst or to the analytic situation.

The feeling of incipient oestrogenous tension is chiefly one of well-being. The patients say that they feel young, alert, that they can work well and think more clearly. For example, case G.S. 8/9/37:

'This morning I felt 17 years old so far as my mood was concerned. I met C. I felt sexually attracted to him which I did not feel when I met him last time.'

The vaginal smear 8/9/37 shows cornification about the 50% level; moderate leucocytosis and mucous output. The basal body temperature is significant only in relation to the entire temperature curve for cycle and will therefore be presented in that form in the charts of the summary.

On September 4th, the same patient says:

'I was energetic and active. I felt quite well.'

The dream of September 5th allows the following interpretation: She wants to be a good looking woman, attractive to men, and able to handle her sexual temptations. This is an obvious expression of incipient heterosexual tension. On the following day, September 6th, the patient describes her mood at a picnic:

'I felt very young and carefree. I liked everybody. I climbed on a tree. I sang. I did not have any selfconsciousness about my body.'

At about the same phase of another cycle, on January 18th, the patient had the following dream:

'Mike came and paid me a lot of attention. I was aware that he was a writer and I was flattered that he had singled me out. He embraced me and fondled me a great deal and I responded.'

The vaginal smear 9/6/37 and 1/18/38 showed 50% cornification, moderate leucocytosis and mucous output.

The psychic energy corresponding with oestrone production can be characterised as follows: It is active, directed from the individual as libido center toward the object, just as FREUD originally described object-libido [11, 12]. The active libidinous desires are directed toward sexual objects in the patient's sphere of action. This active libido may be expressed not only as heterosexual tendencies but also by increased strength of the ego in maintaining self-regard, object-relationship, and more active defenses of the ego toward the outer world. It increases during this phase of the cycle and supplies the ego with an active quality. The ego in this phase of the cycle is more charged with an active energy which seems to prove FREUD's conception [12] that Eros is the energy which unites the parts to a higher organisation. Detailed study of the psychodynamics of individual cases in relation to their menstrual cycles, which could demonstrate what is meant, must be deferred to a later publication.

Although the active charge of the ego is productive and agreeable, it can, when no gratification or transformation into satisfactory activities is permitted, be converted into a disagreeable tension, – restlessness and irritability, which are an expression of the dammed-up, originally libidinous charges. With increasing hormone production the ungratified active charge may achieve psychological expression in the form of aggression directed toward the male. Thus in our material which is chiefly pathological, there is only a brief period when the initial low hormone content is associated with an agreeable libidinous state. It often develops into a tense emotional state in which the psychological material is characterised by aggressive tendencies or by anxiety. The emotional state may be dominated by fear of being attacked sexually. The following dream of case L. (9/12/38) demonstrates unmistakably that increased heterosexual tension may be accompanied by fear:

'Some huge fossil belonging to the reptile family, mounted, standing upright in the museum. Some remark or other brought it to life and it began to crawl over the land. People fled before it in terror. Very slimy and shining ugly green. I think it punctured the tire of an automobile and then proceeded to attack the occupant. The dream woke me up.'

The vaginal smear 9/12/38 indicates that this was the peak of oestrogenous activity in the cycle.

In this dream, even though the snake symbolism is disguised, it is clearly enough a penis symbol in which even the function of erection is easily recognised when the dream describes how this fossil became alive and then dangerous. The ambivalent attitude of the dreamer toward the penis is very clear – admiration is expressed by exaggeration of its size and power; fear and revulsion is expressed by its becoming ugly and revolting. The tension in the dream increased so much that the dreamer awoke. Patient R.E. on 2/11/38 relates the following dream, very typical for her:

'The thing I was afraid to think about or to talk about, the thing that stands out clearly is that there was a bed and no one was in the room except for my father and myself. He was trying to urge me to have intercourse with him. He was shoving me to the bed and I was moving toward it. I was willing. Then suddenly it occurred to me: "It is my father". I was ashamed. It was frightening. He was right after me. I do not want to think of it.'

The vaginal smear 2/11/38 shows about 90% cornification and minimal evidence of aggregation and folding. It is probably a smear of the preovulative phase.

Very often increased oestrone production leads to aggression which in dream material may appear as penis envy, or as an intense wish to castrate the male or to incorporate the penis and become a male. Clear tendencies toward masculine identification and masculine competition are often observed in the preovulative state. How much oestrone tension a woman can stand without turning it into aggression depends upon various factors which can only be discussed in connection with the psychodynamic structure of each case individually. It is self evident that actual sex experiences, gratification or disappointment, may influence the psychological reaction. For example, patient V.M. reported a dream on 12/1/37:

'A man rolls a cigarette, a large one. Then the cigarette is being sliced off, like plates or drops. I was conscious of its dryness.'

The vaginal smear 12/1/37 consists of purely cornified cells with only an occasional red blood cell and indicates extreme oestrone production, which usually precedes ovulation.

It needs no deep interpretation of the above dream to sense the hostile, castrative, depreciative attitude toward men. This is emphasised more strongly by the associations. At the same time the patient seeks gratification by promiscuous sexual relations. It is obviously a preovulative tension.

We now present the preovulative phase of a single patient from its inception right through ovulation. Patient G.S. on 12/17/37 expresses a heterosexual wish but with a helpless feeling and wants to be helped.

The vaginal smear 12/17/27 shows beginning cornification.

On the night of 12/18/37 the patient dreams:

'My nose or someone's nose was smashed, or perhaps a skull. Immediately on awakening I thought of a face all swathed in bandages. It was our coalman whom I had seen in a coffin when I was a young child.'

The vaginal smear 12/18/37 shows increasing cornification to about the 75% level.

The destructive aggressive tendency is easily recognized as a character of preovulative tension. On December 19th she dreamed:

'Of a head that was cut off or hanging connected with a holiday candle.'

The vaginal smear 12/19/37 shows cornification at about the 90% level with abundant mucous and progressive reduction in the number of leucocytes – clearly preovulative.

In this dream the aggressive tendency of the previous dream is repeated. The patient described her emotional condition of 12/20/37 as follows:

'I feel rotten. I have a dull headache. I was disgusted with you. I was furiously angry.'

And on 12/21/37 she reported a dream:

'I felt a temper tantrum, breaking things and shaking with rage. My *oldest sister K.*, my *youngest sister R.*, and I were together. R. was critical. K was studying what was the matter with me. I yelled to R.: "You are afraid of me. You think that I am insane. If I were insane I would not show it to you." I felt weak in the dream. I had the feeling I was dissipating my energy in fruitless rage.'

The vaginal smear 12/21/37 shows 100% cornification, leucopenia, beginning aggregation and folding. This is a smear which signals impending ovulation.

Ovulative state. As we observed in the last few examples the psychological changes related to the production of oestrone developed gradually or in sudden leaps to their highest point, when the ripe follicle may burst and ovulation occurs. However, before ovulation does occur, lutein activity begins. The very first evidence of function of the corpus luteum is a change in direction of metabolic activity, and is reflected by corresponding change in the psychodynamic tendencies. The examples, cited above showed the heterosexual interest with its various emotional expressions, such as love, fear, and hostility. When the function of the corpus luteum hormone – progesterone – begins, this exclusive interest in man changes immediately. The heterosexual tendency appears combined with passive, receptive instinctual tendencies. The psychoanalytic material reflects the libidinous interest in one's own body. The emotional interest is self-centered. The woman appears more passive and dependent.

Patient V.M. on 3/15/38 has the following dream:

'I was coming down the steps with Jack carrying a creature which I decided was a baby. It was not the proper way to carry it. The baby was not properly dressed. I was sure it was a girl. But to my surprise it was a boy. I felt badly since I wanted a girl. I felt so badly, I considered cutting off its penis. I could not accept it as my child, having a penis.'

The vaginal smear 3/15/38 shows complete cornification, folding and aggregation coresponding to ovulation.

This dream expresses a great conflict tension, the solution to which is castration of her own child. The dream solution shows the direction of the instinctual conflict, which is here aggression toward the penis. We distinguish in this manifest dream first, the first dream thought, which shows ambivalence toward the child. In the second dream thought the wish to have a daughter is expressed (the associations emphasised the wish to have a daughter more beautiful and more feminine than the patient herself). These 2 dream thoughts show a content which we correlate with the lutein activity. Then the conflict shifts to the aggression toward the boy, toward the penis. The aggression toward the penis is the predominant direction of instinctual tendency in this dream because it offers the dream solution. Therefore, the incipient lutein activity and stronger oestrone tension was diagnosed: *preovulative tension.*

On 6/24/38 patient R.G. reported:

'Yesterday evening I had a bad spell of eating and today too. Today I ate a very adequate lunch and slept an hour and awoke hungry. I thought of my brother. I felt I wanted to destroy his genitals. Well, it is a real wish. To pull him out. The thing that bothers me so much is that I still have the wish to do it. I connect it with the fact that my mother used to tell me that she'd cut my thumb off when I used to suck it.'

'It is as if I almost want to feel depressed.'

'This day after the analytic hour was the worst day I ever had. After I finished lunch I had a terrific craving for candy. I got quite depressed.'

The vaginal smear 6/24/38 shows 80% cornification with minimal folding and aggregation, indicative of the incipient luteinization, but chiefly preovulative.

This example of craving together with the wish to incorporate the penis shows the reaction of this patient to the preovulative state: to the increased oestrone and incipient lutein function.

Our observations so far permit the statement that our patients can handle their hormone balance psychologically much better as long as only one of the hormones is active. In the case of a normal woman with normal sex life increased heterosexual tension is usually relieved by sexual gratification. Thus the preovulative tension will not achieve a level at which symptoms develop. Most of our cases however do not find complete sexual gratification even when they have heterosexual relationships. The emotional expressions of this state turn into great tenseness or depression, irritability and sensitiveness, weeping spells and rage reactions. An insatiable need for some type of gratification develops. Cravings and incorporative wishes of all kinds appear and lead to sadistic and masochistic tendencies which occur chiefly when both oestrone and progesterone are active. When ovulation actually occurs the tension is suddenly relieved and relaxation takes place. We now present some examples of ovulative change.

Ovulative change. The psychoanalytic material and corresponding endocrine findings of case G.S. from 12/17/37 to 12/21/37 were cited above as an example of aggressive tendencies which developed during the period of increasing preovulative tension. The dream of 12/21/37 q.v. shows homosexual content also, corresponding to incipient corpus luteum activity; the smear was called immediately preovulative. On 12/22/37 she reported the following dream:

'Young girl. She talked in a very facetious way. She must, must be me. This girl talked with a man who had flaming red hair, curly lashes. He was interested in this girl and made a date with her. I talked to the girl. I told her about a case. Someone was pregnant and the man did not assume responsibility. I told her men don't like to do this. She answered, "Is that so? Do you mean this really?" In the same dream somebody said, "He is very *very hurt*".'

The vaginal smear 12/22/37 shows marked desquamation and leucocytic infiltration typical of the first postovulative day.

In this dream it is obvious that sexual temptation is directly connected with the danger of being impregnated and then abandoned. 'He is very hurt' is the expression of her wish for revenge as well as the projection of her own being hurt. The dream shows marked heterosexual wish, expression of oestrone activity, and fear of pregnancy, expression of lutein activity, and therefore might be interpreted as clearly preovulative. During the analytic hour on 12/22/37 the patient feels relaxed. She starts her associations jokingly:

'Oh, my dear – It is a hard job to overcome an inertia against talking.' During this hour she talks about her admiration for her body, how she used to stand in front of the mirror admiring herself. She talks in a relaxed, receptive mood about her need for being loved. But she brings up bitter associations about men who do not love her as she wanted to be loved. The mood and content of the hour clearly show the postovulative relaxation and narcissistic gratification. On 12/23/37 the patient says:

'I functioned well yesterday. I loved myself very well, on the basis if nobody else loves me I will love myself. Yesterday evening I was pleased with my body. My husband made overtures but I felt removed from him. I loved my breast. I did not want him to touch it. Though my body was burning for love I withdrew.'

This recital of her emotions shows that her libidinous interest was withdrawn from the outerworld and centered on her own self, which is not an individual characteristic of this patient but may be found more or less clearly expressed in all cases after ovulation occurred. The management of this erotisation by withdrawal from the heterosexual partner has however individual significance, the consequences of which can be seen on the next day. The relaxation and happiness was of short duration, for on the night of 12/23/37 she dreamed:

'Jim's mother was walking with Jimmy. We were on the railroad tracks – I and Jim. Suddenly the child dropped his mother's hand and dashed toward the tracks, threw himself on the rails and rolled about. When my sister on the other side saw the child she shrieked.'

The vaginal smear 12/23/37 is clearly postovulative.

In this dream the patient's aggression toward her own child is evident. The associations during the analytic hour showed that the dreamed suicide attempt of the son is a substitute for her own suicide wish. She identified herself with her son. The apparent aggression developed toward her own pregnancy and is really an aggression toward herself. The aggression which was directed toward the man's penis during previous days 12/19 and 12/20 is now directed, after incorporation of the penis, i.e. pregnancy, toward the son, and therefore toward herself. The introversion of the aggression is indicative. It supports the general observation that the psychic energy which was directed toward the object world during the preovulative phase is turned toward the patient's self in the postovulative phase of the cycle.

It is interesting to compare this ovulative state with the following cycle of the same individual. We have already cited the pleasant erotic sensation associated with minimal oestrone activity which persisted from 1/18/38 to 1/20/38 of G.S. On 1/20/38 she had many symptoms: perspiration, irritation of the rectum. In fantasy she identified herself with prostitutes and became extremely angry and hostile toward all authorities.

The vaginal smear 1/21/38 shows complete cornification.

On 1/22/38 she forgot the main part of her dream. The fragment which she remembered had homosexual content. During the analytic session she was excited. Her fantasies were aggressively directed toward the penis which she wanted to pull and incorporate.

The vaginal smear on 1/22/38 was clearly ovulative, showing complete cornification, minimal folding, with leucopenia, similar to the smear on 12/21/37.

After the analytic session the patient had a dream which contained an involved argument with her mother about the feminine role. The dream showed an intense dynamic conflict between the wish to be like her mother, (i.e., accept the motherly role) and the overwhelmingly powerful sexual desires which expressed themselves in prostitution fantasies which is the opposite of motherliness. The dream permitted the conclusion that although there was an increasing tendency toward accepting the mother role, heterosexual tension was nevertheless maintained, therefore the diagnosis of preovulative state was made.

On the next day 1/23/38 she felt weak, 'like a baby – my hands look washed out – I ate a great deal, slept a great deal.'

The vaginal smear on 1/23/38 was clearly postovulative and showed marked desquamation of cornified cells and leucocytic infiltration.

On 1/24/38 her dream showed identification with her child but not in the suicidal aggressive manner of the preceding month, rather in a positive, satisfactory attitude of being proud of the son. The last part of the dream expressed various hostile impulses in connection with pregnancy.

The vaginal smear 1/24/38 showed definite luteal phase with reappearance of a few normal cells and increased mucification of all cells.

Thus postovulative relaxation on 1/23/38 was accompanied by a regression, being weak like a baby, sleeping, and eating like a baby. The oral dependency, the need for love, as well as the awareness of her own genitals were manifest in symptoms and in conscious feelings. They express the need to be close to the mother like a baby, to be protected by love and gratified by food. The change from the aggressive incorporative, preovulative tension to postovulative relaxation and oral regression (identification with infant) can be observed in this cycle which shows some psychological improvement as compared to the previous cycle.

These 2 subsequent ovulative periods of 1 patient may suffice to demonstrate that the instinctual tendency changes its direction after ovulation took place. While it was active, and directed toward the sexual object during the follicle-ripening phase, it becomes passive and directed toward one's own self after ovulation. Further examples of other patients with quite different personality structures make it evident, that the change in direction of the instinctual tendency is not characteristic of any individual case but is found generally.

A patient, R.E. with severe phobia, and passive infantile personality had 2 dreams in the same night, 11/1/37.

'My husband, my sister and myself were at a show and on the screen 2 shots were fired. Someone was getting killed or there was a war or something. Anyhow some shots were fired. I heard somebody in the audience sort of scream in Jewish "Oi veh" as though she couldn't stand the shooting on the screen. The voice was very familiar to me. I turned around. It was my mother standing in the aisle hollering at the top of her voice. I was very embarassed. I sort of pulled her toward where we were sitting on the aisle. I felt embarrassed and kind of funny about having people know it was my mother screaming that way. I asked where my brother was that stays with her. She pointed to him sitting in a seat all by himself. She said "He's sick". He had his hand holding his forehead and I got scared and went up to him and asked him what was the matter. I don't remember whether he was sick or he was sleeping, and I don't remember and don't know the end of it.'

This dream shows the fearful defense against heterosexuality. The aggressive scene in which the mother is desperately wailing is the typical representation of her early experience of the parents' coitus. In the dream it is partly projected to the screen, which decreases the own fear of being attacked sexually. The next dream thought considers the brother. (She experienced the sexual attack of the brother in childhood.) But now he is sleepy or sick – he is now not dangerous. Thus she can act in a motherly fashion and take a kindly interest in his

condition. This last part of the dream shows a motherly attitude. The next dream in the same night shows impregnation symbolism on an infantile, oral level.

'I was in my sister's house eating fried fish and a baked potato. I was on very good terms with her. All of a sudden I heard a loud noise outside, people hollering and screaming, and I thought it was my mother so I ran out to see who it was. There were some people on the street fighting –, police officers with guns in their hands and clubs. I couldn't find my mother. I thought it was her doing all the screaming. I looked around for her. I came back to my sister-in-law's, but the baked patato was gone.'
'Only the fish was left. But she had eaten the baked potato. I asked her if she had enough fish for supper. She showed me a platter with enough fish for supper and in the dream I wondered why I was speaking to her when I'm supposed to be angry at her. Then I remembered that some woman with whom I played poker said "You'll be speaking to her soon." That thought of what this woman really said came to me in the dream. So that was the end of it.'

In its manifest content the dream showed only a slightly disguised childlike conception of impregnation[6]. The first dream expressed the heterosexual tendency and beside this some motherliness; the second dream expresses the same tendencies, but the wish to be impregnated is stronger.

The vaginal smear 11/1/37, showed 100% cornification, some folding and aggregation typical of the *ovulative phase*.

At the analytic hour on 11/1/37, oral regression seemed to dominate. The patient came like a child with a chocolate bar in her hand, eating, and offered some to the

---

[6] Children have their own concepts as to how children are conceived and they cling to these fantasies very often even after they have full enlightenment as to the natural processes. FREUD refers to these fantastic concepts of the children as infantile sexual theories. One of the most wide spread conceptions is that children are conceived after the mother eats something such as potatoes, beans, fish, etc.

analyst. On 11/2/37 the analytic material showed increased fear of being attacked sexually. She recalled a dream fragment in which her husband had protected her against sexual aggression of other men and associated it with the sexual attack on her by her brother when she had been a child and to which she had reacted with the fear of being pregnant. This material is thus an elaboration of the problem expressed on the previous day.

The vaginal smear on 11/2/37, showed 100% cornification plus folding and aggregation as on the previous day, still ovulative phase.

On 11/2/37 the patient could not take a basal metabolism test because she felt she was suffocating. On 11/3/37 she came into the analyst's office cheerful and relaxed. She recited the happenings of the previous day in a normal way, described her suffocation, her tenseness, her extreme irritability toward her husband. The entire session was filled with uninterrupted, free-flowing cheerful but rather empty talk. When the analytic session was finished she arose from the couch and asked proudly for praise because she 'associated so freely' without being urged.

The vaginal smear, 11/3/37, was postovulative and showed leucocytic infiltration of the previously leucopenic vaginal mucosa.

The state of intense preovulative tension persisted from 10/31 to 11/3. The heterosexual tendency of this period was masked by fear while the progesterone activity was expressed by wish for impregnation and regression to oral state. In another cycle of the same patient, on 1/18/38, the dream material was interpreted as *fear of impregnation*. During the analytic hour she felt peaceful, quiet, contented, tired and without fear.

The vaginal smear 1/18/38 showed complete cornification with minimal folding, probably a smear of the ovulative day.

The postovulative relaxation was clearly marked. On the next day 1/19/38 she reported:

'I had a dream about playing poker. We were going to play poker in one of the women's houses. My brother's wife was going to watch me. Even in the dream I knew I was afraid to be alone. She took the baby along. She was going to give her some milk for lunch. I asked her "Is that all you are going to give her? Why that isn't enough. It's very hungry." My brother loved the baby a good deal and if anything happened to the baby, if she didn't get enough to eat it would be my fault and I'd be blamed by him. So I asked the hostess if she had any eggs and she said they don't eat eggs in her home. I was sorry that I didn't take one along with me from my mother-in-law's because I knew that she had eggs.'

The vaginal smear 1/19/38 shows marked desquamation of cells and a slight regression from the complete cornification of the previous day, clearly postovulative.

The dream has a slight heterosexual content. The patient cannot indulge in sexuality because she is jealously watched but in the dream her brother's baby is her baby. Here we see the same wish to have a child, as we found it in the material on 11/1/37 and 11/2/37. Here is repeated again the competitive attitude toward the mother. When she is the mother, she feeds the baby more and better than the real mother does. She also shows the tendency to identify herself with the child whom she feeds as she wants to be fed and taken care of.

The ovulative change of patient V.M. may be presented here. Her dream of 12/1/37 we have already reported q.v. as an example of increased heterosexual tension in the preovulative phase. On 12/2/37 she reports:

'I hate my mother. She likes to talk about intimate things. I don't want her to be that close to me. I have an unpleasant feeling in my vulva when my mother talks of intimate things.'

The vaginal smear 12/2/37 was clearly ovulative and showed complete cornification, leucopenia and an occasional red blood cell.

The change of heterosexual tendencies into a clear awareness of her own body and into conflict with her mother might be characteristic of the ovulative and early postovulative state. This material exposes, however, still too much active hostile feeling toward the mother and the dream as well as the associations during the analytic session fail to show relaxation. Even though the 'mother conflict' is estimated as corresponding to lutein activity, on the basis of this hostile tension, the diagnosis of preovulative tension with increased corpus luteum function was made. On the next day, however, she reported the following dream (the patient is analyzed by a man).

'You and I were sitting in an operating room. You said that an operation would take place, and that the cost would be 50 dollars. I felt very thankful and thought it was worth any price. I thought that the operation was to be on my throat.'

The vaginal smear 12/3/37 showed continued cornification but beginning aggregation indicative of ovulation.

Comparing this dream with that of 12/1/37 the difference in direction of the psychic energy is obvious. On 12/1/37 the patient dreamed that a man's penis was being sliced, while on 12/3/37 she yields to a passive masochistic feminine tendency. Gratitude instead of vindictiveness is an evidence of relaxation which permits the conclusion that the characteristic postovulative emotional state had developed. The psychoanalytic hour offered further evidence for relaxation. The flow of associations started playfully:

'Humpty dumpty sitting on a wall. Wiener frankfurter my favorite food.'

In another cycle V.M. on 10/13/37 felt tense. Her dream expressed a strong defense against the feminine sexual role and an intense wish for masculine identification.

The vaginal smear 10/13/37, was ovulative and showed 100% cornification, with some folding and aggregation.

On the next day 10/14/37 the patient was depressed and calm. She wanted to be taken care of, to be nursed by her husband. This passive dependent attitude expresses the regression which we consider characteristic of early postovulative phase.

The vaginal smear 10/14/37 showed increased desquamation and aggregation, clearly postovulative.

This brief selection of psychological material of the ovulative state demonstrates the main correlation. Other cycles investigated show the same correlations but the underlying psychodynamics assumed a more camplicated form. This material has displayed the increasing intensity of conflicting psychodynamic tendencies during the preovulative state, when both oestrone and progesterone were present in the organism. It should be emphasized that the basic unconscious conflicts of the individual come closer to consciousness during this period of the cycle. Very often dreams and the conscious emotional attitudes do not adequately discharge the tensions. Symptoms increase in intensity and new symptoms develop. The characteristic symtomatology of this period we shall defer to a later publication.

The ovulation is characterised by the sudden decrease of oestrogenous activity and by the increased activity of corpus luteum. Hence, after ovulation the active heterosexual libido decreases and the passive libidinous tendencies appear with greater intensity. Emotionally this state is mainly characterised by the relaxation of the preovulative tension, which was caused by the conflicting tendencies of oestrone and incipient lutein activity.

Our examples have demonstrated the relaxation which follows ovulation. This relaxation has various emotional concomitants. Sometimes the patient becomes talkative or even hypomanic. Preovulative and postovulative talkativeness are distinctly different. Tense, speedy talk with increasing sensitiveness, with the patient suffering from the feeling of being compelled or driven to talk is characteristic of the pre-ovulative state. Satisfied, pleasant, relatively passive free flow of associations distinguishes the postovulative state. The most valid psychological sign of ovulation is a relaxed feeling of well-being which is accompanied by positive, pleasant feelings about the subject's own body, for example: V.M. on 12/7/37 feels well and relaxed. She enjoys herself passively during the analytic hour and tells:

'I saw my breasts, I wanted to be recognized as a woman. The sexual feeling I had was going through my breasts. I put my arm around myself and I remember the sensation in my breasts, the sensation of shame.'

On the basis of the narcissistic sensations, the diagnosis of 'postovulative' was made.

The vaginal smear 12/7/37 was definitely postovulative and showed marked desquamation and aggregation of cornified cells.

The very similar material of G.S. on 12/22/37 was already cited – as falling in love with her own body. On 10/5/37 she describes her emotional state in another postovulative period as follows:

'I feel young, alert, and unantagonistic.'
The vaginal smear, 10/5/37, showed increased aggregation and secretion. Very few cornified cells; clearly postovulative.

A gratified warm feeling follows the great tension. In the postovulative condition the body is flooded with libidinous feelings. This erotisation of the patient's own body may be conveyed to other persons too: A need for closeness, for love in a general sense is the emotional expression of this hormonal state.

The relaxation may express itself as a sudden regression, such as we saw in G.S. on 1/23/38 when she felt her body 'weak and passive like a baby', sleepy and hungry; or in V.M. on 10/14/37 who acted out her wishes for dependence and her desire to be nursed and taken care of; or in R.E. 11/1/37 who acted out the regressive oral condition by coming with a chocolate bar in hand to the analytic session.

The immediately postovulative state is also characterised by an increased libidinous charge of the propagative organs. This charge is frequently strong enough to result in a conscious awareness of the patient's own genitals. It may also be expanded to include the entire body. The reaction to this feeling is normally pleasant. It may give rise to strong feminine exhibitionistic tendencies, to the wish to dance alone, e.g. in V.M. on 3/17/38. The increased sexual charge may result in masturbation or may give rise to defense against being a woman and arouses inferiority feeling.

Lutein phase. The attitude increases during the ovulation phase, and thereafter the psychodynamic material is either narcissistic or clearly passive receptive, typical of the female and the small child. The passive receptive tendency determines the psychodynamic situation as long as progesterone dominance persists. Progesterone is the hormone chiefly concerned with preparation of the uterus for nidation and with maintaining pregnancy. The physiological preparation of the uterus for nidation implies a task for the psychic apparatus to be dealt with in every cycle, namely to solve the problem of being a woman. While the activity of the corpus luteum increases, we observe in the psychological material the attempt of the individual to prepare herself for the propagative role of womanhood. During the study of the psychological material related to the menstrual cycle it was striking to see that under the influence of corpus luteum activity the psychological material shifts to the mother-conflict, to the problems of the relationship with the mother. For example, V.M. reported on 2/22/38:

'A hotel. Lots of strange people. I was afraid of them. My mother was with me. Mother and I picked up drawers and took them to the kitchen. A young man was then laughing at my mother. I went to help her. Somebody laughed at me. I decided not to pay any attention. I began to feel affection for her. I began to feel like rubbing myself against her leg. She seemed to be bothered by it. I did it more openly and then decided she was my mother. She became disgusted with me.

Associations. 'My mother in the dream was much younger. Something about the way she treated me caused a peculiar feeling inside. She was afraid other people would see it. I remember her sitting on the floor playing dolls with me when I was 6 years of age. Her face in the dream was more like then. I have a feeling my mother was very lovely. I never could feel like a woman should feel. I have a very unlovely feeling most of the time. The only time I feel that way (womanly) is in a nightgown that I like. As soon as I look in the glass it cancels the feeling I get.'

The vaginal smear on 2/22/38 showed marked aggregation and folding, with gradual disappearance of cornified cells, typical of luteal phase.

The outstanding feature of the dream is the relationship to the mother. The solution of the dream problem is to separate ihe mother from her heterosexual interests and possess her entire attention, even in the sense of physical gratification. In this material the longing to have positive undisturbed feminine feelings toward her own body is also obvious. This tendency is typical for the undisturbed lutein state.

On 2/23/38 – the *dream* shows homosexual content. One part of it is:

'I finally said the woman can come and sleep with me.'

The vaginal smear on 2/23/38 – typical for lutein phase, all the signs of lutein function increase beyond the previous day.

The emotional state corresponding to lutein activity is not always so happy and gratified as this material indicates. Here the patient was able to develop her fantasy of being accepted and loved by the mother. The same patient on 5/23/38 is depressed, cries, does not know what to do. She feels unwanted and unloved. She complains that the analyst does not love her either. The patient is pleading for the analyst's love –, understanding.

The vaginal smear on 5/23/38 aggregation and folding of desquamated, cornified cells typical of progesterone activity.

On 5/24/38 the patient feels the same disappointment because of lack of love.

She comforts herself with the fantasy and associations that her mother kissed her buttocks when she was a baby.

The vaginal smear on 5/24/38 shows increased aggregation – lutein phase.

We have already followed the cycle of G.S. which started on 12/10/37 through the very aggressive preovulative phase, through ovulation on 12/22 – 12/23/37 which was marked by an intense but short-lived narcissistic relaxation; after which the patient became tense and depressed again. On the night of 12/24/37 she has the following dream:

'We were on our way somewhere and had been admitted to a home. We were going through the house, and talking in a friendly fashion to the children in the house. One part of the house appeared locked against us, but we were able to wander through the other rooms which were light, spacious and somewhat cluttered up. It appeared to me that it was necessary for us to go. Suddenly my mother appeared in a bathrobe. She had J., my son, in a bathtub filled with water. She appeared very intense. The other people and I watched with interest what occurred and were surprised. My mother kept pressing the child down in the water. He was completely submerged, struggled for a while and then lay quite still under the water, as though lifeless.'

The vaginal smear on 12/25/37 showed marked aggregation with only an occasional cornified cell and was typical of the luteal phase.

In these general interpretations of the correlations between emotional state and hormonal state, case histories have been purposely omitted. At this point, however, it is necessary to state that in this case the aggressive impulses toward the pregnancy and the infant were indeed the central conflict which resulted in depression. In spite of this, reviewing the dream material of this cycle we recognize that the conflict of the patient is not apparent in the psychological material of the preovulative phase. The aggressive impulses in the dreams of the preovulative state were directed toward the man; (dreams on 12/18/37 and 12/21/ 37) they increased to rage in the dream 12/ 21/37 and then the ovulation occurred accompanied by emotional relaxation. After the ovulation the aggression turned toward herself and toward her child in the dream (12/23/37). In this last dream the conflict with the mother is obviously expressed. She was afraid of her mother, because she was rejected by her. In the manifest dream the mother kills her child in water in a bathtub. The aggressive impulse is here passively experienced. The passive direction of the instinctual tendency, the repetition of the conflict with the mother and with the child are those contents of the dream which we correlate with the intensified function of the corpus luteum. It is comprehensible that after this dream patient feels tense and remarks: 'I was aware of all my nerves, even those in my ears.' The awareness of her female body burdened by fear of the mother's aggression toward her and by the guilt for her own aggression toward her child charge the problem of mother-child with fear, aggression and guilt.

The complicated interrelationship between mother and daughter (from the beginning of life) is the subject of psychoanalytic investigation of individual development. The conflicts vary in depth and structure in every case and change during the course of psychoanalytic therapy. It is not germane to this paper to describe the different types of conflict or their changes during analysis – tending toward reconciliation with the mother – except for the following point: as long as the unconscious relationship to the mother is hostile the oral material becomes aggressive and tensions develop which destroy all the pleasant passive-dependent narcissistic feelings which were found to be characteristic of the postovulative state. Thus hostility leads to more or less severe depression during the lutein phase as for example in G.S. 12/25/37 and in V.M. 5/23/38 q.v.

The psychological material corresponding to the activity of the corpus luteum would in the usual psychoanalytic terminology be described as belonging to the pregenital, oral level of libido organisation. From the cycles we have studied, we may describe the course of instinctual tendency as follows: after maintaining active heterosexual libido directed toward the object on a genital level for a period of time (oestrone phase), the libido changes its direction and appears as a passive receptive tendency which, during the preovulative state may conflict with the heterosexual object libido. The passive receptive tendency becomes stronger after ovulation. The earliest object of the passive receptive libido was the mother who satisfied all needs of dependence, the need to be loved, sheltered and fed. We dare say that passive oral-receptive tendencies appear in the psychological material of an adult woman only when progesterone is present. Of course it is possible to observe 'oral material' in the follicle-ripening phase of the cycle as well, for then the aggressive incorporative tendencies serve the purpose of masculine identification. The distinction between passive receptive and aggressive incorporative oral tendencies[7] is important in recognising the various phases of the cycle. The former belongs to the postovulative, the latter to the preovulative phase.

The passive receptive tendency of the corpus luteum phase has its normal emotional representation on the genital level: this is the wish to be impregnated, the wish to have a child. The tendency toward nursing and feeding appears often parallel with this wish. Thus the passive receptive genital desire manifests itself in connection with an active oral –, 'oral-giving' tendency: with the desire to feed. Both intellectual tendencies unfold after successful identification with the mother. Hence in dreams and in the other psychological material they

---

[7] This distinction of the oral tendencies in oral receptive and oral aggressive, as well as the distinction of the oral dependency was worked out mainly by Dr. FRANZ ALEXANDER in his Vector conception [1, 2, 3]. These investigations confirm his findings on a larger scale.

appear together with the wish to be like the mother. Between these extremes (1) the wish to be a baby and be nursed and fed by the mother, and (2) the wish to be a woman, be impregnated and become a mother, we find all the varieties of female development. The biological preparation for pregnancy is reflected in the psychological material as pregnancy fantasies or dreams and appears sometimes as the early expression of corpus luteum activity even in the preovulative state. Such early pregnancy material is however projected to the mother as for example in R.E. on 11/2/37 and in R.G. on 6/26/38 q.v. Such pregnancy material is referred to mother's pregnancies and may be expressed by birth fantasies or womb fantasies. It may repeat the conflicts and traumata caused by birth of siblings, as for example in R.E. on 1/19/38.

The psychological material corresponding to late progesterone activity shifts from the conflict with the mother to the problem of being a mother and to the relationship with the child. Pregnancy material is then concerned with the problems of their own pregnancy (not that of the mother), the fear and desire. The wish to nurse, feed, and take care of the child is characteristic of very late corpus luteum activity. This material can rarely be demonstrated apart from other factors which influence the cycle at this time. One such example is provided by G.S. on 1/28/38 (the earlier part of this cycle has already been cited).

'I seem to have been told that I could get clothes for a small child, but I forgot about it when I saw the child. I made preparations to cut its nails. The person in charge of the clothes came along and told me that I keep forgetting to take care of the clothes. Then we came to a place which looked like a kindergarten.'
The vaginal smear on 1/28/38 consists mostly of normal cells indicating very low hormone content.

Progesterone dominance persists only a few days unless pregnancy occurs. Otherwise the new follicle starts ripening and reflects its activity in the psychological material. With reappearance of oestrogenous

activity there is again a period in which tendencies corresponding to both corpus luteum and follicle-ripening function influence the emotional state simultaneously, for example in V.M. on 12/8/37 (the ovulative state from 12/1 to 12/3/37 has been presented before) the following dream is reported (*male analyst*):

'I am in your office waiting for you. I wanted you to pay attention to me. I looked in the mirror. My hair was all white. My skin was smooth, my figure slender. I was dressed in a long velvet cloak. I thought you were punishing me by not looking at me, so I decided to go to the North Side. I went into a store on Milwaukee Avenue. I felt somebody changed things and I was tired out. I thought I would be late and that I should phone you. I decided to call you up at home. You were not there. Finally I went to your home. You lived in a little frame cottage. A little boy was in the window. I decided to save him and I did.'
The vaginal smear on 12/8/37 shows together with the extreme aggregation typical of the luteal phase minimal cornification which is evidence of a newly ripening follicle – premenstrual.

In the beginning of the dream the satisfaction with her own body is expressed. She feels feminine and attractive. This part of the dream expresses the feelings which are associated with progesterone production. It is obvious that she directs her attractiveness toward a man with a normal heterosexual feeling. The heterosexual tendency is also expressed by fear of prostitution tendencies. The dream thought – 'when my father does not love me I am like a lost child, in danger' – is another expression of the heterosexual tendency. There is sufficient heterosexuality to diagnose this as a premenstrual state.

We have already reported the lutein phase on 5/23/38 to 5/24/38 of V.M. showing conflict with her mother. On 5/25/38 still in a depressed and dependent mood, the patient reported the following dream (*male analyst*):

'I changed my profession and got into school teaching. I went across the hall and put my hand on a child. I went down the corridor and saw my own son who did not belong here. Then I was here telling you about it. I became very angry because you did not give me a chance to express myself. A man and woman came in and you were angry at their coming. I began to cover up so she would not think that anything was going on. Then I decided I did not need to be scared because another man was there too.'

The vaginal smear on 5/25/38 shows initial cornification – premenstrual. The patient in this dream sought a solution for her dependence.

The only possible solution was to be a good mother and protective to her son. But the heterosexual wish toward the analyst-father whose attention she wants for herself interferes with her wish to be a good mother. The dream is therefore concerned with the mother-child relationship (lutein phase)

and expresses heterosexual tendencies (newly ripening follicle).

The first evidence of premenstrual change is the consequence of a slight influx of oestrone which usually remains at a low level for some days. During this period the heterosexual content of the psychological material does not overshadow the material which is related to nidation. With further atresia of the corpus luteum and the consequent diminishing progesterone output, there is again a change in direction of metabolic processes. This is reflected in the psychological material. The psychological complexities of the premenstrual-menstrual phase, except at its very beginning, require more detailed description than can conveniently be included in the compass of the present paper. These complexities however

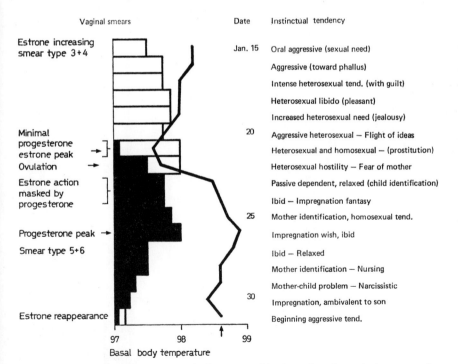

Fig. 2. Basal body temperatures, vaginal smears and instinctual tendency during one ovulative phase of patient G.S.

Diagram I

Hormone	Instinctual tendency	Neurotic elaborations of tendency

Oestrone	Active object libido on genital level: heterosexual desire	1. Aggressive incorporative: penis envy, castration wish
		2. Masochistic: masochistic concept of female sexuality
		3. Defense reactions:
		  a) fear of being attacked
		  b) masculine protest

Follicular hormone		

Progesterone dominant
Corpus luteum hormone
	Passive receptive tendency on genital level Desire to be loved and wish for impregnation	Passive receptive tendency on regressive level: oral receptive and oral dependent wishes, may be directed toward
		  a) mother
		  b) homosexual object
		  c) heterosexual object

Diagram II

Phase of cycle	Hormone state	Psychological material
Follicle ripening	Initial oestrone function	Heterosexual tendency, usually pleasant, feeling of well being
Late preovulative	Increasing oestrone plus minimal progesterone	Relief by sexual gratification or increasing tension – conflicting tendencies (see Diagram I)
Ovulative (immediately after ovulation)	Diminishing oestrone plus in-creasing progesterone	Relaxation of conflict tension. Erotization of female body, passive-receptive. Pleasant emotional state
Postovulative, luteal	Progesterone dominance	See Diagram I, especially passive receptive tendencies and object libido toward mother or homosexual object
Late luteal, early premenstrual	Diminishing progesterone plus resultant reappearance (unmasking) of oestrone effects	Recurrence of heterosexual tendency on mostly receptive level, and pregnancy fantasies

can be correlated with the simultaneous hormonal complexities of this phase of the cycle as we plan to show in the second part of this publication.

Summary

We have presented and discussed the psychological and physiological material of that part of the menstrual cycle which centers about ovulation: the preovulative, ovulative and postovulative periods. The presentation of material of the premenstrual-menstrual phase will occur in the second part of this publication. We present above a graphic summary of the ovulative phase of the cycle of one of our subjects, G.S. Jan. 15–30 as a type of all cycles in which ovulation occurs (fig. 2).

Careful study of vaginal smears and basal body-temperatures on the one hand, and of the psychoanalytic records on the other, led us to infer the correlations presented in the diagrams I and II. In the light of the foregoing material, the diagrams are self-explanatory.

The content of these two diagrams may be repeated shortly in the following correlations:

(1) The oestrogenous phase of the cycle corresponds to an emotional condition characterized by active heterosexual libido. This appears normally as a wish for heterosexual gratification but it may turn into aggression toward the man or into a fearful defensive attitude. The psychological material during this phase of the cycle reflects the psychodynamic aspects of the relationship to man. (2) The function of the corpus luteum corresponds to the erotization of the female body. In this phase of the cycle the libido is turned from the outer world toward the individual which appears more passive and dependent. The psychological material during the stage of the corpus luteum reflects the erotization of the female body and the preparation for motherhood. (3) The ovulation is characterized by sudden decrease of the oestrogenous activity and by the influx of the narcissistic erotization according to the greater activity of lutein hormones. Emotionally this state is mainly characterized by the relaxation of the preovulative tension which was caused by the conflicting tendencies between the increased oestrone and incipient lutein activity.

Conclusions

(1) The day-by-day study of vaginal smears and basal body temperatures provided a useful and enlightening method for analysis of gonad function of adult women. (2) The psychoanalytic method could also be employed for a day-by-day study of the cycle of propagative function on the psychological level. (3) The simultaneous use of the two methods provided clear correlations between the physiological and psychological processes. (4) The investigation suggests that in the adult woman, it was possible to relate instinctual drives to specific hormone functions of the ovaries; (a) Heterosexual tendency is correlated with oestrone activity. (b) Passive receptive and narcissistic attitude is correlated with progesterone activity. (5) Whenever the metabolic gradient correlated with the specific gonadal hormones changes its direction or slope, the psychological material shows a change in direction of the instinctual drive. (6) This method affords an approach to the study of the biological foundations of instincts.

References

1. ALEXANDER, F.: The logic of emotions and its dynamic background. Int. J. Psycho-Anal. *16:* 399 (1935).
2. ALEXANDER, F. and WILSON, G. W.: Quantitative dream studies. Psychoanal. Quart. *4:* 371–407 (1935).
3. ALEXANDER, F.: The influence of psychological factors upon gastro-intestinal disturbances, Psychoanal. Quart. *3:* 501–588 (1934).
4. ALLEN, E.: Sex and internal secretions (Williams and Wilkins, Baltimore 1932).
5. BURR, H. S.; HILL, R. T., and ALLEN, E.: Detection of ovulation in the intact rabbit. Proc. Soc. exp. Biol., NY *33:* 109–111 (1935).
6. EVANS, H. M. and SWEZY, O.: Ovogenesis and the normal follicular cycle in adult mammalia. Mem. Univ. Calif. *9:* 119–185 (1931).
7. FRENCH, T. M.: Reality and the unconscious. Psychoanal. Quart. *6:* 23–61 (1937).

8. FRENCH, T. M.: Reality testing in dreams. Psychoanal. Quart. 6: 62–77 (1937).

9. FREUD, S.: The Interpretation of dreams (Allen and Unwin, London 1932).

10. FREUD, S.: On Narcissism: An introduction; in Collected Papers, vol. 4, p. 30 (Hogarth Press, London 1925).

11. FREUD, S.: Three contributions to the theory of sex, nervous and mental diseases (Publishing Company, New York 1930).

12. FREUD, S.: The ego and the id (Hogarth Press, London 1927).

13. HISAW, F. L.; GREEP, R. O., and FEVOLD, H. L.: The effects of Oestrin-progestin combinations on the endometrium, vagina, and sexual skin of monkeys. Amer. J. Anat. 61: 483–504 (1937).

14. MORTIMER, H.; WRIGHT, R. P., and COLLIP, J. B.: The effect of the administration of estrogenic hormones in the nasal mucosa of the monkey. Canad. med. Ass. J. 35: 503–615 (1936).

15. MYERS, H. I.; YOUNG, W. C., and DEMPSEY, E. W.: Graafian follicle development throughout the reproductive cycle in the guinea pig, with especial reference to change during oestrus. Anat. Rec. 65: 381–395 (1936).

16. PAPANICOLAOU, G. N.: The sexual cycle in the human female as revealed by vaginal smears. Amer. J. Anat. 52: 519–616 (1933).

17. PRATT, J. P.: The human corpus luteum, Arch. Path. 19: 380–425, 545–562 (1935).

18. ROCK, J.; REBOUL, J., and SNODGRASS, J. M.: Electrical changes associated with human ovulation. Amer. J. Obstet. Gynec. 36: 733–746 (1938).

19. RUBENSTEIN, B. B.: The relation of cyclic changes in human vaginal smears to body temperatures and basal metabolic rates. Amer. J. Physiol. 119: 635–641 (1937).

20. RUBENSTEIN, B. B.: Estimation of ovarian activity by the consecutive day study of basal body temperature and basal metabolic rate. Endocrinology 22: 41–44 (1938).

21. RUBENSTEIN, B. B.: The fertile period of women. J. Contracept. 2: 171–173 (1937).

22. SEWARD, G. H.: The female sex rhythm. Psychol. Bull. 31: 153–192 (1934).

23. SHERWOOD, T. C.: The relation of estrogenic substances to thyroid function and respiratory metabolism. Amer. J. Physiol. 124: 114–116 (1938).

24. STERBA, R.: Handwörterbuch der Psychoanalyse (Internationaler Psychoanalytischer Verlag, Wien 1936).

25. WITSCHI, E. and PFEIFFER, C.: The hormonal control of oestrus, ovulation and mating in the female rat. Anat. Rec. 64: 85–107 (1935).

26. ZUCK, T. T.: The relation of basal body temperature to fertility and sterility in women. Amer. J. Obstet. Gynec. 36: 998–1004 (1938).

Emotions and Gastroduodenal Function[1]

Experimental Studies on Patients with Gastritis, Duodenitis and Peptic Ulcer

B. Mittelmann and H. G. Wolff
With the technical assistance of Margaret P. Scharf

Retrospective comment by Dr. L. Gottschalk. This paper stands out as a landmark in psycho-somatic medicine and research for its imaginative combination of clinical studies and ex-perimental observations as well as for its broad range of innovative approaches and provocative hypotheses concerning psychophysiological gastric relationships. Among the investigative approaches and psychophysiological phenomena which these authors deserve credit for ex-ploring are the following: (1) The 'novelty effect' of the experimental situation on psycho-physiological gastric function. (2) The usefulness, in hypothesis formation, of obtaining psycho-logical-gastric relationships in the patient's life history followed by explorations in interviews of the actual psychophysiological associations occurring in each individual patient. (3) The investigation of other areas of physiological function concomitant to the gastric psychophysiol-ogy, namely, studies of concomitant changes in finger temperature and respiration. (4) The comparison of gastric function in normals and in patients with peptic ulcer, gastritis, and duodenitis. (5) The exploration of psychophysiological relationships occurring with a full range of affects (anger, resentment, fear, anxiety, guilt, embarassment, humiliation) and other psycho-logical states (feelings of security and confidence, relaxation, and pain) – both naturally occurring and experimentally induced – as well as such psychophysiological associations occurring during sleeping and dreaming. (6) The early exploration of the question of the specificity of affect and stomach function. Mittelmann and Wolff noted in their studies that 'resentment, guilt, frustration, and anxiety' was usually associated with gastric hypermotility and hypersecretion, but that among their normal group there were individuals in whom the induction of such emotional reactions was commonly associated with hypomotility and hyposecretion. (7) The early observation that patients with these upper gastrointestinal disorders tended to have a personality facade of independence, self-sufficiency, and perfectionism which overlaid feelings of insecurity, frustration, resentment, guilt, and anxiety. Mittelmann and Wolff noted that the arousal of resentment, anger, guilt, and anxiety was associated with gastric hypermotility and hypersecretion, a decrease in finger temperature, and rapid and shallow respiration and that the mobilization of feelings of emotional security and relative equanimity was associated with more normal, baseline physiological functioning. Similar psychosomatic changes occurred in their normal subjects as in the group with the pathological conditions, but the changes in the patho-logical group were reported to be greater in magnitude and duration.

Looking at this paper in retrospect, one must acknowledge the thoroughness and pioneering quality of these investigators. One should, also, note two aspects of this work which later led to controversies which have yet not been completely resolved. First, these investigators used a concept of 'anxiety' which is somewhat different from that used by other investigators in the field and this usage may account in part for divergent findings from other workers. Instead of regarding anxiety as irrational fear or as fear stemming from internalized psychological conflicts rather than from real external threats, Mittelmann and Wolff clearly indicated in a footnote that their use of anxiety related to a much different construct. They said (p. 131): 'In this commu-nication "fear" is used to indicate an emotional reaction to danger in which feelings of alarm,

[1] From the New York Hospital and Departments of Medicine and Psychiatry, Cornell University Medical College, New York, N.Y.

terror, and helplessness verging on abjection dominate; "anxiety" a reaction to danger in which defeat threatens, but in which resistance survives. It is commonly associated with hostility, resentment, guilt and conflict.' Second, neither the historical method nor the experimental procedure used permitted the investigators to determine whether it was, indeed, resentment, anger, guilt, and anxiety that were the key psychological variables associated with the increased secretion and motility and disturbed circulation or whether it was the frustrated dependency and the (irrational?) 'anxiety' about revealing strong dependency needs or the 'anxiety' or fear that unfulfilled dependency needs would not be satisfied. The latter issue subsequently became a focus of controversy between the group of investigators at the New York Hospital (represented by H. WOLFF; B. MITTELMANN et al.) and the more psychoanalytically oriented workers at the Chicago Institute for Psychoanalysis (represented by F. ALEXANDER, T. FRENCH et al.).

Introduction

A relationship between emotional disturbances and peptic ulcer has been indicated by many observers. The beginning, or increase of epigastric distress, nausea, or bleeding after incidents affecting the peace of mind is an old observation frequently made by patients themselves and statistically supported by various studies [17, 27, 29, 31, 36, 47, 55, 59, 61, 66, 67, 77, 82, 96; see also 30]. It has been noted also that anxiety is an outstanding component of these emotional disturbances and that anxiety may not be recognized by the patient. It has been assumed by some that sustained emotional disturbances are capable of so altering the gastroduodenal structures as to lead eventually to ulceration.

The purpose of this study was to ascertain what personality features and emotions predominate in patients with peptic ulcer; what changes in gastroduodenal function are associated with these emotions, and whether such changes may be forerunners of tissue destruction.

I. The Problem

A. Personality Features and Reactions of Patients with Peptic Ulcer – Material

A series of 30 unselected patients with peptic ulcer, including 27 men and 3 women ranging in age from 19 to 64 years, was studied. All but 2 were under 45 years of age. Also 3 males with gastritis and duodenitis were investigated. All lesions were visualized either at surgical operation or by X-ray. Among the patients with peptic ulcers there were 25 with duodenal ulcers and 5 with gastric ulcers. Thirteen 'normal' subjects with no pathological conditions of, or complaints referable to any part of the gastrointestinal tract were also studied.

Pertinent instances rather than statistical analyses are presented, since equal opportunity to elicit evidence and measure changes in gastroduodenal function was not afforded by all patients. Unpredictable personal relationships and accidents either enhanced or decreased such opportunities.

Gross characteristics. These patients presented a wide range of personality features and reactions, with, however, a commonly shared characteristic. Some individuals were gregarious and outgoing, others were reserved and taciturn; some seemingly dealt lightly with their responsibilities, others were meticulous and overconscientious. However, among the men, the characteristic of assertive independence was outstanding in almost every instance. Rarely did any of these patients complain of anxiety, tenseness, or of other emotional distress, nor did they complain of personality problems or their life situations. Complaints revolved about the epigastrium. For the most part they were 'successful' persons and superficial contact might lead to the conclusion that they were well adjusted.

Examination revealed that the reaction patterns of these male patients were similar in the following respects. Behind the facade of independence and self-sufficiency was a background of long standing and severe anxiety, of feelings of helplessness or of being caught, frustration and desperation. Resentment and manifestations of aggression and hostility stood out. Such resentment sometimes was associated with an attempt at resolution through action but more commonly it was not overtly expressed, nor was there a plan for its resolution. The subject was not necessarily aware of its existence. In brief, despite the seeming heterogeneity of characteristics, these persons commonly showed assertive independence and self-sufficiency, covering underlying anxiety and insecurity, and accompanied by feelings of resentment and hostility.

Though resentment was the most apparent emotional reaction, feelings of guilt and self-condemnation were common. Indeed, remorse, guilt and self-denunciation were almost universally associated with anxiety and resentment, and were the basis of much conflict and personal stress. The guilt seemed to stem from hostile attitudes and resentments toward persons for whom these patients desired to feel approval. Self-condemnation and guilt feelings often resulted, seemingly, from harbored hostile feelings, from failure to achieve or give affection, from failure to obtain social esteem, from failure to maintain personal standards, and from loss of self-esteem. Associated with resentment, feelings of defeat without plans to improve the state were common.

The pernicious emotions described in those individuals were not a matter of minutes' or hours' duration but of weeks', months' and often years'.

As already mentioned, the existence of these pernicious emotional reactions was usually unrecognized by the patient. The beginnings of these emotional states, however, were often indicated even early in life by the development of character rigidity. No differences were noted between those patients who had their lesion in one part as compared with those with ulcers in another part of the stomach or duodenum.

Childhood. Untoward childhood experiences may have been a factor in the genesis of the emotional insecurity found in these patients. The failure of the home in every instance to lend a stable background resulted from a variety of causes. Outstanding among these were: the unhappy married life of the parents; the separation or loss of the father during the child's development; early remarriage of the mother after separation from the father; feelings in the child of being rejected by either or both parents or the foster-father; the anxiety of parents who, either by restrictions or 'coddling', created in the child doubts concerning his adequacy. This often resulted in resentment, as did the hostility shown by the less favored children of the family toward the protected one.

In one instance, the early death of the father left the child with an over-solicitous parent. With the subsequent close attachment and identification with an ailing, complaining mother, the child not only felt the loss of a protector, possessed by other children, but through identification with the mother, he himself felt weak and devoid of the culturally linked 'male characteristics'. Subsequently, he strove for 'success' as a means of achieving self-esteem in his attempts do deal with the feeling of weakness.

In several instances, children threatened with fears of abandonment and rejection because of the expressed conflict between the parents attempted to gain approval through perfect performance, usually linked with repression of resentment. The development of such compensatory measures began in early childhood. But in several instances the child did not achieve any degree of security through such methods until puberty or even later (18 to 20 years). For example, when one patient was 2 years old his father emigrated to America. The patient spent his childhood with relatives in Europe who made him do menial work, while his mother earned a livelihood as a traveling merchand. When the patient and his mother finally came to America to join his father, the latter was extremely critical and abusive. The patient felt mistreated and worthless until his late adolescence when he did achieve a defiant independence by establishing himself in business. His gastric complaints developed when he later failed in business and had to turn to his father who refused to help him.

Adulthood. In these adults, as mentioned above, feelings of insecurity and dependence were usually disguised by a show of independence, and the assumption of excessive responsibilities. Feelings of bitter resentment and hostility were offset by feelings of guilt and expressions of oversolicitude, devotion and concern; feelings of desperation or of being caught and helpless were compensated for by exhibitions of bravado, arrogance and defiance. For instance, one patient with peptic ulcer had renounced the usual competitive methods and had become a professional beggar. Yet within this frame of apparent humility the subject exhibited great show of independence, such as refusal to eat except in relatively esthetic surroundings, refusal to wait in line for beneficences and refusal to accept clothes other than those which pleased him.

'Hard work' or sustained, relentless application to the pursuit of business, profession or the culmination of a campaign was a feature of the behaviour of many of these individuals. On first inspection, the individual's stomach complaint might be imputed to stress of continued work without opportunity for relaxation. But even superficial analysis made evident that the drive behind the competitive effort was anxiety and insecurity. The actuating motive for such stress arose from the desire 'to achieve' at any cost, and such desire was whipped into greater and greater intensity by mounting feelings of insecurity.

Another adjustment to feelings of insecurity and anxiety, as noted in one subject, was a preoccupation with respectability and conventionality and desire for social approval. Yet the same individual, apparently inconsistently with this aim, selected a marital partner and sexual companions who had none of these qualities and who were unacceptable to his social group. The selection was based on the patient's belief that he was in a position to bestow a privilege, would gain affection and devotion, and be cared for at little emotional cost to himself.

The conflict created by a desire to maintain a front of independence and strength with the emphasis upon aggressiveness, competitiveness, initiative and possessiveness in men with but little of these qualities resulted in feelings of loneliness and of being deserted, which were reinforced by the patient's blocking of attempts on the part of his family and friends to do anything for him. For example, one fearsome, sensitive, married man with peptic ulcer asserted his independence in a dramatic way by arising each day at 5 a.m. to clean a bathroom and kitchen before starting his usual work activities. His wife in turn was humiliated by his denial to her of responsibilities which were hers.

Assertive independence and the exclusive shouldering of responsibilities were often combined with the patient's refusal to share his fears and sorrows with the marriage partner or with anyone. Such patients had the conviction that they should bear all burdens alone. This form of 'emotional independence' merged with another trait, namely, emotional detachment and the repression of a number of emotional reactions. The individual preserved a calm exterior under all circumstances and showed neither attachment nor resentment openly. The repression of hostility seemingly became associated with the repression of most outward expression.

Such detachment meant to the patient not only emotional independence but also protection against hurt. But on the other hand, among the patients here reported, failure to be given support when it was needed caused profound resentment. Marriage brought into focus such dilemmas in a number of ways.

An example is seen in one anxious, insecure man whose assertively independent behaviour implied that he needed no emotional support from his wife. This frustrated emotional relationship she reluctantly accepted supposing it to be inevitable in her relations with the strong man she married. He, however, when he needed support at a vital point made known to his wife his need for her sympathetic reassurance and in a sense demanded it from her. This sudden shift in their relations confused her and aroused her resentment because he now proved not to be the 'strong' man she married and furthermore, was now demanding warmth and understanding from her when originally he had refused to accept it. The man's disappointment in his wife for her failure to give him what he felt to be unquestionably his due created in him a profound resentment toward her.

Along with the attempts to resolve anxiety by 'I will gain approval by doing it better than anyone else', or 'I am strong and independent and need no help from anyone' was a third means often mingled with the other two. This was seen in the seeking of adoration, praise, flattery, encouragement, approval and unquestioning love.

Thus, a patient selected as a wife a woman whom he supposed to be passive, docile and non-assertive. He married because he was convinced that his wife would shower endless and unquestioning devotion upon him – in brief, was a personality that would offer him no competition, would be completely dominated and would provide him unquestioning love. The wife soon became aware that he had not 'given himself', which aroused on her part an unwillingness to give him the support which he believed his due. The sensitive husband perceived the change in his partner, and felt convinced that he was doomed to frustration should he ask for help. He therefore never turned to his partner for much wanted emotional support, but felt alone, betrayed and hostile. He turned to extra-marital relations, again giving nothing and receiving nothing but adding to his resentment and feelings of guilt.

Seemingly irreconcilable character traits in the same individual were common, as mentioned above. Thus, submissiveness with assertive independence occurred not infrequently. Such a patient took no measures to get out of a situation which was causing him distress, or he started to take measures but submitted as soon as he encountered serious opposition. Submissiveness was most commonly present in relation to the marriage partner, and less frequently it was present in work relationships. In work relationships the self-assertiveness, bravado and aggressive defiance were more often evident.

In an ambitious, seemingly aggressive male an ulcer developed during his courtship of a woman who humiliated him by her attempts to mother him. Her attitude engendered in him a feeling of insupportable weakness and inadequacy.

Another insecure, over-assertive, independent male selected a wife whose attitude and financial position indicated that she would 'take care of him'. When subsequently he was mothered by his marital partner the implied inadequacy aroused his anxiety, insecurity and resentment.

Many varieties of untoward life situation were associated with the onset and exacerbation of gastroduodenal complaints in these ulcer patients. These situations were sometimes dramatic or in the nature of a crisis but more often were without such colorful incident. They were commonly situations of stress which the patient finally had lost hope of solving.

Characteristic situations charged with stress, noted among this series of patients, were briefly as follows: failure to be made the object of unquestioning love; a man being made to feel inadequate by the attitude of dominance of his partner; failure to feel appreciated by family and friends, with feelings of loneliness and of being deserted; being unfairly treated, lied about, abused, disgraced by the wife and denied sexual relations; failure of the wife to build up security in the patient by providing such important symbols of security as the well kept 'home', 'having the food ready', 'making things that I can eat', or 'taking proper care of me'; a rejected husband's failure to return, resulting in the wife in feelings of 'misery', loneliness and dejection; poor relations with the intimate members of the family and blocked emotional outlets due to the necessity of long stays away from home; a wife's refusal to discriminate in her affection between her father and her husband (the patient) with resultant hostility in the patient toward the father and a feeling of helplessness and that 'nothing can be done about it'; a patient's being 'pushed' by his brother and wife and thus made aware of his failure at work; being driven so hard at work that perfect results could not be obtained; having to live with 'in-laws', made to assume a subordinate position and to feel 'less the man', a wife's extravagance undermining such security as the patient achieved by penuriousness and accumulating possessions; a husband's failure to satisfy the love requirement of his wife, the patient; resentment in one man because of the nature of his job which was secure and provided for his future and old age, yet was menial and caused him to recognize his failure to succeed in a competitive world. In general, situations that engendered sustained anxiety and conflict, feelings of being caught, resentment, guilt, self-denunciation and helplessness, were chronologically and intimately related to symptoms.

In contrast to the majority of men the need for assertive independence as a mask for insecurity was not evident in the women of this series. Indeed, a few of the men and all 3 of the women were outspoken in their demands for emotional dependence. The three women were submissive, responsive, truly dependent and anxious to receive devotion and to be dominated by their respective spouses. It so happened that their husbands were unable or unwilling to give them the emotional support which they wanted and which they felt justified in receiving. Thus, the reaction in the women was not unlike that of the men as regards hurt self-esteem, resentment and hostile aggression, but the manner in which this reaction developed was different.

In all of the 30 patients with peptic ulcer it was possible to demonstrate a chronological parallelism between the onset, recrudescence and course of gastroduodenal symptoms and the occurrence of untoward emotional reactions. The inference that this association was not fortuitous is supported by the fact that the history of the epigastric complaints and signs was obtained independently of the biographic data. When the two bodies of data had been assembled 'life charts' were made which then demonstrated the chronological relationship between the two. As indicated above, the situations that prompted these emotions in themselves were not necessarily dramatic or critical. However, because of the emotional frame within which they occurred they had important effects on the patient.

The following case notes illustrate emotional reactions and conflicts and their intimate chronological relationship to the symptoms of peptic ulcer.

Case 1
Epigastric burning and pain were initiated in a man during his first courtship when he was beset by fears that he was homosexual and recurred later after marriage to a woman who made him feel inadequate as a husband. Gastric hemorrhage was precipitated by his wife's refusal to let him provide a home for her.

Personal history. The patient was a 40-year-old lawyer and engineer, the third of 4 siblings. His parents were English and in the theatrical business. The father died before the patient was 2 and his mother remarried. The father was said to have been the 'black sheep' of a good family and had been disowned by his relations. The stepfather, who was devoted to the patient, was a simple, hard working stage carpenter. The patient as a child was energetic and a leader. He did well in school and at 14 began to work after school selling librettos at the Metropolitan Opera House. He discovered at this time that his supposed father was actually his stepfather. This was a shock to him and made him feel very insecure.

He graduated from high school at 19 and began to study engineering at night college. At 23 he ended his technical training without a degree and thereafter had various engineering jobs. He led an active social life, was fond of girls, and was popular with them.

At 27 the patient became engaged to a school teacher slightly older than himself. After his engagement was announced he heard rumors that his fiancee was homosexual. This suspicion caused him to feel accused of being homosexual himself and he broke the engagement. 'Dyspepsia' symptoms started during this period when he doubted his adequacy as a male. At 28 shortly after he broke his engagement to the first girl he married a Roman Catholic of Italian extraction whom he had known since his childhood. She became pregnant during the first month after marriage and left him to return home to her mother. This he resented deeply. ('They are kind, but not the type I care to live with. They are illiterate, except for my father-in-law who has travelled and is accomplished in his work as a tailor for costumes at the Opera.') She stayed with her mother during the remainder of her pregnancy, which terminated in a miscarriage at the end of 10 weeks. He then gave up a good job in order that he might have an apartment for his wife near her mother.

During the next 3 years (age 28–31) he studied law and had a year of clerkship but failed to pass the first bar examinations. He then got a civil engineering job. At the age of 34 he finally passed his bar examinations. Because of the lack of engineering projects, his term of service was ended and it became necessary for him to give up his apartment again and move into the home of his wife's family. When he was 35 years of age, a full term infant, a son, was born during his stay in his wife's family's home. He was embarrassed by the family's attitude toward him and their lack of appreciation of his values. During the next 4 years (age 35–39) there was very little financial success.

('Then there is a difference in religion. I don't care if they don't make an issue of it but they do. I am Protestant and they are Roman Catholic. I've always tried to help them, and at times it has not been appreciated.')

His tense, frustrated state continued and at the age of 39 while having his teeth repaired he became 'nervous' and at this time his gastrointestinal complaints returned in full intensity. Now, despite the fact that he was doing very well at his work his symptoms continued and became worse. Because of his unhappy domestic situation and because of his better financial state, he wished to re-establish his own home but his wife refused to leave her mother.

At the age of 40, during gastrointestinal discomfort, he developed hematemesis which brought him to the hospital. During his stay in the hospital he was very anxious and suspicious and was afraid that minor mistakes in his prescribed diet meant that the hospital was 'no good' and that the doctors were dangerous.

Personality. The patient was an intelligent, energetic, ambitious man, anxious to succeed and provide education and relative ease for his son. He was proud and self sufficient. He would do menial work rather than accept aid and always worked hard and persistently.

('I've always been rather aggressive and I've tried beyond my capacity to succeed. I have never been discharged but usually advanced. I've had responsibility and like it. I never shirk.')

He was athletic, fond of sports but always had to be a 'good player' or he preferred not to play. He got on well with his employers but needed their approval for peace of mind.

('Pain started while I was on risky work in tunnel construction. The chief engineers were not the right type, they didn't believe I was sick. They threatened to discharge me and that made me mad. That was the first time any man ever said anything critical about my work. I gave up this job and took inside work which was more congenial.')

He sought to be the center of attention in a group, was looked upon as a leader and lost no opportunity to speak in public. He was fond of reading and enjoyed music, especially opera. He liked to dance and enjoyed the company of the opposite sex. He was a suspicious person and excessively cautions about himself, however, and afraid of illness and sexual over-indulgence. His anxiety caused him to have frustrated sexual relations with his wife because of a desire to have her fondle his breasts. This he wouldn't allow because he felt it might be bad for him.

('For the last year or two we have had intercourse only once a month. I have weakness, tiredness and depressed feelings after the act. I think my wife wants it more. I would like to be able to satisfy her although she has never complained. I'm not in the mood, I thought it wasn't good for me, I was depressed. We used condoms as contraceptives (tired of vaginal diaphragms). Is there any detriment to the male to have the male breasts fondled by women? Men say it affects their nerves. I asked my wife to do it as an experiment; it brought on pleasant sensations but made me nervous. My wife likes fondling better than I. I can't discuss sex with her. She wanted me to go on fondling her breasts but I said too much was not good for her. Frequent intercourse makes a woman over-sexed and they demand it and injure the man. I have an erection twice a week, though intercourse is resisted because I thought too much was bad. I'm too much concerned with my physical condition. I'm too anxious to succeed and provide for my wife and college for my son. I would hate to have him go to night college like I did.'

'A man should have better understanding of women. My wife is too sympathetic, like Italians. She says she doesn't see how I can be so cool about things. My wife gets unduly alarmed. She is unduly sympathetic toward her immediate family. If they knew what goes on inside an Anglo-Saxon they'd know he suffers more. I'm sympathetic too. I see now I've been wrong in combating my wife.')

Onset and course of symptoms. It was during his first serious courtship at the age of 27 that the patient developed severe abdominal pains. These had their onset in association with the anxiety which was caused by the rumors of his fiancee's homosexuality.

('I had been engaged to a girl and it was a shock to me when I discovered she was homosexual. I couldn't speak to her about it. I did something beneath a man. I attempted natural intercourse and she resisted (I had had intercourse before but never with a virgin).

I accused her by implication and she said, 'Don't disgrace me'. But she was very shrewd. A person of that nature was repugnant then, not now. I was also fond of my future wife at the time. Mother would say the teacher (homosexual girl) was full of the devil. People who told me about her became repugnant to me too. I've learned since then there are many people of that nature. It is not in me to be of that nature. I was humiliated, the neighborhood thought I was that type.')

He thus felt accused of being a pervert for being fond of such a girl. His symptoms of epigastric burning and pain persisted in spite of breaking his engagement, although he promptly engaged himself to a girl whom he subsequently married.

A month after his marriage (age 28), his symptoms reached a peak when his wife deserted him to return to her mother. He continued to have symptoms for the next 5 years, culminating in the first hematemesis at the age of 33. During the next 6 years he felt well despite the fact that it was a period of great occupational and financial stress, which forced him to give up his home and move into his wife's family's dwelling. During this time, however, he passed his bar examination, and his child was born.

('I was married in 1925; the boy was born in 1931. He is a splendid specimen. He will choose his own religion. She and her family are influencing him. Our understanding was to give religious training at home until he is old enough to choose a church. I inwardly resent his going to their church. There would be a scene if I insisted he go to my church too. Neither my wife nor I are very religious. My wife's grandmother lives in the home and is highly religious.')

Six months before his admission to the hospital, aged 39, despite the fact that he was having more success at his work, there was an exacerbation of epigastric pain, nausea, and vomiting. This occurred during an attempt on his part to re-establish his own home. The attempt, however, was opposed by his wife. He desired to have his 'own home', where his wife could take care of him.

('My home life isn't what I'd like, I don't care to live with in-laws; I would prefer my own place.')

He felt isolated and ignored in her family home. In addition to epigastric pain and nausea he felt insecure, inadequate and resentful. Hematemesis caused his admission to the hospital, aged 40. A duodenal ulcer was visualized at this time.

Comment. This man's ulcer symptoms began at a time when his adequacy was challenged and were increased during periods of frustration induced by his wife's attitude toward him as shown by her insistence upon living with her family. His insecurity feelings began in childhood. He had persistent doubt concerning his adequacy as a male and conflict about accepting a passive relationship. Outstanding ambition was coupled with submissiveness and fear of self-assertion. He seldom had symptoms during periods of difficulty about work and finances nor even at the birth of his son. The outstanding emotional reactions associated with epigastric burning, pain and vomiting were anxiety and near panic at the implications of homosexuality in himself; greatly increased emotional insecurity and resentment at his wife's decision to live with her mother; doubts and misgivings as to whether, constituted as he was, he could keep his wife's emotional support; resentment at her family's failure to esteem him and his values.

To avoid repetitious description of many features and reactions the next three protocols are more briefly presented, especial emphasis being given to those facts that make them different from each other.

Case 2

A 32-year-old male laboratory technician was accustomed to unusual attention and affection from his parents. After the death of his father the first symptoms of epigastric burning and pain occurred. At this time he assumed an attitude of assertive independence. His attitude of self-sufficiency in his marriage prevented the satisfaction of his desire for attention and being cared for. His gastric symptoms grew progressively worse and 6 months after his marriage a pyloric ulcer with retention was diagnosed.

Personal history. The patient was a man of 32, born in Ireland, the oldest of 8 children. His father was a quiet, calm, affectionate man; his mother quick-tempered. Both showered affection upon the patient as a child. After pneumonia at the age of 8 he was considered 'sickly' for 7 years. He was coddled at home, received more attention than any of the other children and was punished less. He was kept out of school sports and became closely attached to his parents. He completed high school at the age of 17. After considerable conflict he left home at the age of 20 to come to the United States.

For the first 6 months after his arrival he had difficulty in finding work but then became a laboratory technician, which he has remained since with the same employer. Because of his ambition and good performance he was given a leave of absence and worked through two years of college. Despite repeated promises to himself and his parents he postponed a trip home to Ireland because of his opportunity to get college work. A few days after the completion of his work at the age of 27 he was notified of the sudden death of his father.

('Father died in 1933. I was not at home. It was a shock; I had lived to go back and see him; I'd promised to go home in 5 years [1933] but didn't because of a scholarship at school. Father told me to accept the scholarship and come home later. I was back at school a few days and heard of his death [September 1933].')

The patient was deeply disturbed and filled with a sense of guilt. He felt lost and alone, and his character changed so that he showed an exaggerated degree of independence amounting to aloofness and taciturnity. He began a courtship of a girl he had known for many years. Six months after his marriage he was admitted to the hospital. He entered marriage expecting to act the role of protector and good provider to the extent of refusing to allow his wife to do anything for him. To this pattern he adhered although he admitted his need of being loved and cared for.

Personality. The patient was an ambitious, yet shy, man who felt inferior in a group and made friends with difficulty but got along easily when acquainted.

('It's hard for me to approach people, I'm very shy. I get along after I've met a person if I know they are satisfied with my company. I'm always afraid they might be dissatisfied. In discussion groups I tend to feel inferior, especially with strangers. I work hard; I might accomplish as much with less energy, I rush around from one thing to another – nervous, always on the go – much pseudo-energy. I'm tired when I stop but o.k. when I'm going and am fatigued in the evening.')

He was over-anxious to please and exceedingly sensitive to criticism. He was politic and wished 'peace at any price'.

('The boss has never called me down, seems funny – hard to believe. I might feel better if he did. I know he's the kind who does call people down. I've heard him.')

Despite the fact that he was very angry when criticized he never showed it, and though obstinate as a child and adult he was also submissive under authority.

('I don't have much of a temper, only an inward feeling of temper, not shown. If I'm called down I get an awful inward feeling, depressed and scared. I never show anger.')

His independence evident even as a youth was more apparent after his father's death. It was known that he never allowed anyone 'to do anything' for him. He lent money freely but seldom borrowed because he felt uncomfortable until it was repaid. His wife complained that he wouldn't allow her to show the usual solicitude and attention. He confessed to a genuine desire for love and affection and that his assertive independence started after the death of his father when he felt he had no one to turn to.

Onset and course of symptoms. His epigastric discomfort, occurring some hours after meals and relieved by eating, began shortly after the death of his father when the patient was aged 27. He felt lonely, guilty and hungry for affection. He felt that no one any longer stood in back of him.

('I felt there was no one to turn to, felt left alone, a peculiar feeling. I became independent and wouldn't let anyone do anything for me, though I wanted it for the last year and a half. I have always tried to avoid accepting favors from a superior.')

He threw himself into an active courtship at about this time. He wanted to be married and assume the responsibilities of a wife and children. He feared these responsibilities, however. At age 30, 3 years after the onset of his inconstant discomfort, he became engaged. At this time he began to have gnawing pains in the epigastrium, sometimes with vomiting 2 to 3 h following meals, with no long periods of freedom from pain.

After marriage his symptoms continued, gfadually increasing in severity, especially the vomiting. The patient, because of pride, railed to allow his passive needs a proper outlet. He worked excessively long and hard, and lost 25 pounds in weight. X-ray of the stomach revealed pyloric ulcer and some retention.

Comment. This sensitive, insecure man, guilty over his neglect of his parents, resentful because of emotional dependence upon them, added to his anxiety by assuming the responsibilities of marriage. In order to maintain his self-esteem it was necessary for him to reject affection and to frustrate his own needs for dependence. His guilt and insecurity forced him to assume an attitude toward responsibility which cut him off from the affection he craved.

The patient's emotional insecurity arose in a childhood setting of personal illness with 'coddling' and discriminative attention and devotion. This imposed on the child his parents' anxieties and an awareness of his own inadequacy. This insecurity was augmented by the attitude of the other children in the family who showed their hostility toward him. His need to overcome his feeling of dependence on his parents, notably on his father, caused him to state assertively his independence. He developed an aloof manner in an attempt to achieve this detachment, fearing always that he would become dependent if he allowed himself to grow fond of anyone. After his father's death he felt guilty because of his long stay away from home and was also frightened at 'being alone'. These reactions resulted in a reaffirmation of his purpose to be independent and protect himself against a repetition of such personal injury through close emotional ties. His marriage was a compromise in which he hoped to gain devotion from his wife without jeopardizing his desired emotional self-sufficiency. This failed, however, because he needed more affection than he could accept. Resentment and hostility arose from the fact that he was caught in these circumstances of needing and desiring affection on the one hand, and of fearing to accept it on the other.

A frankly dependent woman with peptic ulcer, described in the next protocol, was selected because she demonstrated frustrated 'need of being cared for', uncomplicated by compensatory efforts of assertive independence or self-sufficiency.

Case 3

A child-like dependent woman of 37 failed to get the attention, devotion and security she demanded of her marriage. Epigastric burning occurred soon after she married. The symptoms disappeared while she lived at home with her parents, separated from her husband, but recurred with increasing severity when she returned to live with him and resumed the responsibilities of her own home. Gastric hemorrhage occurred after a period of quarreling and expressed disapproval by her husband.

Personal history. The patient was a 37-year-old married woman, born in Austria, the older of 2 daughters. In childhood she exhibited jealousy of her younger sister, fought with her and showed by her behaviour an excessive need for her mother's attention and devotion. She sulked at home and misbehaved at school in order to get it. From the age of 4 to 6 she lived with her grandparents while her parents were in the United States, and again from 10 to 20 her home was with or near her grandparents. She completed 6 years of schooling at the age of 13 and was then put to work in a nearby city as a chambermaid.

She came to the United States at the age of 22, found work as a domestic for a year, and then married and gave up her former work. She had no deep affection for her husband whom she married with the aim of gaining financial security. This attitude toward her husband was associated with her sexual frigidity. Despite the latter, sexual relations were frequent. At the age of 24 a son was born. At the age of 31 she returned to Austria for a visit to her parents. A year later she returned to America to her husband.

Personality. The patient was a simple, childlike, dependent woman, who clearly expressed her desire to be cared for and had no hesitancy in demanding attention. She was sulky when her demands were thwarted. She bore resentments for long periods and had few friends.

('I have no friends, I work all day. I was popular and friendly as a young girl.')

Onset and course of symptoms. Soon after her marriage at age 23 she began to complain of epigastric burning and she was never really well thereafter. Her marriage had failed to give her the devotion and security she expected. Her frustration resulted from her husband's precarious financial situation and because he considered that his wife's duty was to attend him and satisfy him sexually. Her epigastric burning and pain increased after the birth of her first baby. She resented her augmented responsibility, the care and devotion required by the infant, and the attention which her husband showered upon the child. When she complained or stated her inability her husband called her lazy and disciplined her by pushing her into work.

('Lately I was so excited, especially the day before yesterday. My husband makes me mad. He teases me, and says I don't do anything about the house. He says I'm lazy. The day before, I was so mad I could go through my husband's neck. He was home with a boil. He said I looked out the window all day and didn't work. He won't help, he says I'll be more lazy. He's not handy at home. He won't allow my boys to help me. He tells them not to be sissies. He refused to let me have a doctor when I fainted. He just said he had to work for the money the doctor would get. He said I'd be all right in the morning.')

All symptoms disappeared during the period she lived in Austria and enjoyed again the warmth and security of her parents' home. Her symptoms recurred with full intensity shortly after her return to this country, aged 32, and the resumption of her domestic duties and responsibilities. Her husband's irritability and disapproval increased. She was admitted to the hospital after passing a large tarry stool.

Comment. This woman married with the hope of gaining emotional and financial security without giving emotional support in return. Her husband failed to give her either of these and in addition criticized her constantly. She developed gastric ulcer during a period of frustration and resentment induced by the attitude of her husband and the increased responsibilities associated with having children. The predominant emotions of this frustrated woman were resentment, insecurity and fear.

Case 4

Epigastric burning and pain developed in a man when his wife neglected him and falsely accused him of 'drinking' and non-support. When she exhibited affection for him his symptoms left, but when she again neglected him his symptoms grew progressively worse, despite adequate diet and financial security. He deserted her with the hope that she would seek his return and this she refused to do. Duodenal ulcer developed after the failure of his plan to regain her affection.

Personal history. The patient was a 56-year-old married man, the sixth of eight children of Irish parents. He attended parochial elementary school until the age of 14. He was devoted to his mother and was greatly distressed over her death when he was 13 years old. At this time he began to 'play truant' from school, and at 14 was put to work by his father as a plumber's helper. He joined an electrical company which continued to employ him at the time of admission. For the first 26 years of this term of service he worked 'outside' and then was given a 'made job in the office'. His father, a policeman, died when the patient was 21, thus saving the patient from being forced against his will to enter the police service.

At the age of 24 he married an attractive, vivacious Irish girl. They had 6 children of whom 5 survived. His wife also had a few miscarriages and several stillbirths. After the death of his second child in infancy the patient, at that time 31 years of age, noticed a change in his wife's attitude toward him. She began to resent his sexual advances and urged him to find satisfaction elsewhere. This he refused to do.

('She never complained about money – she was well provided for. She refused sex relations for 15 years, absolutely in the past 8 years. She says she was a beast long enough. She began to sleep with her daughter. All her life she was that type, even when she was young. She said if I wanted that kind of stuff to go get it. It seemed that started after Bill was born. She had had a couple of miscarriages; then Bill died; she seemed to change.')

When the patient was 48 years old his wife's personality seriously altered in association with her menopause. She became irritable, depressed, refused all sexual relations and had notions of being persecuted. She accused her husband of drunkenness, lack of support, cruelty to the children, and refused to attend to his wants.

The patient's gastric complaints began at this time. With the exception of a short period her attitude persisted, and 5 years later, at the age of 53, on the advice of friends he decided to frighten his wife by leaving her, believing she would be shocked into better behaviour and beg him to return.

('My wife criticized me, tells friends that I go home drunk, that the children fear me, that I give no money. Women looked at me when I went down the street. That's no illusion. Friends told me it was her change of life; it lasted 10 years. She's my age, 56. I'm

fond of her yet, she's a good mother and brought up my children. She told me that I was a big bum, and said nothing good about me. Then I'd get mad. There was the devil to pay when my income was cut.')

However, his departure from home failed to have the desired effect. Rather than changing her attitude it caused her to become adamant and she never asked him to come back. Moreover, she succeeded in convincing many of his friends and acquaintances of his unworthiness. His stomach complaints, which had been present for 5 years, became much worse at this time.

('For the children's sake I kept out of court and promised my wife $ 25 to $ 30 a week. If the court decided to put her away I wouldn't want to. She told her friend I was trying to put her away when I suggested she rest with her sister. That was 5 years ago. That was after the ulcer started. It gets me when I see people with homes and children – I cry, I don't know where to live. Not with my sister, I don't like her husband.')

Personality. The patient was of average intelligence and was energetic and talkative. He radiated the impression of great independence and self-sufficiency. He liked the feeling of 'running things' and worked by getting 'inside information' and 'pulling wires'. He was quicktempered and suspicious, but made friends easily and enjoyed people. He liked to bestow favors and was generous with money. Until his separation from his wife he gave her all of his salary to use for the family. He worked conscientiously and persistently. By indirection, he usually succeeded in showing his desire for attention. He resented his wife's failure to look after him and to take his ulcer symptoms seriously enough to cook the proper food for him. While under observation in the hospital he talked a good deal of wanting to be no trouble, but complained repeatedly of nursing procedures and actually maneuvered the situation so as to receive more attention than the other patients.

Onset and course of symptoms. The patient's epigastric pain after meals had its onset at the age of 48, shortly after his wife, in her disturbed state associated with the menopause, expressed her dislike for him and falsely accused him of alcoholism and other irregularities. Her disapproval of him and her refusal to take care of him continued. Two years later the diagnosis of ulcer was made. At this time, when his wife was informed of the diagnosis, she expressed anxiety about the patient and showed interest and affection. Under these circumstances his symptoms cleared up quickly.

He continued to do well during this period of her changed attitude and while she prepared special food for him. However, as soon as she lost interest and grew weary of preparing a special diet and again resumed her critical attitude, asserting that there was really nothing wrong with him, the symptoms returned.

After the age of 53, at which time he left his wife and was grievously disappointed that she did not seek his return, his epigastric pain grew progressively worse and he vomited despite the fact that he had the proper food according to the dietitian's list. He also had pain that awakened him from sleep.

('I was married at 24 and had known my wife 4 or 5 years. She was full of the devil, carrying on and very active. She was wonderful at first and we were happy until 7 or 8 years ago (1930). She got cranky and peevish, gradually we got quarreling. At first I tried to talk her out of it. Then I was so bitter I couldn't. I knew something would happen. A doctor friend advised me to throw a scare into her. I left but don't know if it was wise. I walked out, I thought she would make up, the family would patch it up but no one did. She says I walked out and if I wanted to I'd walk back. I can't do that. She has told the neighbors terrible things about me. She said I abused the children and refused to support her. I got ashamed to meet the people. I didn't know what she said. She has been a terrible liar for the last 8 years. She would tell people I was drunk when I hadn't even been out of the house.')

When he was visited by his sons his complaints diminished. At that time he felt well and had no pain, but shortly after their departure and the resumption of his lonely state his symptoms recurred. The sons remained loyal to their mother and made their home with her.

Because of intolerable epigastric pain the patient was admitted to the hospital where a duodenal ulcer was visualized by X-ray. While in the hospital under observation, although he asserted his self-sufficiency, his ability to take care of himself and his desire to help others in almost a boastful manner, yet he managed by complaining to receive more attention than other patients and had symptoms whenever he felt neglected.

Comment. The patient's personality difficulty became apparent at the age of 13 shortly after the death of his mother. This expressed itself as a defiant independence, in part a reaction to the deprivation of his mother's affection and in part in response to the domination by his father. His 'independence', however, was a superficial manifestation covering an underlying unacknowledged need for approval and affection. His wife never gave him much emotional support or attention except at times during his illness. His outspoken complaints and demands for attention were for the most part frustrated at home and only partly appeared in the hospital. His dominant emotions during his hospital stay were loss of self-esteem because of the accusations of his wife, resentment at her indifference to his illness, and feelings of helplessness at being deserted and alone, and because he had 'lost everything'.

General Comment

The personality features of these patients were variable and the incidents precipitating the emotional reactions numerous. However, the reactions of anxiety, insecurity, resentment, guilt and frustration obtained in all. Also, compensating efforts to bolster the self-esteem by assertions of independence, self-sufficiency and perfectionism were common. It was evident from the time of onset of the personality disturbances that the ulcer itself was not responsible for the major emotional conflicts or the reactions.

In this series of patients males predominated as is usual with patients with ulcer in contemporary western society. All these men had the conviction that the successful man must be the dominant figure as compared with women, must be more independent, more responsible; must be the aggressor in social and sexual relations, the more highly competitive, possessive and initiating member of the group.

Some interpretation of these values and their relevance to the problem is called for. It is safe to assume that the culturally linked masculine demands for achievement, strength, and the shouldering of responsibility did not start in the individual in his adulthood. In fact, these demands reached the child as an environmental attitude as soon as he became aware of the concepts of man-woman, father-mother, and probably long before the knowledge of genital difference. The so-called female characteristics – receptivity, passivity and dependence, were considered by the male patients as evidence of weakness and were unacceptable. These men, as DRAPER and TOURAINE [28] also pointed out felt inadequate unless they made a show of possessing the socially male-linked qualities mentioned above, whether or not they did possess them. When the drive in these directions was not strong or was associated with conflict, their subsequent feelings of distress, inadequacy or failure resulted in attitudes of resentment and defeat.

On the other hand, attempts to gain security through 'success' in competitive effort were avidly pursued by many of the male patients. FRANK [30] points out that the individual who in early life is emotionally insecure and is goaded by an inner feeling of inadequacy or guilt finds in the competitive game a release for these tensions and a further stimulus to increased tension.

Hence, technological changes, increased speed of production, accelerated tempo of communication and transportation and the pressure of competitive effort necessarily played a part in the work life of these patients. As mentioned above, several patients attempted to resolve their emotional insecurity through extra effort, longer hours, more persistent application and by creating about them an atmosphere of 'busy-ness', pressure, and hard work. Indeed, this manner of solving personal problems fitted well into the industrial competitive pattern in which they found themselves. However, in all instances the pressure truly came from within rather than from without. These men tried to glean from work a security which success in work alone cannot give.

In ALEXANDER'S [2] formulation of the problem of his patients with peptic ulcer he indicated that these individuals had wishes of a receptive nature, such as the wish to be loved, to be fed, to be helped and taken care of by others, as in the child-mother relationship. In many of our patients attempts were made to gain emotional security by establishing such a relation of dependency. In others a threat to emotional support was very important. Furthermore, awareness of these unacceptable wishes often injured the pride and self-esteem of these adults. The difficult interpersonal relations that stemmed from such conflict ended in frustration of these important needs, and invariably produced anxiety, resentment and guilt.

Although this male pattern of assertive independence observed so commonly in the attitudes of these patients permitted of no leaning or asking for emotional support, there is a means which affords such dependence and which these patients frequently grasped. Contemporary western society has set a value upon the care of the sick and justifies complaint, dependence and retirement with illness or pain. Hence, the assertively independent man who in health denied himself the emotional support which his wife could give did, nevertheless, feel free to demand her attention for his digestive complaints. Special foods, diets, and eating times were his due. The stay in the hospital, the prescribed regime of milk, cream and powders given with pedantic regularity lent emotional support compatible with assertive independence because of the social sanction given to being cared for when sick. Thus the complaint gained for the individual the support which the dependent male is allowed in a society where assertive independence is of the highest value.

The steps in the development of resentment and hostility from initial feelings of insecurity and anxiety in several instances were as follows. The insecure and anxious individual gained a degree of assurance by evolving a life pattern of being self-sufficient, independent, or the 'lone wolf', or on the other hand by gaining approval through extra effort, conscientiousness, 'perfectionism', and meticulousness. Under the usual circumstances of his life, such a system seemed adequate, i.e., the individual was relatively comfortable and effective. Then, because of a change in his situation such as a new position, the assumption of new responsibilities in courtship, or marriage, criticism from without was implied or expressed and this again challenged his adequacy. Feelings of insecurity and anxiety were then experienced. One reaction to this challenge was to increase efforts by more work, greater conscientiousness and 'perfectionism'. Another reaction was seen in the bolstering of self-esteem through additional assertions of independence and the shutting off of much needed affection. There developed frustration, resentment and hostility directed toward the person or situation which re-aroused the feelings of insecurity and inadequacy, causing his fragile system to falter or break down.

In short, the patient had evolved an almost adequate pattern for dealing with anxiety and then, through some life incident, was thrown into a disorganized anxious state to which he reacted with hostility. His hostile attitudes toward those whom he wanted to love and the community of which he wished to be a part gave rise in turn to feelings of guilt, remorse and self-condemnation. Coincident with these reactions there occurred epigastric burning, pain, vomiting and hemorrhage.

To infer that all persons with gastritis, duodenitis or peptic ulcer will be found to have special personality features and reactions is unjustified. It is equally unjustified to infer that all persons having such personality features and reactions must have gastroduodenal lesions. However, since these subjects were unselected, they form in all likelihood a representative group of persons with gastritis, duodenitis, and peptic ulcer.

B. Sex Incidence of Peptic Ulcer

The above case notes indicate the importance of threats to self-esteem and emotional security in patients with peptic ulcer. Self-esteem and emotional security are deeply influenced by the relations of men to women. Important changes in this relationship during the last 50 years coincide with a dramatic shift in the sex incidence of peptic ulcer.

A review of the incidence of perforated ulcer at the New York Hospital from 1880 to 1900 revealed that women had perforated ulcer at least as commonly as men, i.e., 6:7. All perforations in these patients were visualized either at operation or autopsy (all autopsies from 1880–1891). Beginning in the period of 1901 through 1906 the ratio of males to females changed. The following figures were found for the years 1901–1939:

	Males	Females	Ratio
1901–1906 (5 years)	10	4	2 ½ :1
1907–1914 (7 years)	55	9	6:1
1915–1930 (15 years)[2]	260	16	16:1
1932–1939 (8 years)	36	3	12:1

JENNINGS [54] investigated the age incidence and sex distribution of a large series of patients with peptic ulcers in the last 150 years and obtained similar ratios. The lesions were not visualized in all instances but the evidence for the diagnosis seemed convincing. Between 1850 and 1900 of every 6 patients with peptic ulcers perforated into the peritoneal cavity 3 were young women under 25, 1 an elderly woman, 1 an elderly man, and 1 a young man. Since 1920 of every 10 perforations 1 has occurred in an elderly woman and 9 have occurred in men, mostly in the middle years or younger. Thus, perforations in young women increased rapidly in the beginning of the 19th century and died out completely and suddenly at the beginning of the 20th. According to JENNINGS, the same changes have taken place in Germany, France,

2 Records incomplete for 1931.

Scandinavia and the English-speaking countries. Uncomplicated ulcers probably fall into the same category as perforated ulcers. A careful collection of statistics further illustrating these points has been compiled by ALSTED [3].

Whether or not there has been an absolute increase in peptic ulcer in relation to the total population is irrelevant to the fact that during the last half century peptic ulcer has become principally a male disorder. Let us return to a consideration of some important factors in the shifting sex relations. Of outstanding significance to our problem is the change in women's attitude toward men. Entirely unpremediated changes in our social pattern have been precipitated by the introduction of cheap electrical, oil, gas, and other energy stores; by making available easy transportation and communication; by the mass production of food and domestic goods [74]. The ensuing changes in women's social status have resulted for the most part fortuitously in a challenge to the male position of dominance which was taken for granted in the 19th century.

Formerly, prestige for women was gained only through affiliation with men and especially through marriage. Indeed, if a woman were not married by her early twenties her position was exceedingly difficult. Her period of maximum striving and competitive effort occurred between ages 17 and 27. If by this time she had not achieved her goal, marriage, she became a subservient figure in the household of her brother's wife or in some other relative's home. The set pattern for female behaviour aroused conflict by denying all overt expression of this competitive effort. A woman could express no hatred or jealousy of her rivals; hostility in all forms was taboo; 'sweetness', tears, giggling, 'vapors', and fainting were her only acceptable emotional outlets. Yet within this narrow frame and within a short period of time she had to win 'success' for her life, that is, a man. Men thus possessed the power to bestow prestige or to withold it.

A man was expected to be 'master' in his household, yet within this pattern of male dominance men were permitted emotional dependence upon their women. Under the cover of his dominant position a man could give free expression to his emotional needs. His idiosyncrasies were indulged and his pecadillos tolerated.

With the gradual change in domestic relationships, however, emotional dependence for a man has become more and more difficult, his freedom limited and his unquestioned privileges curtailed. In subtle ways, as well as in obvious ones, the relations of the sexes within the domestic pattern have shifted. Though women retain their role of management of the home and the disposition of funds, the responsibility for the conduct of the institution usually rests lightly in their hands. Environmental changes have swept away many of women's duties, and ambivalence on their part toward their remaining opportunities for responsibility has become a factor in the changed domestic relationship. Also, women now compete with men at 'work' but they do not wish their financial contributions to be 'counted upon', since there is social justification for the feeling that in giving themselves in marriage and in 'running the household' they have already made an adequate contribution. A woman may become the important financial contributor to the home, in which case she often unwittingly creates in her partner a conviction of inadequacy. If she fails in an occupational venture she is justified by society in retiring and being provided for by her husband, brother or father, while such security for a man has no social approval. If a man fails to 'provide' he may be denied the feeling of security which his wife's emotional support could give him. Her humiliation of him under these circumstances is endorsed by cultural sanctions. Thus, while society's requirements of the male are essentially as stringent as before, the emotional support accorded him in return is less.

Although these changes in the status of

women are presented from the point of view of their effects on men it is obvious that discontent, restlessness and idleness have created for most women serious problems which bring with them their own train of disorders. To be excluded are those few women who find in the creative activity of art, science, or industry a suitable way of life and those, on the other hand, whose energy and equipment are just adequate to the limited requirements of the contemporaneous home. But the vast majority of American women are confronted with an imposed task in the management of the home which does not challenge their energies or equipment, and leaves them frustrated, dissatisfied, fault-finding and resentful.

However, a great difference as regards the effects of such emotional states on men and women is that the latter are allowed free emotional expression as seen in tears, tantrums, and idleness – outlets which the standards of male behaviour and the discipline of the workaday world deny the men. Moreover, besides free expression and emotional catharsis, women have the sanction of society for their unpredictability. Also they appreciate that their dissatisfactions are widespread and shared by most of their sex. Their hostile and destructive moods are thus near the surface and freely released. On the other hand, men may not express their complaints, admit weakness or lean for support on other men except when ill. They cannot find support on the shifting emotional sands of women. Hence, it is for the men that harbored hostility, resentment, guilt and anxiety are so especially costly. In short, these changes in women are so destructive in their effects on emotionally insecure men because they create for them an emotional background of challenge, irresponsibility, and unpredictability.

Coupled with these changes in interpersonal relations between the sexes is an alteration in the world state which makes it no longer possible for a man to feel that if things go badly in his home environment there are still the colonies or the frontier where he may start anew and assert his prowess. In the formulation of the 19th century American male, 'life was a turbulent stream as it flowed at his feet, abundantly laden with the rich salvage of many great treasure ships. To dive in, and swim and buffet and fight for the prize; to regain the shore for breath and rest exhausted and bruised in the struggle; to dive in again, and again grasp at what floated past; and again and again until he secured his share of the booty and drew it safe ashore – that to him and his period was success and the way it was achieved' [73]. The beginning of the 20th century saw the passing of this conception and a growing conviction that there was a paucity of opportunities.

A man's conviction of being hemmed in or of being cornered has been fostered by other features of the 20th century world; thus, the substitution of machines for skilled hand labor with less opportunity for personal creative effort; the increasing struggle for existence of the small *entrepreneur;* the decline of individual free choice in occupation with increasing industrial organization; the increasing size of industrial units with impersonalization of relations between employer and employee; the increasing belief that public acclaim is the only criterion of achievement and that this results from 'lucky breaks' rather than ability and effort.

In brief, with the social changes that have occurred during the present century, men have been confronted with decreasing opportunities for emotional support and for overt emotional expression, yet their responsibilities have remained, and the threats to their self-esteem have increased. These changes assume special significance to emotionally insecure men, such as our patients, who are preoccupied with self-esteem, perfectionism, and conflict concerning emotional dependency. Women, on the other hand, though in conflict, have social sanction for free emotional expression and for attitudes of both dependence and independence.

Since resentment, hostility, frustration, anxiety, and guilt are important in the natural history of peptic ulcer, the shift of peptic ulcer from females to males may be understood.

same way on all subjects. A total of 165 observations was made: 89 on those with duodenal ulcer, 4 on the one with gastric ulcer, 12 on those with gastroduodenitis, and 60 on the 'normals'.

II. Experimentally Induced Emotional and Gastroduodenal Changes

If the above described emotional states are relevant to gastroduodenal dysfunction and peptic ulcer in the particular persons described, situations which experimentally or otherwise induce these states should at the same time elicit gastroduodenal dysfunction and symptoms. Moreover, if there be symptoms and defects already existent, they should be increased in severity. On the other hand, situations which engender security and contentment should restore normal function and eliminate symptoms in those with symptoms and abnormal function.

With the knowledge, then, of the emotions dominant in each of these patients and some of the factors responsible for their being, attempts were made to induce in the laboratory emotional and gastroduodenal changes like those resulting from the individual's experiences in his workaday world. The following analysis of gastrointestinal function is based on the data so assembled.

Subjects

Gastric secretion, or gastric secretion and motility together were studied in 26 subjects. Nine of these had ulcer of the duodenum, one a gastric ulcer, and three, gastroduodenitis. All diagnoses were verified either by surgical or X-ray visualization. The remaining 13 subjects were 'normal': that is, they had no pathological condition of, or complaints referable to, any part of the gastrointestinal tract. Instrumentation and the study of the emotional states were carried out in the

Method of Investigation

The subjects arrived for the observation in the morning after a fast of at least 12 h. When gastric secretion alone was to be recorded, one rubber catheter was introduced into the stomach through the nose, causing relatively little discomfort. To obtain records of both secretion and motility, 2 tubes were introduced. Three and one half inches of condom rubber to act as a balloon were attached above the openings of one tube, which was passed first. This was followed by the free tube either through the same or through the opposite nostril. Curling of the tube in the stomach was obviated by having the subject lie on his right side as soon as the tip of each tube reached the cardia. By fluoroscopy it was seen when the ends of both tubes reached the pyloric antrum of the stomach without curling backwards. The subject then lay on his back on a comfortable table and was urged to relax. A pneumograph apparatus was fastened about the chest and a radiometer placed near the fingers of the left hand so that skin temperature could be recorded.

After both tubes were in the stomach the balloon was inflated with air to 100 mm water pressure and connected by rubber tubing to a U-tube water manometer, which contained a writing point supported on a floating cork. Increases of pressure on the air within the balloon caused by contractions of the stomach caused the water column of the manometer to raise the writing point, which was placed against a moving kymograph. Thus, the upstrokes on the records represent gastric contractions, and the downstrokes, relaxation. The effect of respiration on the stomach is represented by the smallest fluctuations superimposed on the gastric motility. A simultaneous tracing was made of the movements of the chest wall by means of the pneumograph attached to a similar manometer system. A time marker recorded the minutes. The gastric secretion was withdrawn throughout the observation by continuous suction with a 50 ml syringe through the free tube, samples being segregated at 5 or 10-min intervals. In one of the normals who had no free HCl on fasting, secretion was stimulated by the introduction of beef broth or coffee into the stomach. Finger temperature readings were made every 1 to 5 min [65]; room temperature was maintained between 21° and 25°C.

After 1 ½ to 2 h the period of observation was terminated. The volume of each specimen was measured, the amount of visible and separable mucous noted, and the amount of bile, if present, was estimated by the intensity of its color. The free HCl and total acidity were ascertained by titration with N/10 NaOH using Toepfer's solution and phenolphthalein, respectively, as indicators. Pepsin determinations were made by the Mett method. Two glass tubes of 2 mm internal diameter, open at both ends and containing coagulated egg albumin, were placed in 1 ml samples of the gastric juice with 15 ml of 0.05 N HCl, and incubated at 37°C for 24 h. The peptic power is expressed as the square of the average number of millimeters of albumin digested at the four ends of the two tubes. Normal gastric juice digests from 2 to 4 mm, corresponds to a peptic power of 4 to 16 'units' [42]. Occult blood was detected by the benzidine method, and because of the frequent positive results in all subjects, was considered to be caused by trauma from intubation or suction [83]. Gross bloody discoloration of the gastric juice and the presence of clots were found under special experimental circumstances in some of the patients with peptic ulcer and were regarded as hemorrhage resulting from these procedures.

Observations on Emotional States

In preliminary 'control' experiments, the subjects were urged to remain as relaxed as possible for 1 ½–2 h. They were not always able to feel secure and comfortable, however, because of anxious anticipation or annoyance over the novelty of the experimental situation or anxiety and tension over personal problems. By explanation and reassurance a period of relative well-being was usually established. In subsequent experiments, after a shorter period of relative relaxation, the subject was interviewed about emotionally charged life situations gleaned from the previous personality study. The interviews were of two varieties. The first aimed at arousing in the subject the emotional reactions he displayed in his experiences outside the laboratory, in order to ascertain the gastroduodenal variations that accompanied such states. The second type had the opposite effect, and eliminated preexistent stress, with the result that gastroduodenal alterations were reversed toward the normal. The behaviour of the subject and changes in the quality of his voice were observed during interviews. Stenographic notes were taken of his utterances. Characteristic poignant phrases indicating the core of the interviews have been included in the protocols. The presence of the author, M.S., making such notes, apparently had no untoward effect on the subjects, since they had become accustomed from the beginning of the experiments to her presence. Note was also made of the subject's statement as to his mood and 'feelings'. In short, the stimulus used experimentally to induce stress was gleaned from a formulation of the individual's method of maintaining his emotional security. This was based on an appraisal of biographic data, personality features and an analysis of the situations outside of the laboratory which had been associated with symptoms. From such a formulation a method of challenging or undermining the individual's security was devised and introduced. A brief statement of such dynamic data for each individual is presented with the protocols. Thus the subject during the experiments passed through three phases: (1) Reaction to a new and unpleasant laboratory situation. (2) Adjustment to this situation with indifference to its novelty. (3) Accentuation of already existent emotional states of different degrees of intensity by interviews focussed upon the factors that most predictably shook the subject's emotional security. Also, in some instances the individual's security was augmented by means of the information gleaned from his personality study.

When all observations on the subject were completed, the records obtained during relaxation were compared with those obtained during induced or existent affective stress. Thus, experiments with and without interviews were utilized to interpret the changes in gastric function that occurred during emotional states.

Results

Acidity in 'Normals' and Patients with Peptic Ulcer, Gastritis, or Duodenitis

The level of free HCl in experiments on persons in a relatively relaxed and contented state varied considerably from one individual to the next both in normals and among patients with peptic ulcer or gastritis. No 'fasting' free HCl was found in any observation in one half our 'normal' patients. Among the other half there was found sufficient acid to neutralize up to 92 ml N/10 NaOH. In these individuals, however, values from 80 to 92 associated with anxiety and resentment.

Patients with gastritis, duodenitis or peptic ulcer had free HCl in almost all of the observations. In these patients values over 100 were also associated with induced or already existent anxiety, resentment and guilt. Relative relaxation in this group was associated with levels of free HCl below

100 (values between 20 and 80). A few, however, in whom free HCl values were consistently as low as 0–40 during relaxation, had free HCl values from 40–100 during anxiety, resentment and guilt.

Comment. Hyperacidity (values most frequently over 100) and hypersecretion have been observed in peptic ulcer or gastritis patients [13, 23, 39, 46, 70] while 'normal' acidity levels are reported by many to be below 100 [14, 24, 45, 93].

Peristalsis in 'Normals' and in Patients with Peptic Ulcer or Gastritis

The peristalsis during phases of relative contentment both among normals and among patients with gastritis or peptic ulcer was commonly found to be quiescent or to be evident usually in periods of 15–30 minutes' duration. 'Quiescence' is the term used to describe periods when contractions were at a minimum in amplitude (1 cm or less on the kymographic records). Contractions of high amplitude (6–12 cm on the records) each of approximately one minute's duration (or less) ('hunger contractions') [16, 20, 21, 79, 80] were followed by longer periods of quiescence. The time of occurrence, frequency, duration and amplitude of such periods of contractions varied from one subject to another. Peristalsis for some period and of minor intensity was never absent in any subject. Contractions of all amplitudes commonly occurred at an average rate of 1 per min.

Acidity and Motility Patterns

In many subjects during periods of relaxation both the motility and acid secretion were fairly stable from day to day. In others, however, the phenomena varied. Either there was no period of active peristalsis observed or its duration and the time of its occurrence varied. At times physiological fluctuations occurred that seemingly had no emotional accompaniments. Their significance remained obscure.

Interviews were started when the same initial physiological phenomena were observed during the short control period as occurred during the longer preliminary experiments without interviews. On such a base line the effects of various experiences were recorded.

The characteristic changes in physiological function during the affective states of resentment, anxiety, guilt, and frustration were an increase in free HCl secretion and a change in peristalsis from periodic to continuous activity of considerable magnitude. These changes were found to be similar in nature in patients with peptic ulcer, gastritis, or duodenitis on the one hand, and in half of the normals, on the other. Increase in acidity during anger, anxiety and guilt, and frustration was not always accompanied by a simultaneous increase in peristaltic activity. When there were physiological changes they were sometimes more evident in one function than in the other. The difference in reaction between the normal subjects who responded to these pernicious emotions[3] with increased acidity and peristaltic activity and the pathological group was one of degree. Among the patients with gastritis, duodenitis or peptic ulcer the changes were usually of greater intensity and duration.

In one-half [6] of the normal subjects no free HCl was present after fasting, or even after the stimulation of beef broth injected into the stomach, either during relaxation or during situations which were designed to induce a variety of affective states. It is possible that in these individulas there was an actual inhibition of HCl secretion due to the stress of the experimental situation. All secreted HCl after histamine injection. It was unclear what the dominant affective state was in these subjects, and whether the experimentors were able to create situations which actually induced anger, anxiety, guilt and frustration. Hence, whether there are individuals who have no appreciable stomach reactions in association with these

emotions, or whether they never existed, cannot be answered now. The study of affective states associated with such hypoacidity, with and without complaints, is the subject of investigations now being pursued, and will receive no further consideration in this presentation.

The finger temperature fell in about two-thirds of the subjects in whom there were induced emotional changes associated with increased secretion and heightened peristaltic activity. In most instances the fall was slight, from 1° to 3°C, but in a few it was as much as 9° below the finger temperature level recorded during relaxation and security. Also, some of the controls who had free HCl during relaxation or induced anxiety, anger, guilt, and frustration, had major falls in finger temperature. Some subjects with major alterations in gastric function during induced stress and subsequent sleep, had drops in finger temperature during distressing interviews, but these were not sustained during sleep. On the other hand, a drop in finger temperature was observed during an interview which induced relaxation, feelings of security and a decrease in gastric acidity and peristaltic activity.

In short, falls in finger temperature often occurred with increased acidity and motility in patients with gastritis, duodenitis, and peptic ulcer as an accompaniment of anger, guilt, frustration, and anxiety. However, these changes in peripheral circulation seldom approached in magnitude the changes in gastroduodenal function. Occasionally, cold hands persisted as stomach function returned to normal, or hands warmed up as heightened acidity and motility function persisted. Thus, though falls in finger temperature were common, they did not always follow closely changes in gastroduodenal function.

In the following detailed reports illustrative experiments and pertinent personality features of the subjects are given.

[3] Pernicious, because they always give rise to conflict.

Results on patients with duodenitis, gastritis, and those with peptic ulcer are presented with the results obtained in the experiments on normal subjects*.

III. Interpretation

In patients with peptic ulcer, evidence of long standing and severe anxiety, hostility, resentment, guilt, and frustration, has been adduced, and shown to be relevant to the presence and aggravation of peptic ulcer. Furthermore, it has been shown that certain situations that induce or accentuate these destructive emotions also induce in the stomach increased acidity, increased secretion, increased peristaltic activity, and increased blood flow. Under these circumstances symptoms may be induced or accentuated, and there may be evidence of tissue damage.

How may these functional changes in the stomach be interpreted? Since they so closely resemble the changes that occur with the smell or sight of food, may they not have the same physiological significance – namely preparation for eating? [75, 100a].

That there is a long standing awareness of the link between eating and certain emotions is shown by the derivation of common English words denoting feeling, for instance: fret, A.S., to eat, to devour; disgust, L. to taste badly; remorse, L., to gnaw; bitterness, A.S., to bite; nag, A.S. to gnaw; rancor, L. to be rancid. The word stomach has had numerous meanings such as inclination, liking; anger, violence of temper; sullenness, resentment, obstinacy; pride, haughtiness. As a verb stomach has meant, to bear without open resentment; as an adjective, filled with resentment. In Chinese the word *Ch'ih* meaning to eat, is included in compound words meaning to suffer distress, to suffer loss, to be startled, to be jealous, to stand the strain, to find a situation unendurable.

The subsequent comments aim to present a concept by which this linking of the

stomach and emotions may be interpreted, and to indicate by what mechanisms the linking may be effected.

Neural Mechanisms and Emotional States

CANNON [17, 18] studied the bodily changes during a crisis situation using the cat as a model. When held before a dog in such a manner as to prevent injury or flight, the changes noted in the cat were as follows: The animal stood on extended legs, head high, teeth exposed, back arched, and tail erect and bushy. The blood pressure was elevated, and the pulse rate and pad sweating were increased. There was increased force of skeletal muscle contraction, increased adrenalin output, and a raised level of blood sugar. Gastric motility decreased often after initial vomiting, associated with hypoacidity and hyposecretion. Peristaltic activity in the small intestine also stopped.

CANNON suggested that the sympathetic division of the autonomic nervous system dominated in this state and acted to mobilize stored energy to serve the animal during an emergency. Its muscles and circulation prepared for fight or flight, rid of gastrointestinal encumbrances, and ending digestive activity, the organism seemed to be focussed upon a desperate effort to save its life.

Monkeys who were threatened with sticks, black rubber hose and a monkey-catching net, presented many similar aspects of sympathetic activity but there was also parasympathetic activity, as indicated by contracture of denervate skeletal muscle [9].

In earlier studies of emotional expression DARWIN [26] described a cat in a state similar to that investigated by CANNON. DARWIN considered this animal to be

---

* The reader will note that pages 23–52 of the original paper have been omitted to conserve space. (The editors.)

dominated by terror. But he described, in addition, an emotional expression which is noted when the animal is stalking its prey or ready to pounce upon its enemy. At such times the cat does not look fearful, but ready and eager to fight. It is crouched low on the ground, forefeet extended, head and back straight, tail extended behind and lashing back and forth, and with little pilomotor reaction. Since the stalking cat may eat its prey soon after it has pounced upon it, the implication is that the stomach is prepared for digestion, as regards secretions, blood flow, and motility. These suggest that parasympathetic function dominates in the stomach. Yet, the pursuit and kill also call for extra muscular and circulatory activity, or effects actuated by the sympathetic division.

It is evident therefore that in the terrified cat and monkey and in the stalking cat both divisions of the autonomic and the somatic nervous systems participate. The question as to which parts of the nervous system will dominate under stress is of secondary importance; of primary significance is the interplay or combination which will best serve the needs of the animal in meeting a given life situation.

The Specificity of Affect and Stomach Function[4]

In studies by several investigators on man and on cats and dogs it has been demonstrated that fear or threats may be associated with reduction in gastric peristaltic activity and decreased secretion with hypoacidity [19, 58, 100b]. Rage was coupled with similar gastric changes [11, 15, 19, 51]. Disgust induced by hypnosis was associated with nausea and a decrease in acidity followed by a rise [10]. Emptying time was prolonged, sometimes with decrease in peristaltic activity or even with reverse peristalsis [43]. Severe muscular activity as in competitive games may be associated with a hypoacidity [44].

On the other hand, anxiety in man has been shown to be associated with hyperacidity [63] and similarly, intense hostility may be accompanied by hyperacidity and increased peristaltic activity [33]. It was shown [100] in the man with gastrostomy previously mentioned that situations inducing alarm or dejection were associated with pallor of the stomach mucosa and a fall in acid secretion. The effects were apparent in less than a minute after the stimuli were experienced. Situations inducing hostility and resentment, on the other hand, were seen to be accompanied by reddening of the membrane and an unusually high level of acid production. Therefore, in this subject alarm and hostility were associated with opposite extremes in gastric function.

However, the results of the changes in the gastroduodenal functions associated with various affective states are not all in accord [5, 9, 12, 16, 18, 32, 33, 48, 49, 56, 71, 78, 84, 87, 90, 91, 92]. For example, WITTKOWER [98] concluded that, although fear was always associated with the same gastric effects in the same patient, the reaction in some individuals was associated with hypoacidity, in others with hyperacidity. These seeming contradictions may represent a failure on the part of the subject or the observer to name correctly the dominant emotional reactions. Whereas the reactions to life situations are always complex, often intermingling resentment, fear, feelings of helplessness, vengeance, remorse, and even elation, it is necessary to recognize that some one or two emotions dominate. However, it is conceivable that there are individuals who are so constituted that resentment, hostility, anger, and hate

[4] The terms 'fear' and 'anxiety' have been used by various authors to imply different meanings. In this communication 'fear' is used to indicate an emotional reaction to danger in which feelings of alarm, terror, and helplessness verging on abjection dominate; 'anxiety', a reaction to danger in which defeat threatens, but in which resistance survives. It is commonly associated with hostility, resentment, guilt and conflict.

never become dominant, so that fear prevails whenever the individual's security is challenged. In all events, no patients in this study with gastritis, duodenitis or peptic ulcer could be included in this class.

Experience with conditioned reaction experiments on dogs is suggestive [72, 99]. It has been found useful to divide dogs into two extreme types with a large intermediate group. Dogs of the first type readily develop positive conditioned salivary reactions. During or after a period of stress they show an increased salivary reaction to almost all stimuli. These animals are aggressive, active, noisy, and are often fierce fighters. In contrast, dogs of the second type are fearsome, inactive, quiet, cringing, and readily develop negative conditioned salivary reactions. During or after stress, they respond to stimuli by suppressing all salivary secretion. It is to be recalled that secretions in the parotid gland and stomach usually rise and fall together [98].

Among our normal or control group, there were individuals with hypoacidity even after the administration of food when the latter was given under circumstances which apparently induced resentment, guilt, frustration, and anxiety. Studies now being carried on further indicate that there are persons in whom stress is commonly associated with hyposecretion and hypomotility. What the dominant emotion is in such persons must await further investigation. CANNON's formulation [18] suggests that this inhibition of gastric and salivary secretion may be a part of the animal's preparation for emergency.

May not excessive secretion in mouth and stomach under stress, on the other hand, be a manifestation of an attempt to resolve hostility and to gain security through eating? Does not this state of the stomach represent preparation for eating the prey or the enemy? In DARWIN's words [26] 'serviceable actions become habitual in association with certain states of mind, and are performed whether or not of service in each particular case'.

Eating, Aggression, and Security

Apparently some animals during acts of hostile aggression have gastric accompaniments necessary to eating and digestion. The wolf, foxhound, bloodhound, and greyhound may chase their prey perhaps for miles, and after subduing it in a lively struggle, immediately fall to and eat it. Among the cats, the cheetah behaves similarly and consumes its prey without delay. It may be surmised that the gastric mechanism under those circumstances is ready for digestion and exhibits proper motility and acidity. Racing horses, on the other hand, do not eat until several hours after a race, and some are unable to eat for as long as three days. But the horse in his primitive state runs, not to pursue, but to escape the pursuer. He has not chased and caught his prey and, therefore, is not called upon to eat it at the end of a race.

The pattern of man's eating, of course, is different from either of these. Man eats during a period of respite, gradually increasing hunger becoming associated with an increase of gastric motility. However, in our experiments a gastric state which closely resembled preparedness for eating often followed a situation which induced hostility or anger. An illustration of the operation of this pattern under circumstances when the eating impulse could be carried out, is seen in the following: M. H., a fifty-year-old unmarried woman, lived in the household of her brother-in-law, her dead sister's husband. She was fond of her nephew and niece, and unadmittedly devoted to her brother-in-law. The latter had remarried, and M. H. hated the new wife, and had implied to her friends that the second wife had been his mistress even before her sister's death. The setting in which these various people lived was thus charged with intense jealousy and hostility. M. H., a large, masterly woman, usually voiced her resentment to some aspects of the new wife when all were assembled at meal times. On such occasions harbored feelings were given full expression, and hate, jealousy, hostility and tears were commingled. It was noted by all that M. H. then ate enormously, and 'wolfed' her food. Her sister's husband seldom spoke during such outbursts.

In contrast to these situations with their expressions of hostility against the new wife, were those in which fear or near panic resulted in M. H. from implied or expressed criticisms by her sister's husband. After such disapproval from this man, M. H. would rush from the table, vomit, and be unable to eat for some time.

It is noteworthy in this connection that the patients of this study with their dominant reactions of hostility, anxiety and guilt, usually had good or even excessive appetite for food.

Other cultural groups than our own provide illustrations of the joining together of eating and hostile aggression. The Mundugumor [60], a New Guinea tribe, a people who place high social value upon aggression, competition, initiative, and possession, practice on occasion a frank and boisterous cannibalism, 'each man rejoicing at having a piece of the enemy between his teeth'.

FRAZER [35] has described human eating of the fallen enemy to gain his strength or cunning; eating of ferocious animals to gain their character and physical attributes, the bones of old bulls to acquire their ability to live long; eating of images of the 'gods' in the form of prepared cereals or cakes to assimilate their power.

The beginnings of this linking are suggested by the chief expressions of the infant, most of which are connected with eating [40]. Thus, clenching the fists, grasping, biting, following objects with the eyes, drawing objects toward the body, carrying objects towards the mouth, poking objects, and movements of rejection are earliest seen in connection with food getting. These acts are associated with no hostility, unless frustration or delay are encountered, when offensive movements may promptly develop.

Later in life the eating patterns become linked with the drive for sexual satisfaction, as indicated by drooling in animals, and the increased salivary secretion in man during sexual excitement.

Other drives ultimately may become allied with food getting patterns in modes of expression. Facial expressions of resentment, rage, aggression, and hate involve the use of eating muscles, as in baring the teeth, and those used in food rejection, as with spitting with disgust or scorn. The facial expressions of food getting and food rejection are similar to the most outspoken facial, oral, and vocal expressions of rage and resentment. It has frequently been pointed out that the naso-labial folds of persons with peptic ulcer are accentuated. It is suggested that the accentuated folds result from the sustained contraction of the muscles about the nose and mouth from longlasting expressions of resentment, contempt, sneering, curling the lip, hissing and gestures of resentment [53].

Thus, aggression originally associated with alimentation may subsequently come to be allied with such other drives as the getting of possessions, and the drive to satisfy resentment through revenge.

Eating, Dependence, and Security

For the infant and child it would seem as though eating were the greatest source of security, and food deprivation the greatest threat. Eating retains some of its early significance through life. Closely linked to deprivation are feelings of rejection and abandonment. Such threats are usually short-lived and have no significance, but if they persist they may lead early in life to feelings of insecurity or anxiety. Furthermore, because of the infant's helplessness, food must be presented to him by other individuals. Hence, alimentation becomes involved in the infant's relations with persons around him and particularly with the adult on whom he is dependent. The taking of food may persist as the symbol of being 'cared for' and of being loved, and epitomizes figuratively the state of complete dependence.

Eating as a means of gaining security is a well known pattern in which men and women under stress eat excessively and indeed may become obese during difficult periods. Gum chewing and tobacco and cigar chewing in adults often gives composure, reassurance, and freedom from feelings of frustration or tension. Eating also has the significance of family bond and thus of 'home', of fraternization, and of comradeship. However, the links that connect eating and feelings of security are usually lost from awareness and only the pattern remains.

Such unconscious linking of alimentation with desire for dependence as well as with hostile aggression, and with sexuality, has been suggested in dreams, fantasies and symptoms. For example, vomiting expressed rejection of an unacceptable fantasy about the beloved one [37]; refusal to eat expressed reaction against the hostile desire to devour the person responsible for the patient's frustration [1]; over-eating expressed a desire to gain security by implying a state of dependence and of being loved and cared for [1, 52]; fantasies of eating and of being eaten expressed hostile attack and retribution [7, 57].

It is suggested, therefore, that eating becomes allied with attempts to gain security principally in two ways: through the coupling of eating with hostile aggression and of eating with the wish for dependence and being cared for. Thus, the emotionally insecure patients of this study, with gastroduodenal complaints and lesions, aimed to gain security by both hostile aggression and submission. Side by side were found, on the one hand, desperate attempts to gain security by effective offense, and on the other hand, efforts toward being cared for, toward winning approval, and at seeking unquestioning love. Sometimes one method prevailed, some times the other, but at all times there was conflict between them. Indeed, most serious symptoms often occurred when

after the frank expression of hostility the patient was overpowered by feelings of guilt, condemnation, and anticipation of counter-attack.

It is further suggested that the bodily patterns of eating which initially become linked with aggressive hostility in the acts of getting food may become involved secondarily through the resentment and frustration that follow criticism, the denial of affection, of emotional support, and of unquestioning love. The bodily changes associated with eating may, in short, become linked with any experience that challenges the emotional security of the individual, as gross as the pressure of war on non-combatants [50, 64, 89, 95], or more subtly, a threat to the self-esteem such as may occur in the work-a-day relations of shop and home.

Eating, Insecurity, and Tissue Damage

It has been shown that increased acidity and motility with resentment and frustration are associated with vasodilatation in the duodenal and gastric mucosa. These considerations may have a bearing on the genesis of the gastric and duodenal lesions that have been discussed here. It is suggested that increased acidity, motility and vasodilatation of long standing are a menace to the tissues of the stomach and duodenum [see also 101c]. Indeed, such sustained physiological preparation for eating, in the stomach and duodenum of dogs that have been sham-fed for periods of several weeks by means of an oesophageal fistula, was followed by gastroduodenitis and actual peptic ulcer [85].

Vasodilatation followed by congestion, coupled with hypermotility and hyperacidity could be responsible for small mucosal injuries and the clinical picture of gastritis and duodenitis. Induced bleeding under stress, in our patient with an ulcer (subject 8) suggests congestion and extravasation of blood either at the site of an old lesion or a new one.

It has been demonstrated that mucosal injuries result from prolonged stimulation of the vagus nerve [86, 41b] and occur with lesions of the brain stem, diencephalon, and even after frontal lobe ablation [25, 38]. Mucosal erosions also follow the intravenous infusion of acetyl choline, the neurohumoral agent which is [41a] liberated during vagus nerve stimulation. These observations indicate neural mechanisms that may be implicated in the gastric changes that accompany pernicious affective states [94, 101]. Once a small lesion has formed, its continuation or disappearance would be determined by a number of factors. Most such mucosal erosions would probably disappear, but an occasional one by accident of site might persist and develop into an ulcerative lesion of the stomach or duodenum [6].

One reason for the sustained higher level of HCl in patient with peptic ulcer is indicated by studies now being made by STEWART WOLF in the New York Hospital. He has shown in a patient with a gastrectomy that an erosion in itself may incite increased acid production when that lesion is experimentally exposed to the corrosive action of the patients own gastric juice. Inversely, the acid falls to its previous lower level when the exposure of the lesion to the HCl and pepsin is terminated. It is indicated, then, that a vicious circle is established – the erosion induces increased acid secretion and the latter retards healing. These observations assume an unusual significance because they show how a slight initial tissue damage may end in critical hemorrhage or perforation.

The facts of this study emphasize the occurrence in the same individual of the frequently mentioned destructive emotions coupled with increased motility and secretion and circulatory changes in the stomach and duodenum, followed by evidence of gastritis and duodenitis and ultimately of actual ulceration. This sequence in our patients suggests that these are phases of the same process differing only in the amount of tissue damage.

In appraising the data of this study, the relation between the described emotions and the functional changes in the stomach was not interpreted as cause and effect. Instead, both affects and gastroduodenal changes were viewed as coincident aspects of biological behaviour in reaction to life situations; behaviour in some instances compatible with health, and in others resulting in disease.

Summary

1. The personality features and emotional reactions were investigated in a series of 30 unselected patients with peptic ulcer, and 3 patients with gastritis and duodenitis. The personality features of these patients were variable and the incidents precipitating the emotional reactions numerous. However, the reactions of intense anxiety, insecurity, resentment, guilt and frustration obtained in all. Also, compensating efforts to bolster self-esteem by a show of independence, self-sufficiency, and perfectionism were common. It was evident from the long duration of the personality disturbances that the mucosal lesion itself was not responsible for the major emotional conflicts.

2. In all of the patients with peptic lesions it was possible to demonstrate a chronological parallelism between the onset, recrudescence and course of gastroduodenal symptoms, and the occurrence of untoward emotional reactions. The situations that prompted these reactions were not necessarily dramatic or in the nature of crises, but because of the existing emotional frame within which they occurred they had important effects on the patients.

3. To demonstrate that the above described emotional states were relevant to the gastroduodenal dysfunction and peptic ulcers in the particular patients studied, situations were experimentally created which induced destructive emotional reactions and precipitated symptoms when the patient was free of symptoms. Moreover, if such affects, symptoms and tissue defects already existed, all increased in intensity during such experimental procedures. On the other hand, in situations which engendered feelings of emotional security and assurance, gastric function was restored toward normal and symptoms elim-

inated, in those with symptoms and abnormal function.

4. Thus, with the knowledge of the dominant emotions in these patients and some of the circumstances responsible for their being, situations were created in the laboratory which resulted in emotional and gastroduodenal changes like those occurring in the individual's day-to-day experiences. Records were made of the behaviour and utterances of the subject. Also simultaneously, records were made of the motility and secretions of the stomach, and of the finger temperature and respiration. 165 observations were conducted on 26 subjects, 10 of whom had ulcers of the stomach or the duodenum, and 3 of whom had gastritis and duodenitis. 13 subjects were healthy and without complaints. The experiments revealed the following association of affective reactions and physiological function in the patients. Tension, anxiety, resentment, anger, guilt, obsequiousness and desperation, already present, accentuated or induced, were almost always accompanied by an increase in hydrochloric acid, mucous and pepsin secretions. Peristaltic activity became continuous, and contractions increased in magnitude. Respiration became more rapid and shallow, with frequent sighs. There was usually a drop in finger temperature. Often in patients with ulcer pain of a burning and gnawing quality was precipitated and unusual amounts of bile and moderate amounts of fresh, unclotted blood appeared in the extractions. Similar changes occurred in a few instances during sleep following a period of affective stress. During and after interview which engendered emotional security, functional over-activity decreased and approached the normal. A comparison of the individual physiological and emotional changes in normal subjects with those of patients with ulcer, gastritis and duodenitis, revealed similar patterns, but the changes in the pathological group were greater in magnitude and duration.

5. The facts of this study emphasize the occurrence in the same individual of the aforementioned destructive emotions coupled with increased motility and secretion and mucosal circulatory changes in the stomach and duodenum, followed by evidence of gastritis and duodenitis, and ultimately actual ulceration. This sequence suggests that the increased secretion, increased motility and disturbed circulation, mucosal erosion and ulcerations

are phases of the same process differing only in the amount of tissue destruction in the stomach and duodenum.

6. In appraising the data of this study the relation between the emotions as described and the functional changes in the stomach and duodenum was not interpreted as cause and effect. Instead, both affects and gastroduodenal changes were viewed as coincident aspects of behaviour in reaction to life situations; behaviour in some instances compatible with health, and in others resulting in disease.

References

1. ABRAHAM, K.: Selected papers on psychoanalysis (Hogarth, London 1927).
2. ALEXANDER, F.: The influence of psychological factors upon gastrointestinal disturbances; a symposium. I. General principles, objectives and preliminary results. Psychoanal. Quart. 3: 501 (1934).
3. ALSTED, G.: The changing incidence of peptic ulcer (Humphrey Milford, Oxford University Press, London 1939).
4. ALVAREZ, W. C.: Ways in which emotions can affect the digestive tract. J. amer. med. Ass. 92: 1231 (1929).
5. ALVAREZ, W. C.: Introduction to gastroenterology (Hoeber, Inc., New York 1940).
6. ASCHOFF, L.: Lectures on pathology, p. 279 (Hoeber, Inc., New York 1924).
7. BACON, C.: The typical personality trends and conflicts in cases of gastric disturbance. Psychoanal. Quart. 3: 541 (1934).
8. BEAUMONT, W.: Experiments and observations on the gastric juice and the physiology of digestion (Allen, Plattsburg 1833).
9. BENDER, M. B.: Fright and drug contractions in denervated facial and ocular muscles of monkeys. Amer. J. Physiol. 121: 609 (1938).
10. BENNETT, T. I. and VENABLES, J. F.: The effects of emotions on gastric secretion and motility in the human being. Brit. med. J. ii: 662 (1920).
11. BISSEL, A. und SASAKI, K.: Experimentelle Untersuchungen über den Einfluss von Affekten auf die Magensaftsekretion. Dtsch. med. Wschr. 31: 1829 (1905).
12. BLOOMFIELD, A. L.: Psychic secretion in man. Amer. J. digest Dis. 7: 205 (1940).

13. BLOOMFIELD, A. L.; CHEN, C. K., and FRENCH, L. R.: Basal gastric secretion as a clinical test of gastric function with special reference to peptic ulcer. J. clin. Invest. *19:* 863 (1940).

14. BLOOMFIELD, A. L. and KEEFER, C. S.: Gastric acidity: Relation to various factors such as age and physical fitness. J. clin. Invest. *5:* 285 (1928).

15. BOGEN, H.: Experimentelle Untersuchungen über psychische und assoziative Magensaftsekretion beim Menschen. Pflügers Arch. ges. Physiol. *117:* 150 (1907).

16. BRUNSWICK, D.: The effects of emotional stimuli on the gastrointestinal tone. I. Methods and technique. J. comp. Psychol. *4:* 19 (1924); Ibid.: II. Results and conclusions *4:* 225 (1924).

17. CALLAHAN, E. J. and INGHAM, D. W.: A practical method of analyzing the precipitating factors producing peptic ulcer. Amer. J. digest Dis. *5:* 751 (1939).

18. CANNON, W. B.: Bodily changes in pain, hunger fear and rage (Appleton & Co., New York 1929).

19. CANNON, W. B.: The influence of emotional states on the functions of the alimentary canal. Amer. J. med. Sci. *137:* 480 (1909).

20. CARLSON, A. J.: Contribution to the physiology of the stomach. I. Character of the movements of the empty stomach in man. Amer. J. Physiol. *31:* 151 (1912–13).

21. CARLSON, A. J.: Contributions to the physiology of the stomach. XLV. Hunger, appetite and gastric juice secretion in man during prolonged fasting. Amer. J. Physiol. *45:* 120 (1917–18).

22. CARLSON, A. J.: Contributions to the physiology of the stomach. XLIV. The origin of the epigastric pains in cases of gastric and duodenal ulcer. Amer. J. Physiol. *45:* 81 (1917–18).

23. CHENEY, G. and BLOOMFIELD, A. L.: Gastric function in cases of gastric and duodenal ulcer. J. clin. Invest. *5:* 511 (1928).

24. CROHN, B. B. and REISS, J.: Studies in fractional estimations of stomach contents. Amer. J. med. Sci. *154:* 857 (1917).

25. CUSHING, H.: Peptic ulcer and the interbrain. Surg. Gynec. Obstet. *55:* 1 (1932).

26. DARWIN, C.: Expression of emotions in man and animals (Appleton and Company, New York 1896).

27. DAVIES, D. T. and WILSON, A. T. M.: Personal and clinical history in haematemesis and perforation. Lancet *ii:* 723 (1939).

28. DRAPER, G. and TOURAINE, G. A.: The man-environment unit and peptic ulcer. Arch. intern. Med. *49:* 616 (1932).

29. DROSSNER, J. L. and MILLER, T. G.: Natural history and diagnosis of gastric ulcer. Amer. J. med. Sci. *199:* 90 (1940).

30. DUNBAR, H. F.: Emotions and bodily changes (Columbia University Press, New York 1938).

31. EINHORN, M.: The role of psychic load in recurrent attacks of gastroduodenal ulcer. New Engl. J. Med. *208:* 681 (1933).

32. EISENBUD, J.: A method for investigating the effect of depression on the somatic expression of emotion in vegetative functions: A preliminary report. Psychosom. Med. *1:* 376 (1939).

33. FARR, C. B. and LUEDERS, C. W.: Gastric secretory functions in the psychoses. Arch. Neurol., Chicago *10:* 548 (1923).

34. FRANK, L. K.: Cost of competition. Plan Age *6:* 314 (1940).

35. FRAZER, J. G.: The golden bough. A study in magic and religion, Chapt. 50 and 51, pp. 479–499 (MacMillan Co., New York 1923).

36. FREMONT-SMITH, M.: Relationships between emotional states and organic disease. New Engl. J. Med. *208:* 69 (1933).

37. FREUD, S.: Collected papers (Hogarth, London 1925).

38. FULTON, J. E.: Physiology of the nervous system, p. 253 (Oxford University Press, London 1938).

39. GALAMBOS, A.: Direct examination of the gastric juice. Arch. intern. Med. *38:* 654 (1926).

40. GESELL, A. and ILG, F. F.: Feeding behaviour of infants (Lippincott, J. B. and Co., Philadelphia 1937).

41a. HALL, G. E.; ETTINGER, G. H., and BANTING, F. G.: An experimental production of coronary thrombosis and myocardial failure. Canad. med. Ass. J. *34:* 9 (1936).

b. MANNING, G. W.; HALL, G. E., and BANTING, F. G.: Vagus stimulation and the production of myocardial damage. Ibid. *37:* 314 (1937).

42. HAWK, P. B. and BERGEIM, O.: Practical physiological chemistry, 11. ed., p. 308 (Blakiston's Son & Co., Inc., Philadelphia 1937).

43. HEILIG, R. und HOFF, H.: Beiträge zur hypnotischen Beeinflussung der Magenfunktion. Med. Klin. 21: 162 (1925).

44. HELLEBRANDT, F. A. and MILES, M. M.: The effect of muscular work and competition on gastric acidity. Amer. J. Physiol. 102: 258 (1932).

45. HELLEBRANDT, F. A.; TEPPER, R. H.; GRANT, H., and CATHERWOOD, R.: Nocturnal and diurnal variations in the acidity of the spontaneous secretion of gastric juice. Amer. J. digest Dis. 3: 477 (1936).

46. HENNING, N. und NORPOTH, L.: Untersuchungen über die sekretorische Funktion des Magens während des nächtlichen Schlafes. Arch. Verdaukr. 53: 64 (1933).

47. HEPBURN, J. J.: Problem of peptic ulcer. Rev. Gastroent. 7: 103 (1940).

48. HENRY, G. W.: Some roentgenological observations of gastro-intestinal conditions associated with mental disorders. Amer. J. Psychiat. 3: 681 (1924).

49. HENRY, G. W.: Gastrointestinal motor functions in schizophrenia. Amer. J. Psychiat. 7: 135 (1927–28).

50. HINCKS, C. M.: Mental hygiene in the emergency work in Canada. Ment. Hyg. 25: 10 (1941).

51. HORNBORG, A. F.: Beiträge zur Kenntnis der Absonderungsbedingungen des Magensaftes beim Menschen. Skand. Arch. Physiol. 15: 209 (1904).

52. HORNEY, K.: Neurotic personality of our time, p. 124 (Norton, New York 1937).

53. HUBER, E.: Evolution of facial musculature and facial expression, p. 157 (Johns Hopkins Press, Baltimore 1931).

54. JENNINGS, D.: Perforated peptic ulcer. Changes in age-incidence and sex-distribution in the last 150 years. Lancet i: 444 (1940).

55. KAPLAN, B.: Can emotions produce organic lesions in the digestive tract? Med. Rec., NY 143: 379 (1963).

56. KHARMANDARYAN, G. I.; PLATANOW, K. I., and BECHINSKAYA, N. M.: Emotions: Effect on response of stomach; preliminary report. Arch. Verdaukr. 55: 23 (1934).

57. LEVEY, H. B.: Oral trends and oral conflicts in a case of duodenal ulcer. Psychoanal. Quart. 3: 575 (1934).

58. LOMMEL, F.: Die Magen- und Darmbewegungen im Röntgenbild und ihre Veränderung durch verschiedene Einflüsse. Münch. med. Wschr. 2: 1633 (1903).

59. MCGREGOR, H. G.: Emotional factor in visceral disease (Oxford Medical Publications Humphrey Milford, London 1938).

60. MEAD, M.: Sex and temperament in three primitive societies, p. 186 (William Morrow & Co., New York 1935).

61. MEULENGRACHT, E.: Medical treatment of peptic ulcer and its complications. Brit. med. J. ii: 231 (1939).

62. MEYER, J.; FETTER, D., and STRAUSS, A. A.: Relation of pain of peptic ulcer to gastric motility and acidity. Arch. intern. Med., 5: 338 (1932).

63. MILLER, R. J.; BERGEIM, O., and HAWK, P. B.: Gastric response to foods. IX. The influence of worry on gastric digestion. Science, 52: 253 (1920).

64. MILTON, G.: Haematemesis and the war. Lancet i: 316 (1940).

65. MITTELMANN, B. and WOLFF, H. G.: Affective states and skin temperature: Experimental study of subjects with 'cold hands' and Raynaud's syndrome. Psychosom. Med. 1: 271 (1939).

66. MOLEEN, G. A.: Influence of emotional shock on the gastro-intestinal tract in the psychoneuroses. J. Amer. med. Ass. 95: 910 (1930).

67. NORTH, H. M.: The emotions and functional disorders of the viscera. Med. J. Austr. 1: 621 (1937).

68. NECHELES, H.: Theory of the formation of peptic ulcer. Amer. J. digest Dis. 4: 643 (1937).

69. PALMER, W. L.: The mechanism of pain in gastric and duodenal ulcer. II. The production of pain by means of chemical irritants. Arch. intern. Med. 38: 694 (1926).

70. PALMER, W. L. and NUTTER, P. B.: Peptic ulcer and achlorhydria. A further study of the role of acid gastric juice in the pathogenesis of peptic ulcer. Arch. intern. Med. 65: 499 (1940).

71. PAVLOV, I. P.: The work of the digestive glands. Translated by W. H. THOMPSON (Griffin & Co., Ldt., London 1910).

72. PAVLOV, I. P.: Conditioned reflexes. Lecture 17 (Oxford Univ. Press, Humphrey Milford, London 1927).

73. PINKHAM, E. G.: Aunt Elsa, p. 95 (Alfred S. Knopf, New York 1941).

74. Recent Social Trends in the United States. Vol. I: Chapt. 3–10, 13, 14. Vol. II: Chapt. 15, 16, 18, 25, 26, 29. Report of the President's Research Committee on Social Trends (McGraw Hill Book Co., Inc., New York 1933).

75. RICHARDS, C. H.; WOLF, STEWART, and WOLFF, H. G.: Studies on blood flow in the gastrointestinal tract of man. J. clin. Invest. 20: 440 (1941).

76. RICHARDSON, H. B.: Report to be published on the study of the ... family in relation to sickness and health care.

77. ROBINSON, G. W.: 'Personality disorders' causing digestive complaints. Johns Hopk. Hosp. Bull. 68: 203 (1941).

78. ROBINSON, S. C.: Role of emotions in gastroduodenal ulcer. Illinois med. J. 71: 338 (1937).

79. ROGERS, F. T. and HARDT, L. L.: Relation of hunger contractions of the empty stomach to normal digestive movements. Amer. J. Physiol. 36: 354 (1914–15).

80. ROGERS, F. T. and MARTIN, C. L.: A roentgenological study of gastric hunger motility in a series of healthy men. Amer. J. Physiol. 82: 113 (1927).

81. RONALD, J.: The value of therapeutic measures in duodenal ulceration. Brit. med. J. ii: 1033 (1939).

82. RUGGLES, H. E.: Emotional influence upon the gastro-intestinal tract. Calif. West. Med. 29: 221 (1928).

83. RUMBALL, J. M.: Gastroscopy with a statistical report of one hundred patients. Curr. med. Dig. 38 (1941).

84. SIEFERT, A. C.: Role of vegetative nervous system in production of motor phenomena observed in the upper digestive tract. Radiology 28: 283 (1937).

85. SILBERMANN,T.S.: Experimentelle Magenduodenalulcuserzeugung durch Scheinfütterung nach Pavlov. Zbl. Chir. 54: 2385 (1927).

86. STAHNKE, E.: Experimentelle Untersuchungen zur Frage der neurogenen Entstehung des Ulcus Ventriculi. Arch. Klin. Chir. 132: 1 (1924).

87. STEIGMANN, F.: Peptic ulcer syndrome in the Negro. Clinical and statistical evidence on psychogenic as against racial factors in the etiology of this syndrome. Amer. J. digest Dis. 3: 310 (1936).

88. STEIGMANN, F. and FANTUS, B.: Acidity modification therapy in peptic ulcer. Amer. J. digest. Dis. 7: 197 (1940).

89. TANNER, N. C. and JENS, J.: The treatment of peptic ulcer in war time. Practitioner 166: 100 (1941).

90. TODD, T. W.: The stomach as an organ of social adjustment. Sci. Mon., New York 43: 341 (1936).

91. TODD, T. W.: Behaviour patterns of the alimentary tract (Williams & Wilkins Co., Baltimore 1930).

92. VAN LIERE, E. J.; VAUGHAN, P. E., and NORTHRUP, D. W.: Effect of noise on gastric secretion. Amer. J. Physiol. 129: 484 (1940).

93. VANZANT, F. R.; ALVAREZ, W. C.; EUSTERMAN, G. B.; DUNN, H. L., and BERKSON, J.: The normal range of gastric acidity from youth to old age. Arch. intern. Med. 49: 345 (1932).

94. VON BERGMAN, G.: Ulcus duodeni und vegetatives Nervensystem. Berl. klin. Wschr. 50: 2374 (1913). Also: Zur Pathogenese des chronischen Ulcus pepticum; Ibid. 55: 524 (1918).

95. WILLCOX, P. H.: Gastric disorders in the services. Brit. med. J. i: 1008 (1940).

96. WILSON, A. T. M.: Psychological observations on haematemesis. Brit. J. med. Psychol. 18: 112 (1939).

97. WINKELSTEIN, A.: A new therapy of peptic ulcer. Continuous alkalinized milk drip into the stomach. Amer. J. med. Sci. 185: 695 (1933).

98. WITTKOWER, E.: Studies on the influence of emotions on the functions of the organs (including observations on normals and neurotics). J. ment. Sci. 81: 533 (1935).

99. WOLFF, H. G.: Die bedingte Reaktion. Handbuch der Neurologie, p. 338 (Springer, Berlin 1937).

100a. WOLF, STEWART and WOLFF, H. G.: Studies on gastroduodenal physiology in a patient with a large permanent gastric fistula. Correlation of circulatory changes with changes in secretion of gastric juice (to be published).

    b. Studies of gastroduodenal physiology in a patient with a large permanent gastric fistula. Report of case with follow-up after 46 years and observations on the sensibility of the gastric mucosa (to be published).

101. WOLFF, H. G. and THOMAS, E. W.: Gastroduodenal ulcers and autonomic imbalance. Arch. Neurol., Chicago 17: 571 (1927).

Psychoanalytic Study of a Case of Essential Hypertension[1]

F. ALEXANDER

Retrospective comment by Dr. M. Lipkin. This paper is an example of ALEXANDER'S work os personality profiles and the types of conflicts seen in patients with specific clinical syndromea· Many observers had commented on the influence of emotional stress and strain on essentinl hypertension. This new work, presented very persuasively by the respected FRANZ ALEXANDER, convinced many people and inspired a series of studies (SAUL, WOLF, RENNIE, BINGER *et al.*) which led to similar conclusions. For over a decade it influenced many to believe that excessive but inhibited hostile tendencies were typical of hypertensives and a major etiologic factor in the disease.

However, the observation of clinical phenomena is notoriously treacherous, particularly when guided by preconceived opinions. There is a natural tendency to see what is looked for and to overlook the unexpected. Furthermore, the reactions of patients may differ with various physicians; the personality and the environment of the physician may provoke hostility from some, dependency from others. Psychoanalysis, the method of psychological observation used in this study, has inherent shortcomings – the impossibility of replication, the partial reporting by both patient and analyst, the inaccuracy of the patient's recall, the common mixing of observation with interpretation, etc. What one observer calls abnormal aggression, another may consider a normal attempt to achieve a goal. And all people show some aggressive characteristics and some tendencies to be dependent in degrees which vary from time to time. Similarly, the patient's blood pressure at a given moment is the resultant of many forces not all of which could be considered in this study. The range of variations reported is rather small and their significance uncertain.

While there is little reason to doubt that emotional factors play a part in the blood pressure level, ALEXANDER'S hypothesis that inhibited hostility acts as a prime determinant of the appearance and course of hypertensive disease, is unproven. Nevertheless this paper contributed heavily to the awareness of the need for considering the emotions, especially those only amenable to psychoanalytic study, in investigating hypertension. As such, it remains a work of historic interest.

The observations described in this article were made in the course of a systematic clinical investigation conducted at the Chicago Institute for Psychoanalysis. The objective of this clinical study was to explore the psychological processes and the personality structure of patients suffering from essential hypertension. This investigation was undertaken in the hope that a systematic study of the emotional life of hypertensive patients by the psychoanalytic method, continued over a long period, would throw some light upon the still open question concerning the etiological rôle of emotional factors in the development of this widespread condition. At the same time the aim of this study was to establish the possibilities of psychotherapy in essential hypertension.

It is common clinical knowledge that acute emotional tensions have an influence upon the height of the blood pressure[2]. A common experience is that a patient who is

[1] Institute for Psychoanalysis, Chicago.

[2] Compare with the review of the literature of E. WEISS in this issue.

in an apprehensive mood while having his blood pressure taken, shows higher readings than after he has been calmed down by the physician's reassurance. Animal experiments have corroborated the clinical findings and have shown that under the influence of rage and fear, the blood pressure rises [3]. The influence of acute and intensive emotions on blood pressure can be observed in patients whose blood pressure is normal, as well as in those whose blood pressure is chronically elevated. It has also been observed in hypertensives whose condition is caused by renal disease. These observations in themselves do not allow any etiological conclusions concerning the rôle of emotions in the causation of chronically elevated blood pressure. They account only for the transient fluctuation of the blood pressure.

Another important clinical finding described by different authors is that most essential hypertensives show marked neurotic personality traits. Neither does this observation allow any definite etiological conclusions because the neurotically disturbed emotional life and high blood pressure may be parallel manifestations of a third factor (constitution); or the hypertension might contribute to the development of neurotic tendencies; or, the hypertensive state may be the result of a long standing neurosis. The opinions of different authors are divided on this subject.

We expected to obtain different kinds of information from the psychoanalytic study and therapy of such patients. In the first place, the psychological observations obtained by the method of psychoanalytic technique promised a more intimate insight concerning the influence upon the blood pressure, not only of acute emotional states, but also of chronic emotional tensions as they can be observed in neurotics. Furthermore, the psychoanalytic study of cases gives a detailed picture of the personality development from early childhood on, which might throw light upon the development of the hypertensive state. Finally a comparative study of a series of

patients suffering from essential hypertension may answer the question whether or not there is a definite personality structure which is characteristic for these patients. Apart from these theoretical objectives, we hoped to find a therapeutic approach based on etiological knowledge. In the following an attempt will be made to (1) give a dynamic picture of the personality make-up of a hypertensive patient; (2) to correlate the fluctuations of his blood pressure with his changing emotional states; and (3) to establish whether or not there are specific emotional tensions which have a specific influence upon the blood pressure.

I. The Patient's Personality and its Development

A. The present picture

The following observations were made during the analysis of a 47-year-old male patient who was suffering from a pronounced though not excessive essential hypertension of the fluctuating variety. The patient's systolic blood pressure fluctuated between 175 mm and 136 mm and the diastolic between 120 mm and 92 mm. This condition is of 2 years' duration[3].

The patient was a married businessman of Swedish descent with a distinctive educational and family background. He had 4 children, 2 older boys and 2 girls. He occupied an important and responsible but not the highest position in a large concern.

The patient's father died young of an acute infectious disease, his mother of a stroke when 73 years old. The patient drinks coffee occasionally and smokes from 20 to 40 cigarettes a day. The physical examination of the patient revealed a well developed, well nourished, somewhat obese, middle-aged man weighing 209 lb. There was a distinct odor of alcohol on his breath. There was a moderate arcus senilis of both eyes. Liver dullness was 2 to 3

[3] Compare with the following article of LEON SAUL [in the original edition] where the typical personality structure of seven analyzed hypertensives is summarized.

fingers below the costal margin, but no evidence of liver tenderness. The second aortic tone was moderately accentuated. There was a questionable enlargement of his spleen. His urine showed a trace of albumin and a considerable number of pus cells in the centrifuged specimen. Hemoglobin was 90; white blood count 7,600. There was a not undue, very moderate arteriovenous nicking in the retinal vessels with no increased tortuosity of the capillaries. Electrocardiographic examination showed a slow, regular heart beat with a slight tendency to left axis deviation and a moderate amount of slurring and notching in QRS in the 4th lead.

When I saw the patient first, he showed an extremely pronounced self-consciousness, with a vivid sense of inferiority. He constantly compared himself unfavorably with others, had little confidence in himself, tended to undervalue his efficiency, and was always doubtful about the merits of his accomplishments. At the same time, he was very ambitious to excel and turn out perfect work. He was definitely a retiring type, inconspicuous, a conformist, always polite avoiding contradiction. His ambitions to progress and to outdo the others remained restricted to his fantasy and did not appear on the surface. It soon became evident that this overt attitude of modesty and compliance put him under an extreme pressure and created intense inferiority feelings in him. These became most tormenting in relation to his chief. The patient never would contradict his chief, would follow his suggestions, accept blame while talking with him; but after he left the office, he was filled with self-contempt and would tell himself, 'You should have answered. You should have said, No! You should have demonstrated to him that he was not right. You are no good and you never will be any good.' This self-depreciatory attitude usually became so unbearable that he would have the urge to drink. Alcohol dissipated his sense of weakness and inefficiency. As soon as the alcohol began to make its effects felt, his spirit was lifted, he felt courageous and strong. But apart from the effect of the drug, the act of drinking itself had the significance of a rebellious act for him. He secretly enjoyed the feeling that in the middle of the day during office hours he escaped his duties and indulged in a forbidden activity. In this alcoholic mood, he would also indulge in promiscuous sexuality in a rebellious spirit against limitations imposed upon

him by external social standards and by the voice of his otherwise so strict conscience. Obviously these alcoholic and sexual escapades relieved his sense of inferiority because under the influence of alcohol, he dared to commit such offenses as he would never have ventured without alcohol. But soon after he thus successfully escaped the pangs of inferiority feelings, he ran into a new conflict, that of guilt. For after he had committed all these forbidden sexual and non-social acts in order to show his independence, and thus escape his inferiority feelings, his conscience began to work and made itself felt in the form of remorse.

The patient's attitude in his professional life closely paralleled his attitude towards his wife. Here also, overtly he subjected himself to all requirements of the marital state but he secretly rebelled against its restrictions. His promiscuity to a great extent was rebellion against the marital chains. At the same time, he had a deep affection for his wife which no other woman has shared. His extramarital relationships were all of a superficial nature.

In brief, the most conspicuous feature in his make-up was this double attitude of overt subjection to external code and to his conscience, with an extremely strong emotional rebellion against this submission. This internal rebellion, however, did not show itself in any other way than in his drinking and occasional promiscuity, both of which had the emotional significance of a short circuit or a vent to relieve emotional tension – particularly his rebellious feelings against every external and internal restriction to which he submitted himself otherwise to an extreme degree.

B. The Unconscious Dynamic Background of the Overt Picture

During the course of his psychoanalysis the deeper dynamic background of this surface picture has been worked out. His rebellious, aggressive attitudes against the social restrictions of marriage, against his boss, against routine –, aggressive attitudes which he never could express openly and freely, were the reactions to a strong passive, masochistically colored feminine tendency and wish for dependence. With the progress of the analysis, more and more unconscious passive homosexual material came to the surface, both in dreams and in the transference. This feminine tendency had definitely a masochistic tinge. In his dreams he was usually attacked. In other dreams, women appeared in the masculine rôle, even equipped with male anatomy. These masochistic and feminine attitudes also came into expression in day fantasies, in which he imagined his chief attacking, rebuking and abusing him. In this passive masochistic attitude, 2 elements were clearly discernible; (1) a guilt component, and (2) a feminine element. The masochistic passivity was a combination of guilt and feminine submissiveness. By being abused and attacked, he relieved his guilt feelings and at the same time obtained feminine passive gratification. The guilt feelings came from his rebellious aggressiveness and extreme destructive competitiveness, which were reactions to the deep passive feminine attitude. The well known neurotic vicious circle was solidly established in him: His unconscious, masochistic feminine wishes hurt his masculine pride and drove him to rebellion, increased his competitiveness and ambition. These overaggressive tendencies, however, created guilt and fear which made the struggle of life too strenuous, exhausting and repulsive for him and thus intensified his longing for dependence and retreat. The thus increased passive dependent wishes, however, could not be accepted by his ego which was educated according to the accepted standards of his environment, namely, to consider success and efficiency and victory in the race of life as the highest virtues. Under the pressure of this deeply entrenched ideology of success, he had to struggle relentlessly against his deep longing for relaxation and dependence and continue the competitive game of social life. However, in distinction to many other cases who show the same vicious circle of emotional life, he was unable to give expression either to his aggressive ambitions or to his wish for passive dependence. Fear and guilt blocked the expression of aggressiveness and the internally accepted social standards prohibited him from giving in to his wish to escape the struggle of life. His aggressiveness and his protest against passive submission found a feeble expression in the adolescent behavior pattern – in surreptitious drinking and forbidden sexual acts. To some degree he gratified some of his submissive and dependent longings in giving his wife full control of their social life, expecting her to make all important decisions, and assuming towards her the rôle of an adolescent towards his mother, a peculiar mixture of obedience and surreptitious revolt. In his dreams, however, he regressed even further back than adolescence, way back to the early dependent attitude of the child toward the mother (oral dependence). A typical expression of this tendency was dreams in which he escaped the difficulties of life by seclusion and returning to mother nature in a somewhat Rousseau-ic manner. Some of the dreams were classical examples of womb fantasies: he saw beautiful and mystical, wild spots in nature; deep pits filled up with crystal clear water where big penguin-like birds rested peacefully and he together with them. The analysis of these regressive dependent tendencies led us back to a period of his life in which he must have reacted with great rivalry towards his 11 year younger brother, envying the mother's care for the baby and the passive gratifications of the little child.

The dynamic picture was one of an extreme polarization of the emotional life; on the one hand, a wish towards the infantile rôle of dependence and the feminine rôle of submissiveness and passivity, counterbalanced by the opposite attitude of ambition, perfection, and masculine superiority. These two opposite tendencies mutually reinforced each other. The passive regressive tendencies hurt his pride and stimulated his aggressiveness, whereas the aggressive competitive tendencies created fear and a longing toward the security of the passive situation of being loved and cared for.

The here described polarization of these two opposing psychological attitudes reinforcing each other in a vicious circle, is a picture very commonly found in neurotic persons. It has been described by my collaborators and me in peptic ulcer cases [1], and in certain delinquent types [2]. The same emotional conflict was most elaborately and convincingly described by HORNEY [6], who even went so far as to postulate this conflict between competitive ambition versus the wish to be loved and taken care of, to be a nuclear conflict, typical for the contemporary neurotic in our competitive Western civilization. The ubiquity of this conflict in our times does not mean, however, that all neurotics have the same personality structure. The psychoanalytic study of a great variety of neurotic patients taught us to recognize many different ways and means by which different personalities succeed in relieving the emotional tension resulting from this central conflict. Thus, for example, we have learned that peptic ulcer patients usually succeed in expressing their ambitious drives toward accomplishment and responsibility, frequently in aggressive business activities, or in administrative or organizational work. The opposite tendency, which is a reaction to this strenuous ambition: their longing for dependence and being loved and taken care of, is drained by organic symptoms, namely, by the increased functions of the stomach. The stomach is stimulated by the repressed unconscious tendencies to be fed, which since early childhood are emotionally linked with the wish to be loved. Also certain delinquent types freely express their aggressiveness and the wish to be tough and independent which they amply gratify in their adventurous life. Only the careful exploration of the depth of their emotional life can reveal the soft nucleus, the wish for dependence and security. This inconscious wish they satisfy when captured and imprisoned; then they freely indulge in the wish for shelter and retreat. Many prisoners' peculiar attachment to the prison, their inconscious wish to be recaptured and thus to escape from the struggle of life into the security of the prison, has been amply demonstrated by the psychoanalytic study of prisoners [2], and has also been recognized by the intuition of novelists [4, 5].

What made this hypertensive case so different from the peptic ulcer personalities or the delinquent types and other neurotics in which this same vicious circle is a central issue, was the patient's extreme inhibition to satisfy either of his two opposing major trends: apart from the 2 inadequate vents, promiscuity and drinking, he was unable to express any aggressive independent wish, but at the same time he was equally unable to satisfy freely his longing for passive dependence. This strong inhibition to satisfy either of the 2 opposing major sides of his nature, his rebellious independence as well as his dependence, accounts for the impression which he made on the observer of being in a permanent emotional tension: a boiling volcano before eruption, but never erupting.

This inability to espress these two opposing attitudes explains the peculiar neutrality which was so characteristic for his human relationships: always polite and modest yet not extremely submissive and humble, outwardly complying but always giving the impression of a tacit resistance. The analysis revealed, that whenever he complied with the request of another person, especially of a superior, he immediately afterwards in fantasy rebelled against it without being able to give free expression to this internal revolt. It is no exaggeration to say that he was paralyzed in every emotional expression, each of the two polar opposing tendencies blocking the expression of the other.

This emotional paralysis accounts for certain recurrent characteristic dreams in which he undertook to do something (to catch a train, to go play golf, etc.) and was unable to do so (his feet did not respond, or he could not put on his shoes, etc.) these dreams were accompanied by a feeling of utter futility. The deeper inquiry showed that even the only vents by which he could express his rebellion and independence, his drinking and sexual escapades, were condensation products of the two opposing tendencies. In his sexual relationship to women, there was a great amount of secret passive gratification (mainly through identification with the sexual partner); and his drinking, apart from its surface significance of an adolescent forbidden act, at the same time gave him the possibility to flee from all responsibilities of life and indulge in a carefree Nirvana-like sensation. It is no exaggeration to say that the alcohol bottle was the direct substitute for the mother's breast. Like feeding in his childhood, now drinking was able to relive all unpleasant sensations, dissipate all worries, and give him a deep feeling of relaxation and happiness. Because it served both purposes to express rebellion and also to gratify his flight from responsibility to passive relaxation, drinking became a dangerous symptom. This explains why his conscious struggle to give up drinking had to remain ineffective.

C. How the Present Psychodynamic Structure Came About – Bird's eye view of the life history

As will be seen, this emotional tension, resulting from two equally strong opposing tendencies blocking each other, was the psychodynamic situation which could be brought into correlation with this patient's high blood pressure. Therefore it might appear irrelevant for this study to enter the genetic problem as to how this emotional impasse came about during his life history. If it were true, that such a chronic emotional tension might produce a chronic elevation of blood pressure, the history of this condition is of secondary importance. In different cases, the same emotional blocking might come about in different ways; the important question is, whether or not, if present, it necessarily leads to high blood pressure. In order to decide this latter question, above all it must be established, whether or not this type of chronic emotional tension is characteristic for hypertensive patients. SAUL in his article to follow[4] summarizes our observations concerning the characteristic personality structure of hypertensives. His summary shows, however, not only that the actual emotional situation prevailing in adult hypertensives shows great similarities in different cases, but also that the developmental history shows certain parallel features. Therefore I shall try to draw a brief sketch of this patient's emotional development.

Only the most important facts of the life history will be mentioned, only those occurrences and emotional experiences which apparently have contributed to the development of the above described psychodynamic situation.

The patient came of an intellectual refined family, and was born in Sweden. The family came to the States when the patient was 3 years old. He was one of 6 children, an older brother died before the patient was born. The patient was the second of 3 brothers who were born in 3 successive years. Then came a 5 years younger sister, and finally his younger brother, 11 years younger.

As a young boy, the patient was in every respect the outstanding member of the family. His brothers looked up to him more or less as a hero. He could fight the battles of the younger boys. He was inclined to extreme outbreaks of rage, was absolutely fearless, played an astonishing game of football and baseball. In his first 2 years of public school, he resented the routine which was then required and rebelled against one of the teachers quite violently. His being sent home from school for unruly behavior became a regular occurrence. He still retained for a long time his superiority over his brothers and other boys. He was not only the best student in his grade, but probably the best student in the school. The whole family and everybody who was in contact with him, had the greatest expectations of him.

When he was 12 years old, his father died.

He felt he should cry as all the other members of the family did, but he had no true desire for it.

Gradually, the patient lost his leading position in the family. Already in the first college years he began to slip, both in athletics and in scholastic achievements. As a result he developed a severe depression. He was still an excellent student and a good athlete but both of his brothers began to catch up and even surpass him. In his high school days and college days the patient made friendships with socially outstanding boys, much wealthier than he was. When he finished college he obtained a position in a concern owned by one of his friend's families. Leaning over backwards, he accepted in this company a menial position which was connected with extreme discomfort and even degradation. During this time he developed his second severe depression. Soon after he recovered from his depression, he married a socially outstanding girl and through this marriage he entered into a group much wealthier than his family was. Although he obtained a very excellent business position, the patient hat to struggle desperately to live up to the standards of his circle. About in the 12th year of his marriage, he started to drink, which was the only means of getting rid of his apprehensive depressive moods, which with great regularity every morning after awakening, began to torture him. Looking back on his life, back to adolescence, the patient was never free from a strong self-critical depressive state of mind, which gradually grew worse and worse.

Viewing this history from a distant perspective, we see the gradual metamorphosis of an over-aggressive, successful, domineering young man, determined for leadership, into a shy, inhibited, conforming, overly modest and unexpressive person. The aggressive and courageous spirit of his early years appears in the adult only in the form of two neurotic behavior patterns – in promiscuity and drinking – in this typically adolescent way of showing masculinity and a tough independent spirit.

The explanation of this metamorphosis will be found in the analytical material, by means of which we have in part recovered and in part reconstructed those emotional experiences which deflected the course of the patient's masculine development and broke the spirit of this promising young man.

[4] See note 3, p. 141

The history of the emotional development.
For a long period during his treatment, the patient's memory material consisted mostly of recollections of defeats and failures, intimidations and inhibitions. The early period of aggressive leadership did not appear in his associations, was obviously overshadowed by gloomy memories dealing mostly with his internal insecurity, with a continuous struggle against his inhibitions. Although the intimidating experiences which gradually led to the development of an extremely inhibited personality go back to his early childhood, it was not before puberty that they visibly influenced the overt picture and changed his relationship to his brothers from leadership into a slow but continuous falling back.

For a long period the patient did not recall at all the extreme rage outbreaks characteristic of his earliest childhood. This free expression of anger in childhood is in such a contrast to his later inability to express any hostile feeling, that it can only be explained by a later extreme repression of all hostile impulses. This might account for the fact that he forgot this early aggressive attitude to an astonishing degree and that memories about his early aggressive behavior and temper tantrums were recovered only in the progressed phase of his analysis.

One of his earliest memories is that when 3 or 4 years old he climbed up on his father's back, fell and suffered a concussion. About in the same age, he remembered the first spanking by his father who punished him for his violent temper. After this punishment the patient felt extremely humiliated. It was mentioned before that in the first school years he openly rebelled against school routine and was continually punished.

Right at the beginning of his treatment he recalled a series of external events of intimidating nature.

When he was 4 years old he fell into water and was almost drowned. From this incident, he retained up to the present date some fear of diving.

When he was 5 years old, in kindergarten, he locked himself into a closet with another boy, could not get out and became extremely panicky.

When he was five he locked himself out on a playing porch on the third floor, and when he tried to climb down, he fell down one story.

One of his most outstanding memories is of an older man who took him and his brothers out fishing, but then because of his unruly behavior, wrapped him up with a fishline. He never could forget the impotent rage which he felt being bound up this way. Struggle against external pressure was one of the leading motives in his associations.

The most serious intimidations were, however, connected with his sexual feelings. His sexual curiosity appeared early in the prepuberty period and occupied most of his interest. As long as he can remember, he always felt extremely shy and timid toward girls. Everything connected with sex, he considered low and dirty but at the same time he had an extreme longing for it. As an adolescent, he did not dare to touch even the hands of a girl. His first sexual intercourse was with a prostitute, when he was 17 years old. Afterward, he felt morally soiled. He confessed immediately to his mother and did not dare to give in to his sexual impulses again until he was 21 years old. After this time he had casual sexual relationships, but after them always felt terrifically degraded.

In a later period of his analysis he was able to remember probably his first sexual trauma. When 3 or 4 years old, his father caught him masturbating and reprimanded him. About the same time he had a recurrent nightmare of an ogre which appeared at the end of a dark corridor and threatened him.

His father, who died when the patient was 12 years old, played apparently the most important rôle as an object of fear and hostility. He thought that he ought to break the boy's aggressive spirit and rebelliousness against every external pressure and routine and made a point of teaching him how to lose. Patient was about 8 years old when his father began to take him out to the golf course, beat him at golf repeatedly and tried to make him like to be beaten. Patient remembered his senseless rage when he was beaten in any competitive game. It is interesting that even at his present age, the patient has the greatest dislike to go out to play golf with his chief. Whenever the chief asked him to go out to play golf, he wanted to refuse, did not dare to, accepted the invitation, but for days after, the analytic hours would be filled with broodings of the following kind: 'Why did I accept? Why couldn't I say to the boss – "No, I won't go".' In spite of this overt rebellion, his dream material gave ample evidence of the fact that this submission appealed deep down to his passive feminine longings and was a source of unconscious gratification for him.

The most important factor, however, which contributed to breaking his spirit was unquestionably the extreme inhibition of his premature and intense sexual desires by the very strict moral code of his environment and particularly his family. The so common puritanical rejection of everything related to sex was unusually pronounced in his childhood attitude.

Gradually the external intimidation by his father, school discipline, and the moral pressure of his environment, became internalized in the form of a severe conscience, the source of his intensive and continuous guilt feelings. Every manifestation of sexual interest, of aggressiveness and competition became connected with a sense of guilt. He could not win without feeling guilty for it: as a result of this guilt feeling a powerful internal self-thwarting attitude has developed in him. These unconscious guilt feelings explain why, when he later became a business executive, he never could discipline or dismiss anyone without the most severe remorse and self-accusation. He had several dreams in which he first was in the superior position and then compulsively had to identify himself with the underdog.

This self-thwarting attitude was the basis of his extreme self-consciousness, insecurity, inhibition about speaking publicly and persistent fear of losing his leadership. Only this self-inhibiting influence of his overly severe conscience can account for his gradual slipping back in scholastic achievements and athletics, in relation to his brothers. From early puberty on his life consisted of a desperate struggle against this internal self-thwarting tendency trying in vain to retain his former superior position. When his younger brother once made a remark that on one day of the year they are the same age, he threw him on the floor, shouting at him: 'You may be the same age, but you never will have my physical power.'

In school and college this struggle centered around scholastic and athletic achievements, and later during his married life, around income and social prestige. In his adult years his social circle took over the rôle of the competitor which his two brothers played in his youth.

It is not my purpose to give the full case history, only as much as is necessary to substantiate the following dynamic reconstruction of his emotional development.

This aggressive, and intellectually and physically outstanding young boy reacted to the external pressures he met in his early life, such as school routine and other customary restrictions of the latency period, with rebellion. This provoked his father who rationalised his emotional reaction to his son's aggressiveness with some educational theory and tried to break this little rebellious Oedipus. It seems that he succeeded only too well. As has been mentioned before, this submission to his father to which the little boy first gave in under external compulsion, gradually became erotized, or in other words, a source of a feminine gratification. As it can be so often observed, the ego made the best out of a painful situation. At first he was forced to submit and did it under protest; later gradually he began to like it. It must be emphasized, however, that this feminine masochistic attitude remained always unconscious in him. His conscious ego dominated by masculine pride never would admit it openly. This unconscious, masochistically colored, feminine, dependent attitude in combination with the more diffuse and intangible but equally powerful moral pressure, mainly represented by his mother, prepared the ground for the extreme sexual inhibitions and guilt feeling which the boy began to show after his eighth year. These sexual inhibitions hit his masculine self-confidence in its core.

As a continuation of the external intimidations his guilt feeling toward his brothers, forced him towards the *inferior position* which already previously had become erotized in relation to his father. Yet the previous position of superiority and leadership developed in him a sense of obligation to live up to the high expectations which everyone had toward him. Tired by these permanent efforts to maintain his leading position, he developed a keen longing for the comfortable dependent though inferior rôle of the small child. The birth of his younger brother, when he was 11 years old, unquestionably contributed to this regressive longing for the carefree position of the small child. While he had to make desperate efforts to hold on to his leadership and continue to play the rôle of the hero, there was the example of his little brother pampered by the mother and enjoying a comfortable carefree existence. His alcoholism – as became fully evident during the analysis – served the purpose of solving this conflict by satisfying both of the conflicting tendencies. On the one hand drinking meant for him a rebellious act, gave him a spurious feeling of superiority, eliminated his inhibitions, enabled him to give in to his promiscuous sexual tendencies, but on the other hand the alcohol bottle represented the milk bottle and the feeding mother. Intoxication gave him the same relaxed Nirvana feeling which he probably experienced in his earliest infancy during the act of suckling.

II. Relation Between Emotional Tensions and Fluctuations of Blood Pressure

Among all the dynamic forces which participated in this complex dynamic equilibrium, the rebellious aggressive tendencies and the concomitant anxiety stood in direct relationship to the fluctuations of the patient's blood pressure. Although he never could express freely these hostile aggressive impulses, they were not deeply repressed into the unconscious. They appeared in aggressive fantasies or during his depressions in self-destructive attitudes. Whenever they were mobilized, his blood pressure rose, whereas in those periods in which he was relatively calm the blood pressure fell.

I shall submit now the observations concerning the relationship of emotional status and blood pressure readings.

At the beginning and the end of every analytic session the blood pressure of this patient was measured by a mercury sphygmomanometer and compared with the emotional state of the patient and the details of the analytic material. The blood pressure was taken at first by a physician who did not treat the patient and then by the analyst in order to establish the influence of special emotional reactions towards the analyst. However, in the vast majority of readings there was no noticable difference between the two readings. Furthermore, both observers took several readings.

These observations in table I can be summarized as follows: In 201 sessions the patient's blood pressure was taken and compared with his emotional state. In 41 interviews the patient's emotional state was

Table I

I Emotional state: very disturbed 1937		II Emotional state: somewhat disturbed 1937			1938		III Emotional state: calm 1937	
March	1	160/120	March	4	150/104	Jan.	5	150/108	March 19	138/ 92
March	2	158/112	March	5	168/118	Jan.	10	152/104	March 22	136/ 94
March	8	162/104	March 16		140/ 96	Jan.	11	152/104	March 26	138/ 96
March 24		160/104	March 17		160/106	Jan.	12	136/ 98	April	1	142/ 96
March 31		158/112	March 18		146/ 98	Jan.	28	158/106	April	2	140/100
May	7	160/110	March 23		152/102	Feb.	1	156/102	April	3	140/ 94
May	17	164/128	April	23	140/106	Feb.	8	148/100	April	6	136/ 92
May	25	174/124	April	25	138/102	Feb.	9	150/104	April	22	150/110
May	27	160/110	April	28	152/102	Feb.	10	140/102	April	27	164/120
June	1	154/114	May	4	136/106	Feb.	11	144/ 92	May	8	132/ 98
June	2	164/104	May	5	144/104	Feb.	14	148/100	May	24	142/106
June	10	172/122	May	6	154/110	Feb.	15	148/102	June	7	148/108
June	15	154/104	May	18	160/110	Feb.	16	146/100	Sept.	10	128/ 90
June	17	160/106	May	21	150/110	Feb.	21	150/108	Sept.	14	152/106
July	2	142/102	May	26	147/103	Feb.	23	142/ 94	Oct.	4	140/100
Sept.	28	168/112	June	3	136/ 96	Feb.	25	140/ 94	Oct.	12	142/106
Sept.	29	174/120	June	4	150/110	Feb.	28	140/ 98	Oct.	18	146/ 98

Table I (continued)

I Emotional state: very disturbed 1937		II Emotional state: somewhat disturbed 1937		1938		III Emotional state: calm 1937	
Sept. 30	164/110	June 8	148/106	March 1	158/106	Oct. 19	142/100
Oct. 1	158/112	June 9	148/108	March 4	148/ 98	Nov. 2	142/102
Oct. 11	156/110	June 11	154/104	March 7	150/100	Nov. 5	146/ 98
Nov. 3	158/110	June 14	146/116	March 16	144/ 98	Nov. 8	138/ 94
Nov. 17	160/110	June 16	144/106	March 21	138/100	Nov. 11	140/ 98
Nov. 18	160/108	June 18	156/110	March 22	146/ 98	Nov. 12	140/ 98
Dec. 13	166/112	June 29	158/106	March 28	142/102	Nov. 15	140/ 96
Dec. 14	160/112	June 30	146/104	April 6	148/110	Nov. 16	144/102
Dec. 23	170/118	July 1	156/106	April 13	144/104	Nov. 29	148/106
		July 4	152/106	April 15	142/100	Dec. 3	148/100
1938		Sept. 9	146/104	April 18	150/112	Dec. 15	148/110
Jan. 6	168/114	Sept. 13	146/106	April 22	156/108	1938	
Jan. 14	156/106	Sept. 16	150/104	April 23	150/106	Jan. 4	140/108
Jan. 24	166/112	Sept. 20	152/110	April 24	154/106	Jan. 17	140/ 90
Feb. 4	150/106	Sept. 21	162/112	May 5	152/108	Jan. 18	146/ 96
Feb. 7	150/106	Sept. 27	152/106	May 9	144/108	Jan. 19	140/ 96
April 20	158/104	Oct. 25	170/120	May 11	152/106	Jan. 20	136/ 98
April 25	152/102	Oct. 26	156/114	May 19	154/104	Jan. 21	136/ 92
April 27	158/106	Oct. 27	154/110	May 20	154/106	Feb. 2	144/ 92
May 1	166/116	Oct. 28	152/108	May 24	152/120	Feb. 17	134/ 92
May 2	156/112	Oct. 29	146/108	Oct. 3	158/110	Feb. 18	142/100
May 21	162/110	Nov. 4	150/108	Nov. 3	146/104	Feb. 24	142/ 96
Oct. 11	166/110	Nov. 9	146/100	Nov. 7	156/102	March 8	146/100
Oct. 12	146/104	Nov. 10	144/102	Nov. 8	166/108	March 10	146/ 98
Oct. 13	170/110	Nov. 19	162/112	Nov. 9	144/ 96	March 11	142/ 96
Oct. 14	148/106	Nov. 22	148/102	Nov. 14	148/ 96	March 17	144/ 98
		Nov. 24	148/104	Nov. 16	146/104	March 18	136/ 92
Average:	160/111	Nov. 26	148/104	Nov. 17	150/100	March 29	136/ 98
		Nov. 30	152/106	Nov. 18	150/112	April 14	136/100
		Dec. 1	150/108			April 19	138/104
		Dec. 2	140/108	Average:	149/105	May 4	138/106
		Dec. 6	152/104			May 10	142/104
		Dec. 16	152/110			May 12	142/100
		Dec. 20	164/112			May 16	146/102
		Dec. 21	164/102			May 26	132/ 96
		Dec. 24	152/108			May 31	132/100
						June 1	148/102
						Sept. 8	132/100
						Sept. 9	138/106
						Oct. 4	140/ 98
						Oct. 5	140/ 98
						Oct. 6	144/ 96
						Oct. 7	132/ 92
						Nov. 4	140/102
						Nov. 15	150/106
						Average:	141/ 99

Table II. In sober state

I Emotional state: very disturbed 1937	II Emotional state: somewhat disturbed 1937	1938	III Emotional state: calm 1937
March 1 160/120	March 4 150/104	Jan. 10 152/104	March 19 138/ 92
March 2 158/112	March 5 168/118	Jan. 28 158/106	April 1 142/ 96
March 31 158/112	March 16 140/ 96	Feb. 1 156/102	April 2 140/100
May 25 174/124	March 17 160/106	Feb. 8 148/100	April 3 140/ 94
May 27 160/110	March 18 146/ 98	Feb. 9 150/104	April 6 136/ 92
June 2 164/104	April 25 138/102	Feb. 10 140/102	May 24 142/106
June 15 154/104	May 6 154/110	Feb. 11 144/ 92	Nov. 2 142/102
June 17 160/106	May 18 160/110	Feb. 14 148/100	Nov. 5 146/ 98
Sept. 28 168/112	May 21 150/110	Feb. 15 148/102	Nov. 8 138/ 94
Sept. 29 174/120	May 26 147/103	Feb. 16 146/100	Nov. 11 140/ 98
Sept. 30 164/110	June 3 136/ 96	Feb. 23 142/ 94	Nov. 12 140/ 98
Nov. 3 158/110	June 4 150/110	Feb. 25 140/ 94	Nov. 15 140/ 96
Nov. 17 160/110	June 8 148/106	March 1 158/106	Nov. 16 144/102
Dec. 14 160/112	June 11 154/104	March 4 148/ 98	Nov. 29 148/106
	June 14 146/116	March 7 150/100	Dec. 3 148/100
1938	June 16 144/106	March 22 146/ 98	Dec. 15 148/110
Feb. 7 150/106	June 18 156/110	April 13 144/104	1938
April 20 158/104	July 4 152/106	April 22 156/108	Jan. 17 140/ 90
April 25 152/102	Sept. 20 152/110	April 23 150/106	Jan. 18 146/ 96
April 27 158/106	Nov. 4 150/108	April 24 154/106	Jan. 19 140/ 96
	Nov. 9 146/100	Nov. 7 156/102	Jan. 21 136/ 92
Average: 161/110	Nov. 10 144/102	Nov. 8 166/108	Feb. 2 144/ 92
	Nov. 19 162/112	Nov. 9 144/ 96	Feb. 17 134/ 94
	Nov. 22 148/102	Nov. 14 148/ 96	Feb. 18 142/100
	Nov. 26 148/104	Nov. 16 146/104	Feb. 24 142/ 96
	Nov. 30 152/106	Nov. 17 150/100	March 8 146/100
	Dec. 1 150/108	Nov. 18 150/112	March 10 146/ 98
	Dec. 2 140/108		March 11 142/ 96
	Dec. 6 152/104	Average: 150/104	March 17 144/ 98
	Dec. 16 152/110		March 18 136/ 92
	Dec. 20 164/112		April 14 136/100
	Dec. 21 164/102		May 12 142/100
			Oct. 6 144/ 96
			Nov. 15 150/106
			Average: 142/ 98

very disturbed, in 99 interviews *somewhat disturbed,* and in 61 interviews the patient was subjectively *calm.*

His average blood pressure on the basis of all readings was 149/105. During the very disturbed interviews, the average blood pressure was 160/111 and in the calm interviews 141/99. There were only two very disturbed sessions in which he had a rela-tively low blood pressure, and both occur-red on a day after he had consumed a con-siderable amount of alcohol. Otherwise the blood pressure functioned almost as a barometer of his emotional state, being high when the patient is emotionally dis-turbed and lower when he is calm.

Because the patient came to a great number of the analytic sessions after consuming alcohol the question arose as to the direct effect of alcohol upon the blood pressure. In order to eliminate this complication, in the following chart only those blood pressure readings are considered which were taken when the patient was entirely sober.

As is seen in table II here there is no exception from the rule, namely that during the very disturbed sessions his blood pressure is relatively high (average 161/110 mm) during the calm sessions considerably lower (average 142/98 mm).

These observations show a clear correlation between emotional disturbances and change of blood pressure. It is important that in those days when the patient felt calm, did not show emotional conflicts, his blood pressure was only a little above normal. Therefore one is justified in saying that whenever a marked elevation of his blood pressure above normal was observed, it regularly coincided with a disturbed emotional state.

During the majority of the interviews the blood pressure remained about the same at the end of the session as it was at the beginning. In a number of sessions the blood pressure dropped or raised considerably – 15 to 20 points. It is noteworthy that the examination of the analytical material during the sessions when the blood pressure dropped, showed marked relief from emotional tension, whereas in the hours when it rose, it showed increased resistance and discomfort.

The nature of the emotional state which was connected with elevation of the blood pressure can be briefly characterized as a depressed, tense, apprehensive mood, sometimes mixed with some aggressive irritation which, however, the patient never expressed openly but only referred to it in a descriptive calm fashion. When depressed, the patient turned against himself, depreciated himself and his work in many different ways. Such depressive states usually were connected with fearful apprehension. He was concerned lest on account of his inefficiency – which to be sure was merely

imagined – he would lose his job and would not be able to support his family. Then his only escape would be suicide. In other sessions his self-destructive attitude was mixed with anger and embitterment directed against his superior but he never expressed these feelings in an emotional, dramatic fashion. Ideas of physically attacking his chief were not uncommon. In the course of his associations these aggressive thoughts regularly led to anxiety and then to self-accusations and self-depreciation. The consecutive phases of this emotional process could be clearly observed, how his hostile impulses created guilt and fear, then became inhibited and then like a boomerang turned back against his own self.

There is no doubt that the dynamic nucleus of his emotional difficulties consisted of hostile impulses. These led to fear and guilt and as the next step to his depressions. His emotional condition could be best characterized as a state of inhibited hostile aggressive impulses.

In the last part of his analysis, the patient lost entirely his depressions, and his emotional tension appeared only in the form of a tense feeling and some vague irritability. Most significant is the fact that during a period of two months during which the patient's emotional difficulties were reduced to a minimum, when he had no apprehensions about his job, felt calm and contented, his blood pressure did not show the usual extensive fluctuations: his systolic pressure, with the exception of one day, did not surpass 150 mm; in the last three weeks of this period his diastolic pressure with the exception of one day never exceeded 100 mm. This is therefore significant, because viewing the whole period of the analysis, the variations of his systolic pressure were between 175 mm and 136 mm and of the diastolic pressure between 120 mm and 92 mm.

This analysis is still in progress. One cannot, therefore, as yet draw definite therapeutic conclusions from it, especially not concerning the hypertensive state. So much can be stated, however, that in the course of the analysis the patient has almost entirely recovered from his depressions and has his alcoholic tendencies under much better control. The analysis still cannot be considered as completed because although the depressions and apprehensions have disappeared, and the irritation towards his chief has completely subsided, the patient is still under considerable emotional tension, the ideational content of which is much less defined, however, than it was before. This tension consists mostly in a rebellious feeling against every external routine, and limitation. This emotional tension is definitely less than it was before, it has more openly an aggressive connotation and is not turned against himself in the form of depressions and self-accusations. So far as the blood pressure is concerned, in the last eight months the trend was toward a slow but definite decrease of both systolic and diastolic pressures. The day by day fluctuations have been around a somewhat lower level and their range is definitely smaller, with the exception of a period of a few weeks when an extremely traumatic external event upset the patient's emotional equilibrium to a considerable degree. A definite therapeutic conclusion will be possible only if the analysis succeeds in further diminishing the patient's chronic emotional tensions.

Summary

The day by day blood pressure fluctuations of a 47 year old male suffering from a chronic depression, chronic alcoholism and essential hypertension, have been compared with the daily psychoanalytic material. The patient's overt personality has been described and the underlying psychodynamic personality structure reconstructed and explained in the light of the emotional development which led up to the adult personality.

A definite correlation has been found between emotional tensions and fluctuations of the blood pressure. The nature of the emotional tensions has been identified as inhibited, but not deeply repressed aggressive impulses directed partly inward against the patient's own person in the form of depressions, partly turned outwards in the form of hostile feelings. These emotional states were mixed with an apprehensive worrisome state of mind. Finally it was observed that during a period in which the patient was in an exceptionally calm state, his blood pressure was definitely lower and showed considerably smaller fluctuations. During the last period of treatment, with the diminution of the emotional tensions, there was a slow but definite decrease of the day by day fluctuations, and a slow downward tendency of the average blood pressure level.

References

1. ALEXANDER, F.; BACON, C.; WILSON, G.; LEVEY, H. B., and LEVINE, M.: The influence of psychological factors upon gastrointestinal disturbances: A symposium, Psychoanal. Quart. *3:* 501–588 (1934).
2. ALEXANDER, F. and HEALY, W.: The roots of crime (Knopf, New York 1935).
3. CANNON, W. B.: Bodily changes in pain, hunger, fear and rage (Appleton-Century Company, New York 1934).
4. DOSTOJEVSKY, F.: Crime and punishment (Grosset and Dunlap, New York 1927).
5. FALLADA, H.: The world outside (Simon and Schuster, New York 1934).
6. HORNEY, K.: The neurotic personality of our time (Norton and Company, New York 1937).

Possible Etiologic Relevance
of Personality Factors in Arterial Hypertension[1]

G. Saslow, G. C. Gressel, F. O. Shobe, P. H. DuBois and H. A. Schroeder

Retrospective comment by Dr. R. Harris. Following on the early clinical psychiatric studies of hypertensives by Alexander and Binger, Saslow and his colleagues attempted a more rigorous study of the role of psychological factors in the development of high blood pressure. Their study introduced: (1) Careful definitions and quantification of the psychological variables, habitual patterns of reaction to crisis and of inter-personal relations, and (2) two control groups without hypertension, one with personality disorders and the other neurotic disorders.

Their findings of greater degrees of *obsessive-compulsive behavior* and *subnormal assertiveness* in the hypertensives have come to be widely cited in the literature of hypertension, and later studies have reported similar results.

One may perhaps quarrel with their classification of hypertension. They include in their 'essential' group endocrine and renal disorders, and eleven of their fifty 'essentials' were associated with pregnancy. Perhaps their 'neurogenic' category corresponds more closely to conventional definitions of essential hypertension. Incidentally, the absence of differences between their neurogenics and others (endocrine, renal and mixed) was later replicated by Ostfeld and Lebovits, and remains a puzzling problem. Why should the personality characteristics of patients with and without a physical disorder which is presumably adequate to account for elevated pressures be so similar?

The authors' discussion bears repeated reading. It contains: an excellent statement of what is required to 'prove' a psychosomatic hypothesis; a reminder of the distinction between necessary and sufficient causes; and citations from many kinds of observations to buttress the plausibility of an etiological relationship.

Numerous students of this subject have concluded that personality malfunctioning is unusually frequent in hypertensives. The general pattern of maladjustment in interpersonal relations (in such persons) has been variously considered to be habitual unexpressed or displaced hostility [1, 4, 21, 23, 24, 27, 30]; life-long emotional lability with frequent depression, anxiety, or both [10, 23]; lifelong anxiety, perfectionism, compulsiveness, difficulty with authority [4, 6]. The studies have rarely involved more than a few subjects, and have rarely included nonhypertensives for comparison; hence the comparative frequencies of occurrence of various possibly relevant personality patterns in hypertensives and nonhypertensives are not known.

As part of a comprehensive study of hypertension, we have decided therefore to examine this matter afresh. After careful review of our own and others' experience, we have taken our departure from the following points:

1. The presence or absence of a relevant crisis in the habitual pattern of life of the subject is not likely to be a helpful indicator. Weiss [27] was not satisfied that he could establish the presence of such crises in more than a few of 93 subjects; but Dunbar [6] considered that such crises had been detected in 90 per cent of her subjects. Our own experience is like Weiss's: the

[1] From the Departments of Neuropsychiatry, Psychology, and Internal Medicine of Washington University, St. Louis, Mo.

detection of hypertension need be associated with no crisis that is temporally or otherwise significant.

2. The presence or absence of specific patterns of the earliest childhood conditioning is not likely to be a helpful indicator. Such patterns are exceedingly difficult to establish, and even more difficult to establish as to comparative frequency in a representative sample of hypertensives and nonhypertensives. Thus ALEXANDER [1] reported 1 case, SAUL [24] described 7. 'Theoretical' predictions of such frequencies have been based upon the prolonged study of a few subjects [11, p. 99], in the related field of gastrointestinal psychosomatic disorders; but apparently such predictions are premature generalizations, for they are completely contradicted by a careful study of the same problem by KLEIN [18]: very few of her 100 subjects had had the predicted life-long preoccupation with the intestinal tract; or had had diarrhea, constipation, or feeding or eating difficulties in childhood. In any case, such specific patterns if present presumably have correlates in the later recurrent patterns of interpersonal relations and of reaction to crisis; these are easier to study, and have not yet been studied, as to comparative frequency of occurrence.

3. It does not seem probable that a specific 'personality structure' will be found to distinguish hypertensives from subjects with other accepted 'psychosomatic affections' (asthma, ulcer, colitis, etc.). HALLIDAY [11, p. 51], who in one place writes as if a specific personality structure (symbolized by 'preoccupation with security' or 'preoccupation with work' etc.) does correspond to a given psychosomatic affection, contradicts himself in subsequent places [e.g. p. 52] where he points out that the same person may have several psychosomatic affections during his life either simultaneously or in irregular succession and that it is hardly conceivable that his 'personality structure' is multiple or changes each time. Careful reading of HALLIDAY's examples of specific personality structures shows that, in persons with psychosomatic affections, we are dealing with a) a general pattern of interpersonal relations, involving over-inhibition, over-conformity; displaced, delayed, or inadequate overt emotional expression, and the like; and b) diverse verbal symbolizations of this pattern related to the diverse early verbal conditionings associated with inculcation of the general pattern. That there is such a general pattern in such persons is our own experience, and likewise that of LUDWIG [20]. There are other observations of the occurrence of more than one psychosomatic affection in one subject [3].

4. It seems to us reasonable, therefore, as a firstorder approximation, to compare the frequencies of certain types of personality functioning in hypertensives as a group with the frequencies in two other groups from which the more common other psychosomatic affections are excluded (asthma, colitis, rheumatoid arthritis, migraine, ulcer). The inclusion of other psychosomatic disorders in the control population might serve only to blur distinctions indicated by the crude methods with which we must begin.

5. From what has been said above, it seems reasonable also to compare the groups in terms of, a) habitual patterns of interpersonal relations, or habitual patterns of reaction to crisis, b) patterns which could be described fairly explicitly, and c) (for purposes of statistical analysis) patterns which show several discriminable degrees of severity of disability.

6. Since patterns of personality disorder (and presumably of habitual personality functioning) differ in frequency in diverse groups that differ in population density of community of origin, dominant stock in the cultural pattern, education, occupation and socio-economic level, color, and sex [14], the 3 groups compared were matched for these or similar characteristics. Individual matching was not feasible. The degree of group matching achieved is shown in table I.

Table I. Composition of the groups studied

	Group I (50 subjects)		Group II (49 subjects)		Group III (44 subjects)	
	No. of subjects	Percentage*	No. of subjects	Percentage*	No. of subjects	Percentage*
Age						
20–35 yr. [1]	9	18	21	43	12	27
36–50 [1]	25	50	15	31	18	41
51+[1]	16	32	13	27	14	32
Sex						
Male	16	32	15	31	16	36
Female	34	68	34	69	28	64
Color						
White	44	88	43	88	38	86
Negro	6	12	6	12	6	14
Education						
3–8 yr.	31	62	27	55	28	64
9–12 yr.	12	24	16	34	11	25
13+ yr.	7	14	6	12	5	11
Habitat						
Rural[2]	10	20	13	27	15	34
Mixed[3]	2	4	4	8	6	14
Urban[4]	38	76	32	65	23	52
Culture						
American	39	78	42	86	42	95
European	11	22	7	14	2	5
Occupation						
class[5] 0	1	2	1	2	0	0
1	7	14	13	27	16	36
2	8	16	9	18	3	7
3	4	8	0	0	0	0
4	23	46	21	43	22	50
5	7	14	5	10	3	7
6	0	0	0	0	0	0

* Percentage to nearest whole number.

[1] For convenience, only these age groups are used in the table. In the computation of coefficients of correlation, age was coded in 11 steps.

[2] More than 10 years of early life in a community of less than 2,500 population.

[3] One to 10 years of incidental residence in a rural area, but not on an operating farm.

[4] Never lived on a farm or in a rural area.

[5] Occupational class (listing modified from KINSEY and his co-workers [17]: 0, dependent, if adult other than a spouse, and completely dependent; 1, day labor and semi-skilled labor; 2, skilled labor, lower and upper white collar group; 3, professional group, business executives, the extremely wealthy; 4, a minor or spouse dependent upon supporting adult of class 1; 5, a minor or spouse dependent upon supporting adult of class 2; 6, a minor or spouse dependent upon supporting adult of class 3.

156 SASLOW/GRESSEL/SHOBE/DUBOIS/SCHROEDER

7. The groups should be matched approximately as to age, since the frequency of hypertension varies with age.

8. There are different types of essential hypertension: neurogenic, endocrine, renal, mixed, etc. [25]. These groups need to be considered separately, before we can be sure they are homogeneous as to personality functioning.

9. There are different stages of essential hypertension [16]. These need to be considered separately until we can be sure they are homogeneous as to personality function. The present report does not take adequate account of this variable.

10. It is possible that an unknown number of our nonhypertensive subjects are 'prehypertensives.' The effectiveness of the cold-pressor test in detecting prehypertensives is uncertain [22]. Hence, for the present, groups have not been matched so that 'hyperreactors' have been identified and excluded from groups II and III (nonhypertensives).

Method

Some 50 consecutive subjects with essential hypertension were studied (group I). They were referred to us after necessary medical studies had been made, and the diagnosis established. The sources of referral were, a) internists on the staff of Washington University School of Medicine, b) the teaching medical wards of Barnes Hospital, and c) the Hypertension Clinic of the medical school. All necessary medical studies were carried out by the hypertension research group under the direction of one of us (H.A.S.). The patients met the criteria, a) of having sustained blood pressure values exceeding 140 mm of mercury systolic, and 90 mm of mercury diastolic, b) of having essential hypertension, c) (after psychiatric evaluation) of being nonpsychotic.

The composition of group I was tabulated, in relation to age, sex, education, etc. Attempt was then made to match this composition with about 50 subjects (group II) chosen consecutively. In addition to meeting the matching criteria, the subjects in group II, a) had had careful medical study, b) had had several blood pressures recorded during such study, with no

readings exceeding 140 systolic, 90 diastolic, c) had been diagnosed as psychiatrically ill in a clinic for psychosomatic medicine conducted by one of us (G.S.), or in our work with hospital psychiatric referrals or private psychiatric patients (G.S., F.O.S.), d) were not psychotic, e) did not have one of the more common accepted psychosomatic disorders (asthma, ulcer, etc.). Many of this group had been studied and treated psychiatrically just before the present investigation began; the necessary data were obtained from their clinic, office, and hospital records, wherever these records were adequate.

In a similar way, we attempted to study about 50 subjects (group III) who, in addition to meeting the matching criteria, had, a) chronic medical or surgical disorder, in which psychologic factors are considered to have low etiologic relevance[2], b) were not psychotic. Sources of referral were medical and surgical services of Barnes Hospital. All of this group were interviewed specifically for this investigation, while they were in hospital. Their records did not have the necessary data.

Comparative composition of the groups, in terms of the matching criteria, is shown in table I.

The personality ratings of many of the group I subjects had been carried out before work was begun on groups II and III. This occurred as a natural consequence of having started with the hypertensives, more of whom needed to be studied before we could set up a set of matching criteria, as in table I, against which prospective members of groups II and III could be judged as suitable for study. About half the ratings were made as group judgments (G.C.G., F.O.S., G.S.); the rest were made by only one of us. During group discussions, only rarely did differences of opinion about a rating exceed one unit on the scale for a given pattern. The data used for rating were obtained in psychiatric interviews. For groups I and III from one to four interviews were used, as a rule; where necessary, more. For group II (patients undergoing or who had undergone psychotherapy), many

[2] Examples of the disorders present in subjects of group III, are: bronchiectasis, cystic disease of lung, Hodgkin's disease, hypoplastic anemia, sickle cell anemia, cirrhosis (nonalcoholic), lymphoma, pernicious anemia, Addison's disease, chronic otitis media, carcinoma.

more interviews were available; we did not notice that there were any significant changes in our ratings depending upon our use of the first few interviews, or the use of the entire set of interviews. No overall tabulation of the data was begun until the investigation was nearly completed. The careful classification of the subjects with hypertension (as to type of hypertension) was carried out with Dr. SCHROEDER's assistance, towards the end of the investigation.

For the personality ratings, we experimented with a number of habitual patterns of reaction to crisis, and of interpersonal relations, of which only the following seemed feasible to use: hysteria, anxiety, depression, obsessive-compulsive behavior, subnormal assertiveness, impulsiveness. We dropped excessive insecurity, inhibited impulsiveness, precipitating crisis, and various others.

The patterns were rated on the scale 0, 1, 2, 3, 4. Samples of the definitions of the patterns at the different rating levels follow.

Impulsiveness

0. Very infrequently acts on impulse, and only in minor matters.

1. More impulsive than average of his fellows, life-long pattern. Gets on fairly well. Infrequent outbursts with consequent loss of spouse, friends, jobs.

2. Regularly has difficulty, with spouse, subordinates, co-workers, superiors etc., because of impulsive actions. Rare anti-social actions (e.g. stealing, sexual deviations) but in general manages to stay within social bounds.

3. Life-long history of impulsive actions, with severe childhood conflicts with authority, some police experience, frequent change of sex partner or of job, or similar actions. No remorse. Considered not desirable by most in the community.

4. Life-long anti-social behavior, with no remorse. Frequent and severe difficulty with the law (stealing, sex 'crimes', homicide); chronic alcoholism; behavior compatible with that of primary or secondary psychopathic personality [16].

Subnormal Assertiveness[3]

0. Regularly expresses his views, differences, dislikes, in nearly all interpersonal relations; occasional antagonism provoked by him.

1. Shows appropriate assertiveness regularly in at least one major area of interpersonal relations (family, work, school, church, army, etc.); but as a rule in most other areas experiences impulses to differ, to be hostile, etc. without appropriate overt activity; can easily verbalize the felt resentment, anger, disappointment, etc., at such times.

2. Rarely shows overt assertiveness; when he does, experiences distress (anxiety, guilt), tends to overshoot the mark, and subsequently withdraws to habitual pattern or for a time becomes excessively ingratiating, submissive, apologetic, etc.

3. Has hardly ever shown overt assertiveness since childhood; is aware of feelings of anger or hostility, but has difficulty verbalizing these even to physician.

4. Practically never shows overt assertiveness, denies any awareness of hostile feelings or attitudes, but makes excuses for persons who mis-use him (as authority figures).

Obsessive-compulsive Behavior

0. No history elicited of habitual or recurrently episodic meticulousness, over-conscientiousness, ruminative thinking, repetitive acting, or ritualistic behavior.

1. Habitual or recurrently episodic meticulousness, etc. (as above), which do not decrease subject's general effectiveness, and do not produce symptoms.

2. Habitual or recurrently episodic meticulousness, etc., with noticeable associated decrease in general effectiveness or associated presence of symptoms. The repetitive and other patterns can be interrupted without production of great anxiety.

3. Well-established repetitive thinking, acting, etc., with obvious disorganization, or anxiety symptoms resulting directly from interruption of the patterns.

[3] We have used this relatively impersonal term to connote a group of phenomena having to do with the individual's 'trend toward increased autonomy' (ANGYAL, A.: Foundations for a Science of Personality. New York, Oxford University Press, 1941): spontaneity, initiative, aggressiveness, difference, anger, hostility and hatred; and their overt expression. The ratings emphasize the facts that so many of our subjects have decided inability to show overt expression of impulse that is appropriately graded, directed, and timed, and that they live in a state of habitual recurrent blocking of impulses to act, punctuated by covert or overt explosions of dysfunction.

4. Disabling obsessive-compulsive neurosis, as handwashing neurosis, with inability to carry on life pattern like that of subject's peers.

Depressive Behavior
0. Very infrequent sadness, in relation to habitual mood.
1. Mild but definite episodic sadness or reduced activity level ('sad', 'blue', 'down in the dumps'). Decrease in social life, slight changes in sleep pattern, or in appetite. Changes not obvious to casual friends.
2. Marked changes in appetite, sleep, energy level, social activity, self-esteem, outlook for the future, mood, ability to concentrate. May be much crying. Occasional suicide ideas, no serious attempts. Able to sustain major obligations (work, family, etc.), but with decreased efficiency. Changes noticeable to casual lay observer.
3. Changes more severe than in 2. Except under special circumstances, unable to sustain major obligations. Marked reduction of interaction with people. Maintains contact with reality.
4. Psychotic depression: maximal withdrawal from interactional activity. Little speech. May need to be fed.

Anxiety
0. Anxiety symptoms (heart pounding, sweating, fear, overbreathing, blurred vision, etc.) only in close temporal relation to a severe on-going disruption of the habitual pattern of life (crisis), such as bereavement, loss of job, loss of career, etc.
1. Anxiety symptoms in close temporal relation to on-going moderately severe crisis, e.g., jilting in a casual affair, definite but not serious fall in scholastic standing, subject's child ill with influenza, etc. Symptoms appear excessive in duration and intensity, in relation to the crisis as met by similar subjects.
2. Frequent anxiety symptoms in relation to recurrent ordinary hazards, difficulties, frustrations, memories of unhappy events, anticipations of anniversaries of unhappy events. Symptoms soon cease when stimulus ceases; source of symptoms fairly easily demonstrated.
3. As above, but with anxiety symptoms of much longer duration after being set up; relationship to evoking situation not easily demonstrated; definite free periods between anxiety episodes still exist.
4. Constant chronic anxiety state.

Hysteria[4]
0. Very infrequent hysterical symptoms.
1. Five to 10 episodes of hysterical symptoms, intermittent, with long free periods. Subject never considered the symptoms a serious illness.
2. Life-long history of frequent episodes of vague illness, with complete recovery despite absence of definitive diagnosis or of specific treatment; chronic complaints involving more than one of the types of dysfunctions listed in the footnote. Not more than one episode of invalidism or hospitalization for such dysfunctions.
3. Never healthy; many episodes of severely disabling illness involving several types of dysfunctions, but with no definitive 'organic' diagnosis established or even likely. Usually there have been several surgical procedures, long periods of invalidism, or hospitalization for study.
4. Complete continuous invalidism with history as above; conspicuous 'belle indifférence'; disabling phobias; pseudo-psychotic symptoms.

Results

Group I has been subdivided into 2 groups: Ia (neurogenic hypertension) and Ib (other types of hypertension). Table II shows the number of subjects (N) in group Ia, Ib, and I (Ia plus Ib) who were assigned ratings of 0, 1, 2, etc., for each of the personality patterns considered.

It should be noted that the patterns rated have little to do with either the age at detection of hypertension or the duration of hypertension; with very few exceptions, the patterns defined were present at the rated levels long before the detection of hypertension.

[4] In the absence of a generally accepted definition of the term, we have taken it to mean a life-long disorder, characterized by multiple transient dysfunctions (motor, sensory, autonomic, emotional, intellectual, social, pseudo-neurologic, pseudo-psychotic), most of which are easily identified (on study) as consequent upon definable changes in the life situation.

Table II. Number of patients with hypertension: distribution of ratings

Rating	Hysteria	Anxiety	Depression	Obsessive-compulsive behavior	Subnormal assertiveness	Impulsiveness
			Group Ia[1], neurogenic hypertension			
0	10	1	7	3	2	20
1	3	2	7	1	1	2
2	3	7	7	9	6	1
3	6	10	3	9	10	1
4	2	4	0	2	5	0
			Group Ib[2], other types of hypertension			
0	13	3	8	3	3	23
1	2	3	5	4	3	1
2	6	8	8	4	5	1
3	4	10	5	15	13	1
4	1	2	0	0	2	0
			Group I[3]			
0	23	4	15	6	5	43
1	5	5	12	5	4	3
2	9	15	15	13	11	2
3	10	20	8	24	23	2
4	3	6	0	2	7	0

[1] Twenty-four patients.
[2] Twenty-six patients.
[3] Total of group Ia and Ib (50 patients).

We have tested the hypotheses that differences between groups Ia and Ib exist in each of the patterns rated. For a difference to be considered statistically significant at the 5% level, the critical ratio (CR), or difference between the means of the ratings for a given pattern, divided by the standard error of that difference, should exceed 2.45. In no case was the critical ratio greater than 1.29. Hence no significant difference between the two subgroups of hypertensives is apparent, for any of the patterns rated. This is a completely unexpected result, in that nearly half (11 of 26) of the 'other types of hypertension' were endocrine, in relation to pregnancy.

Table III shows the means of the ratings for each pattern in the two subgroups, the difference between the means for each pattern, and the critical ratio of each difference.

From this point on, groups Ia and Ib will no longer be considered separately but will be lumped together as group I for purposes of subsequent comparisons.

Table IV shows the number of subjects (N) in group II (personality disorder without hypertension) and group III (chronic somatic disorder) who were assigned ratings of 0, 1, 2, etc., for each of the personality patterns considered.

In order to test the degree of association between each of the rated patterns in groups I, II, and III, and the presence or absence of hypertension, point biserial coefficients of correlation were computed. The point biserial is an algebraic variant of the ordinary Pearsonian coefficient of correlation. It is used to indicate the degree of association between a continuous variable and a dichotomous variable, when no assumption is made as to the normality

Table III. Comparison of group Ia (neurogenic hypertension)
and group Ib (other types of hypertension)

	Hysteria	Anxiety	Depression	Obsessive-compulsive behavior	Subnormal assertiveness	Impulsiveness
Mean rating, Ia	1.46	2.58	1.25	2.25	2.63	0.29
Mean rating, Ib	1.15	2.19	1.39	2.19	2.31	0.23
Difference between means (D)	+0.31	+0.39	−0.14	+0.06	+0.32	+0.06
Critical ratio	0.81	1.29	0.44	0.19	0.98	0.30

Table IV. Number of patients without hypertension: distribution of ratings

Rating	Hysteria	Anxiety	Depression	Obsessive-compulsive behavior	Subnormal assertiveness	Impulsiveness
Group II[1], personality disorder						
0	22	4	12	16	15	40
1	7	9	12	19	11	6
2	6	16	13	4	11	1
3	6	13	11	10	9	1
4	8	7	1	0	3	1
Group III[2], somatic disorder						
0	34	13	28	23	30	35
1	6	18	10	9	7	7
2	4	12	6	7	5	1
3	0	1	0	5	1	0
4	0	0	0	0	1	1

[1] Forty-nine patients.
[2] Forty-four patients.

of the distributions. In computing the coefficients, the presence of hypertension was arbitrarily assigned the numerical value of 1 and absence of hypertension was assigned the value 0. Consequently, positive coefficients indicate a higher mean rating of a pattern for the hypertensives, while negative coefficients indicate the reverse. In the same way, the presence of personality disorder was assigned the numerical value 1, absence of personality disorder the value 0.

To test the significance of these correlations, we have used the standard error of a zero coefficient of correlation ($r = 0.0$), which, for these samples, is 0.10. A correlation coefficient (in table V) greater than 0.30 would be considered to indicate a statistically significant degree of association.

Table V shows the point biserial coefficients of correlation between (hypertension-absence of hypertension) and (personality ratings) for a) groups I and II, and b) groups I and III (columns A and B).

In groups II and III there is no hypertension. As has been stated, group II patients are psychiatrically ill and group III patients have chronic somatic illness, without personality disorder. For these patients the correlations were computed between (personality disorder-absence of personality disorder) as the dichotomous variable, and (personality ratings) as the other variable; these correlation coefficients are shown in column C.

The ratings of obsessive-compulsive behavior and of subnormal assertiveness differentiate significantly hypertensives from thosephaving personality disorders without hy ertension; the other ratings (hysteria, anxiety, depression, impulsiveness) do not so differentiate. The ratings of all the patterns except impulsiveness differentiate significantly hypertensives from those with chronic somatic disorders.

As between the 2 groups of patients without hypertension, namely those with personality disorders (group II) and those with chronic somatic disorders (group III), 4 patterns were found to differentiate significantly: hysteria, anxiety, depression, subnormal assertiveness. Two patterns, obsessive-compulsive behavior and impulsiveness, do not differentiate these two groups significantly.

As has been stated, in differentiating the hypertensives from the personality disorders without hypertension, the patterns that are most differentiating are obsessive-compulsive behavior ($r = 0.44$) and subnormal assertiveness ($r = 0.38$). The correlation coefficient between these two variables is 0.49, which shows that these two rated patterns have a considerable degree of communality. Nevertheless, the multiple correlation coefficient between (hypertension – absence of hypertension) and these two patterns considered in combination is 0.49, which indicates that combinations of the rated patterns may be found which may be more differentiating than any one pattern in isolation.

Table V. Point biserial coefficients of correlation between personality ratings and the clinical entities studied[1]

	A[2] Coefficient of correlation for hypertensives (group I) and personality disorders (group II)	B[3] Coefficient of correlation for hypertensives (group I) and somatic disorders (group III)	C[4] Coefficient of correlation for personality disorders (group II) and somatic disorders (group III)
Hysteria	− 0.04	+0.41	+0.41
Anxiety	+0.08	+0.58	+0.51
Depression	− 0.03	+0.41	+0.47
Obsessive-compulsive behavior	+0.44	+0.53	+0.14
Subnormal assertiveness	+0.38	+0.67	+0.38
Impulsiveness	− 0.03	− 0.02	+0.01

[1] In columns A and B hypertension or absence of hypertension is the dichotomous variable. In column C the dichotomous variable is presence or absence of personality disorder.
[2] Ninety-nine patients.
[3] Ninety-four patients.
[4] Ninety-three patients.

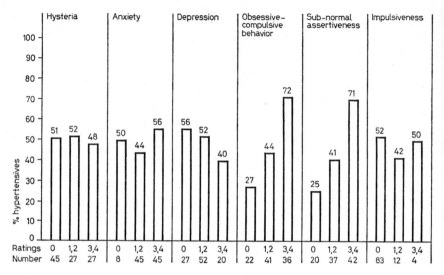

Fig. 1. Relation of presence of hypertension to ratings of six personality patterns. Fifty patients with hypertension and 49 with personality disorder without hypertension.

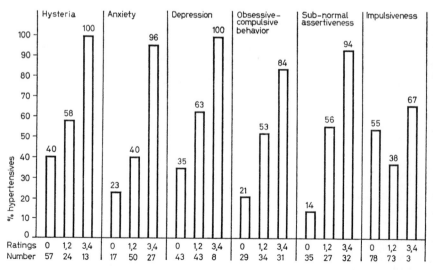

Fig. 2. Relation of presence of hypertension to ratings of six personality patterns. Fifty patients with hypertension and 44 with chronic somatic disorders.

The best combination of patterns for differentiating group I (hypertensives) and group III (chronic somatic disorders) appears to be depression and subnormal assertiveness, which yield a multiple correlation coefficient of 0.69. Approximately the same multiple is yielded by the combination of anxiety and subnormal assertiveness. However, these multiples are only 0.02 higher than the zero-order correlation coefficient of 0.67 between subnormal assertiveness and hypertension.

While the possibility of using the multiple correlation technic for increasing the differentiating power of the rated patterns has not been fully explored, the intercorrelations among the patterns are such that no great increase is to be expected. This, however, is a subject for further investigation.

Since it was impossible to match the three groups perfectly for age (table I), the variability associated with age was held constant, by means of the partial correlation technic, for those patterns significantly

associated with hypertension. While the corresponding coefficients of correlation dropped slightly when age was partialled out, the greatest decrease was from 0.44 to 0.40 for the correlation between obsessive-compulsive behavior and hypertension. In no case was a correlation coefficient decreased to a significant degree. In our data, therefore, the relationship between the ratings and hypertension cannot be attributed to age.

In figures 1, 2, and 3 below are represented graphically the data which have been described in statistical terms in table V. The ratings were grouped in the classes 0; 1, 2; 3, 4; in order to provide as large samples as possible over the extent of the rating scale; but the statistical analysis indicates that the general facts shown graphically would be the same, no matter how the ratings were grouped. The graphs were made up as follows (fig. 1, left corner): 27 subjects from groups I and II were rated 3 or 4 for the pattern hysteria. Of these 27, 13 or 48 per cent were hypertensives (group

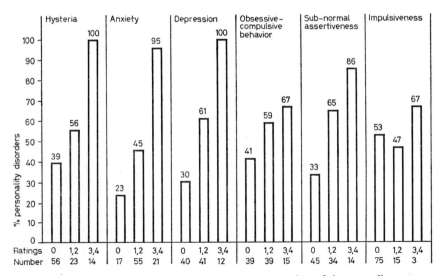

Fig. 3. Relationship of presence of personality disorder to ratings of six personality patterns. Forty-nine patients with personality disorder and 44 with chronic somatic disorders.

I). Twenty-seven subjects from groups I and II were rated 1 or 2 for the pattern hysteria. Of these 27, 14 or 52% were hypertensives. Forty-five subjects from these two groups were rated 0 for the pattern hysteria; of these 45, 23 or 51% were hypertensives.

Thus approximately 50% of the subjects in groups I and II who were rated at any level of the pattern hysteria, were hypertensives; the rest were not. This amounts to saying that the rating for the pattern hysteria does not differentiate significantly the hypertensives from those with personality disorders without hypertension; a conclusion put more concisely in table V where the relevant coefficient of correlation is shown to be –0.04, which is not significant.

What has been said of hysteria, applies to anxiety, depression, and impulsiveness (but not to obsessive-compulsive behavior or to subnormal assertiveness) for groups I and II in figure 1.

Figures 2 and 3 are to be interpreted similarly. The necessary data for the three figures are in table II and IV.

Comment

The significant association of hypertension with obsessive-compulsive behavior and subnormal assertiveness is in agreement with HALLIDAY'S [11, p. 52] general experience, and many of our observations are in general agreement with those of BINGER and his co-workers [4].

The latter report indicates that one or both of these patterns were present to a handicapping extent in 22 of the 24 hypertensive subjects studied. Nineteen of their subjects had conspicuous difficulty in asserting themselves, but only 3 are described as obsessional. Decided inability to grade assertiveness, severe degree of anxiety, depression, and hysteria are noted also in a fair percentage of their subjects.

Additional rough checks on the adequacy of our method are indicated by the facts that: a) the complex patterns rated, though highly intercorrelated, discriminated effec-

tively the three rather different groups studied; b) a pattern found relatively infrequently among adults in our society, 'impulsiveness', occurred in the three groups with a uniformly low frequency; and c) the ratings differentiate between hypertension and somatic disorders and between personality disorders and somatic disorders more effectively than between hypertension and personality disorders. Only 2 of the personality ratings differentiate significantly between groups I and II, while 5 of the ratings do so between groups I and III, and 4 do so between groups II and III. Furthermore, the significant point biserial coefficients are highest between groups II and III and lowest between I and II. The cited facts are evidence that hypertensive persons resemble those with personality disorders much more closely than they resemble persons with somatic disorders, as has recently been the general psychiatric supposition and the experience of HALLIDAY [11, pp. 54–55].

A surprising observation is the absence of significant differences in the ratings for neurogenic and for other types of hypertension (endocrine, renal, mixed). The report of BINGER and his co-workers [4] also indicates great similarity in the personality patterns of subjects with various types of hypertension.

It should be emphasized that the described positive associations between presence of hypertension and certain personality ratings do not signify an etiologic relation between the significant patterns and hypertension, but only that there is concomitant variation of the two variables. In order to explain the concomitant variation in terms of etiologic relationship, one requires a) a hypothesis in terms of which the concomitant variation is meaningful, b) compatibility of the hypothesis with other known facts about the disorder underlying hypertension, c) operational statement of the hypothesis so that consequences can be inferred and investigated. We might postulate a) that persons with the implied makeup of hypertensive persons are recurrently and frequently inhibiting impulses to overt action, b) that blood pressure rises in some of these persons at such times, just as other dysfunctions, obviously occur at such times, c) that in time, and in some such persons, the blood pressure rises begin to outlast the duration of inhibited impulse[5] and d) that finally hypertension is sustained instead of intermittent. Such postulates would be compatible with (1) the habitual nature of the personality patterns in question; (2) the frequent observation of a period of lability of blood pressure antedating sustained hypertension; (3) the high correlation between even transient elevation of systolic pressure and later sustained hypertension with its complications [28]; (4) the observation that, in known hypertensive persons, conflictful interviews may be associated with blood pressure changes of much shorter duration than the associated renal circulatory changes [29]; (5) the ease with which even brief (methodologically reversible) experimental hypertension becomes irreversible [7, 8]; (6) evidence that other factors play a partial causative role: renal and humoral (as in the work of GOLDBLATT and of HEINBECKER [12]), genetic [2], culturally determined outlets for overt expression of inhibited feeling [29] [here a 'hypertensive' was normotensive when doing much physical work but hypertensive when living as a (sedentary) artist]; (7) the possible importance of largescale cultural factors: thus cultures are known which are as conflict-ridden as our own [13], but in some such where medical observations have been possible, hypertension has not been reported [5]. It is possible that the high level of daily physical work is a factor relevant to the low frequency of hypertension in such cultures, if we reflect upon the significance of the observations made upon the artist-muscle builder patient of WOLFF et al.; (8) the variable direction of hypertensives' pressure changes, depending upon maintenance of the internal conflicts or submission to one alternative, as when admitting defeat [29]; (9) experimental evidence that subjection

of animals to recurrent mutually exclusive drives (i.e., to recurrent inhibition of impulses to overt activity) may bring about not only general disorganization [15] but, in particular circumstances and in genetically emotionally labile organisms, sustained hypertension [7].

According to such a hypothesis, the personality factors in hypertension, widely distributed as they are in our society and striking as they are in hypertensives, appear to be only of partial etiologic relevance but neither necessary nor sufficient.

The same statement, that there are factors etiologically relevant to the disorder, but neither necessary nor sufficient, can be made of mechanical factors (only some patients with coarctation of the aorta develop essential hypertension, some patients with both coarctation and hypertension become normotensive after successful surgery of the aorta), renal-chemical factors (not all patients with severe renal impairment develop hypertension), renal and blood viscosity factors (only one-third of patients with polycythemia vera develop essential hypertension [19]), genetic factors [9], and so on.

The compatibility of the hypothesis with HEINBECKER's conception of the significance for diastolic hypertension of relative overactivity of the eosinophile cells of the anterior pituitary could be tested by

[5] The blood pressure changes need not occur simultaneously with the recurrent inhibition of impulse. Conflict interviews with 'normal' subjects may be associated with no change in pressure during the interview, but may be followed by excessive rise in pressure subsequently in the cold-pressor test, i.e., when such a person meets a non-specific pressor stimulus (CRANSTON, R. W.; CHALMERS, J. H.; TAYLOR, H. L.; HENSCHEL, A., and KEYS, A.: Effect of a psychiatric interview on the blood pressure response to cold stimuli. Abstract in Fed. Proc., Part I, Federation of American Societies for Experimental Biology, vol. 8, p. 30, March, 1949. Presented at American Physiological Society Fifty-eighth Annual Meeting, Detroit, Michigan, April 18–22, 1949).

chronic experiments of the type reported by FARRIS *et al.* [7], as part of which histologic and other relevant studies could be performed. The postulates stated could also be tested by observations of the effect on the hypertension of demonstrated modifications of the significant personality patterns; by careful studies of the behavioral (operational) correlates of supposedly identical 'anxiety' in different cultures (perhaps these correlates are widely different); by careful studies of the association between change in prevalence of hypertension and change in personality patterns in a cultural group (with hitherto low prevalence) that is undergoing rapid acculturation [5] and by still other methods independent of the present one.

Summary and Conclusions

The degree of association between presence of hypertension and certain personality patterns has been studied, in a) hypertensive persons, and b) two control groups. Statistically significant degrees of association are found for 'obsessive-compulsive behavior' ($r = 0.44 \pm 0.10$) and for 'subnormal assertiveness' ($r = 0.38 \pm 0.10$). This association implies concomitant variation, rather than proves etiologic relationship.

A hypothesis is stated, in terms of which the observed concomitance appears meaningful. The hypothesis appears compatible with much now known about the underlying disorder, and can be tested in various ways. The personality factors may be looked upon as etiologically relevant, but neither necessary nor sufficient.

Neurogenic hypertensive and other types of hypertensive subjects have not been shown to differ significantly in the rated patterns.

The experimental method reported in this paper appears to afford a means of objectifying complex relationships suggested by much more laborious study of far fewer subjects and should prove useful in similar investigations.

References

1. ALEXANDER, F.: Psychosomatic study of a case of essential hypertension. Psychosom. Med. *1:* 139 (1939).

2. AYMAN, D.: Heredity in arteriolar (essential) hypertension: A clinical study of 1,524 members of 277 families. Arch. Intern. Med. *53:* 792 (1934).

3. BAUER, W.: quoted in A. O. LUDWIG, Some psychosocial factors in cases of severe medical disease. Appl. Anthropol. *7:* 1 (1948).

4. BINGER, C. A. L.; ACKERMAN, N. W.; COHN, A. E.; SCHROEDER, H. A., and STEELE, J. M.: Personality in arterial hypertension. Psychosom. Med. Monographs, New York, American Psychosomatic Society, 1945.

5. CAROTHERS, J. C.: A study of mental derangement in Africans and an attempt to explain its peculiarities, more especially in relation to the African attitude to life. Psychiatry *11:* 47 (1948).

6. DUNBAR, F.: Psychosomatic diagnosis, Chap. 5, pp. 248–293 (Hoeber, Inc., New York 1943).

7. FARRIS, E. J.; YEAKEL, E. H., and MEDOFF, H. S.: Development of hypertension in emotional gray Norway rats after air blasting. Amer. J. Physiol. *144:* 331 (1945).

8. FLASHER, J. and DRURY, D. R.: Persistence of hypertension after removal of the causative ischemic kidney. Abstract in Fed. Proc. *8:* 47 (1949). Presented at American Physiological Society, Fifty-eighth Annual Meeting, Detroit, Michigan, April 18–22 (1949).

9. FRIEDMAN, M. and KASANIN, J. S.: Hypertension in only one of identical twins. Arch. Intern. Med. *72:* 767 (1943).

10. GOLD, L.: Mental characteristics associated with 'essential' hypertension. Psychiat. Quart. *17:* 364 (1943).

11. HALLIDAY, J. L.: Psychosocial medicine, p. 99 (Norton Co., New York 1948).

12. HEINBECKER, P.: a) The pathogenesis of Cushing's syndrome. Medicine *23:* 225–247 (1944); The pathogenesis of diastolic hypertension. Paper presented at meeting of the Central Neuropsychiatric Association, St. Louis, Mo., October 21 (1949).

13. HENRY, J.; HENRY, Z., and SHACHTEL, A. H.: Rorschach analysis of Pilagá Indian Children. Amer. J. Orthopsychiat. *12:* 4 (1942).

14. HYDE, R. W. and KINGSLEY, L. V.: Studies in medical sociology: I. The relation of mental disorders to the community socioeconomic level. New Engl. J. Med. *231:* 543 (1944); II. The relation of mental

disorders to population density. Ibid. *231:* 571 (1944); HYDE, R. W. and CHISHOLM, R. M.: III. The relation of mental disorders to race and nationality. Ibid. *231:* 612 (1944).

15. JAMES, W. T.: The formation of neurosis in dogs by increasing the energy requirement of a conditioned avoiding response. J. comp. Psychol. *36:* 109 (1943).

16. KARPMAN, B.: The myth of the psychopathic personality. Amer. J. Psychiat. *104:* 523 (1948).

17. KINSEY, A. C.; POMEROY, W. B., and MARTIN, C. E.: Sexual behavior in the human male, pp. 77–78 (Saunders Co., Philadelphia 1948).

18. KLEIN, H. R.: A personality study of 100 unselected patients attending a gastrointestinal clinic. Amer. J. Psychiat. *104:* 433 (1948).

19. LAWRENCE, J. H.: The control of polycythemia by marrow inhibition: A ten-year-study on 172 patients. J. amer. med. Ass. *141:* 13–18 (1949).

20. LUDWIG, A. O.: The practical importance of modern concepts of psychosomatic relations. New Engl. J. Med. *238:* 175 (1948).

21. MILLER, M. L.: Blood pressure in relation to inhibited aggression in psychotics. Psychosom. Med. *1:* 162 (1939).

22. PAGE, I. H. and CORCORAN, A. C.: Arterial hypertension: Its diagnosis and treatment (The Year Book Publishers, Inc., Chicago 1946).

23. RENNIE, T. A.: Personality in hypertensive states. New Engl. J. Med. *221:* 448 (1939).

24. SAUL, L. J.: Hostility in cases of essential hypertension. Psychosom. Med. *1:* 153 (1939).

25. SCHROEDER, H. A. and STEELE, J. M.: Studies on 'essential' hypertension: 1. Classification. Arch. intern. Med. *64:* 927 (1939).

26. SCHROEDER, H. A.: Personal communication.

27. WEISS, E.: Psychosomatic aspects of hypertension. J. amer. med. Ass. *120:* 1081 (1942)

28. WHITE, P. D.; LEVY, R. L., and STROUD, W. D.: Transient hypertension: The relative prognostic importance of various systolic and diastolic levels. J. amer. med. Ass. 1059 (1945).

29. WOLFF, H. G.; WOLF, S.; PFEIFFER, J. B.; RIPLEY, H. S., and WINTER, O. S.: Hypertension as a reaction pattern to stress: Summary of experimental data on variations in blood pressure and renal blood flow. Ann. intern. Med. *29:* 1056–1076 (1948).

30. WOLFE, T.: Dynamic aspects of cardiovascular symptomatology. Amer. J. Psychiat. *91:* 563 (1934).

Emotional Stress
in the Precipitation of Congestive Heart Failure[1]

W. N. CHAMBERS and M. F. REISER

Retrospective comment by Dr. J. Sapira. When the research performed in the following paper was begun it was known that tension and anxiety were associated with deleterious changes in cardiovascular function. Why then, was emotional stress so infrequently reported as a precipitant of congestive heart failure? CHAMBERS and REISER realized that superficially mundane life events could have great emotional meaning for an individual patient and they incorporated this concept into their experimental design. Thus, they were able to demonstrate that the 'discrepancy' (between the expected and the reported frequencies of emotionally-related exacerbations of congestive failure) was more apparent than real.

A second finding was that the doctor-patient relationship appeared to have therapeutic value in and of itself. This is worth emphasis and reiteration in light of the following historical consideration: This research was done predominantly in the late 1940's at a time when potent oral diuretics were yet to be discovered and when many components of the sodium retention sequence were not even known, let alone related to each other. Now and perhaps unfortunately our present ability to pharmacologically intervene with a high degree of effectiveness appears to have caused some physicians to minimize or even abandon the use of the doctor-patient relationship as a therapeutic modality.

Perhaps the following work needs to be replicated by each generation of physicians, not because of suspect results, but rather to allow the rediscovery of its essential validity.

It has been demonstrated repeatedly that emotional stress may be accompanied by measurable changes in pulse rate, stroke volume, cardiac output, peripheral resistance, and arterial blood pressure [2, 4, 6] and that anxiety may significantly increase the amount of work required of the heart [4]. Such stress may be accompanied by physiologic alterations which decrease myocardial reserve through interference with the functional adequacy of the coronary circulation, or through interference with the intrinsic cardiac mechanisms governing heart rate and impulse conduction [1, 5, 8]. It has been shown further [7, 10] that the circulation in individuals with both normal and diseased hearts recovers from exercise inefficiently (thus prolonging the period of increased work) during states of emotional tension.

In the patient with structural heart disease and diminished cardiac reserve, events which either (a) increase the demand for cardiac work beyond the capacity of the myocardium, or (b) decrease the myocardial capacity below the current or basal work demand, result in the development of congestive heart failure. Emotional stress, being such an event, might well be expected to participate in the precipitation of congestive failure in individuals with diminished cardiac reserve. It is included in the list of precipitating factors in several of the standard texts [3, 9], but there have been

[1] From the Division of Clinical Physiology, Department of Medicine, and the Department of Psychiatry. University of Cincinnati, College of Medicine, Cincinnati, Ohio.

no systematic studies to determine the frequency with which emotional stress is of etiologic importance in general clinical experience. It has long been recognized that catastrophic or overwhelming emotional trauma (such as the death of a spouse or a narrow escape from accidental death) may be followed by an episode of failure in the cardiac patient. The fact that such major events occur relatively infrequently has led to the tacit assumption that anxiety or emotional tension operate only infrequently as contributory or precipitating factors in most cases of heart failure.

Such an expectation, however, seems too conservative when considered in relation to the psychodynamic observation that superficially routine life events may, because of past experiences and learning, have specific meaning for the individual. Such meaningful experiences are attended by specific, unconscious emotional attitudes which, though not apparent in the overt behavior of the person, may nonetheless be accompanied by significant physiologic responses. Since stress of this type is so commonly encountered in our complex society, it might well be expected that emotional

factors contribute significantly, more frequently than had previously been thought, to episodes of cardiac decompensation. It seemed worthwhile then to inquire systematically into the factors contributing to the development of congestive failure in a representative group of patients.

Material and Methods

Twenty-five patients admitted consecutively to the Cincinnati General Hospital for treatment of congestive heart failure were studied and constitute the 'consecutive' series. Later, 5 additional patients were selected for more detailed investigation and follow-up.

There were 14 men and 11 women in the consecutive series. The average age was 58 years for both sexes. The youngest was 30 years and the oldest 83 years. There were 14 white and 11 Negro patients. With few exceptions, these patients came from the poorest social and economic group. There were 9 patients with chronic alcoholism in the group, 8 of whom were men. It was of interest that neurotic personality disorders were clearly recognizable in 23 of the 25 patients. Table I summarizes the primary cardiac diagnoses and complicating medical conditions in the group.

Table I. Clinical diagnosis of 25 consecutive cases of congestive heart failure

	Total number of cases	Auricular fibrillation	Digitalis intoxication	Acute myocardial infarction	Pulmonary infarction	Occlusion of descending aorta	Acute bronchitis	Thyrotoxicosis	Malnutrition
Hypertensive cardiovascular disease	11	5	1	1*	1*	1*	2	1*	I (ascorbic acid)
Arteriosclerotic heart disease	8	5	2					1	I (thiamin)
Rheumatic heart disease	4	2	1						
Syphilitic heart disease	1					1			
Chronic cor pulmonale	1		1						

* Co-existant in same pt.

All of the patients in this series had severely reduced cardiac reserve and 5 of them died within 4 weeks after admission to the hospital. Six patients were seen during the initial episode of congestive heart failure. Twelve patients had had chronic failure of varying degrees for from 7 weeks to 9 years before admission. Seven patients had had repeated acute episodes of congestive failure.

In all cases the anatomic diagnosis of the heart disease and the functional diagnosis of congestive failure were established by the usual clinical studies of the medical service[2]. The history of previous congestive failure was, in most instances, documented from records of previous admissions to the hospital or visits to the out-patient clinic.

Each patient was interviewed for an average of three 1-hour sessions by one of the authors (W.N.C.), an internist with no formal psychiatric training. The technique of associative anamnesis was used primarily and was supplemented when necessary by direct questioning. Whenever possible, the interviews were begun on the first day of hospitalization and were continued on consecutive days.

Regular discussions of the material, as it was being gathered, were held with the psychiatric observer (M.F.R.) for the purpose of reaching tentative psychodynamic formulations and receiving suggestions concerning technique and goals of further interviews. Members of the patient's family and close associates were also interviewed. Extensive use was made of social service workers for these contacts. From these studies of the patient and his environment an attempt was made to reach an understanding of the specific emotional meaning to the individual of his life situation at the time cardiac decompensation had developed.

Finally, from the combined data of the clinical and psychosocial investigations, an attempt was made to reconstruct the pathophysiologic dynamics associated with the development of cardiac decompensation, and, if possible, to isolate from the multiple noxious factors, the single one which appeared to be responsible for finally destroying the balance between cardiac reserve and demand for work. In other words, the term 'precipitating factor' is used in this study to denote 'the straw that broke the camel's back'.

Following the medical study and a series of psychiatric interviews, the examiner wrote up his findings with the material classified and outlined according to the following form:

I. Clinical diagnosis
   A. Medical
   B. Psychiatric
II. Medical history
   A. Past history
   B. Family history
   C. Present illness
III. Psychiatric history
   A. Chronological personal history
   B. Genetic and dynamic formulation of personality structure
      1. Genetic trauma
      2. Dynamic factors
   C. Overt personality
   D. Psychological testing
IV. Analysis of contributing factors
   A. Organic
   B. Functional
V. Analysis of precipitating factors
   A. Organic
   B. Functional
VI. Physical examination
VII. Laboratory and physiologic investigations
VIII. Course in hospital
IX. Follow-up
X. Evaluation of total information available
   A. Evaluation of housestaff histories
   B. Evaluation of psychiatric data
      1. Type of interviews
      2. Patient's reaction to interviews and interviewer
      3. Contribution of total situation to type of material obtained
      4. Therapeutic coloring to investigation
      5. Number and length of psychiatric interviews
      6. Number of interviews required for making presumptive formulation
      7. Number of interviews required for factual confirmation
      8. Information from relatives
XI. Formulation.

[2] The clinical diagnosis in each case was based upon the findings and diagnostic impressions of the Medical Service, Cincinnati General Hospital, the type of study being indicated in detail in case 1. In addition, a complete physical and functional evaluation was carried out by one of the authors (W.N. C.) and was reviewed by the investigative team.

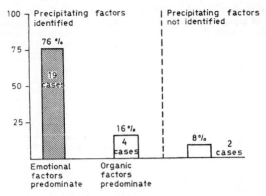

Fig. 1. Incidence of precipitating factors in 25 consecutive cases of congestive heart failure.

These data (exclusive of the examiner's final formulations) were reviewed separately by the psychiatric observer, who then independently constructed his final formulations and impressions. As the final step, the two observers met for comparison of their separate impressions and final, joint formulation of the results.

The 5 additional selected patients were referred for study and treatment because of the obvious participation of emotional factors in the course of their disease. There were 4 women and 1 man in this group. Their ages were 31, 49, 50, 54, and 36 respectively. There were 3 patients with hypertensive cardiovascular disease and 1 with chronic glomerulonephritis; 1 case of syphilitic heart disease and hypertension; and 1 case of rheumatic heart disease and auricular fibrillation. All had moderately advanced to severe degrees of cardiac involvement with markedly diminished cardiac reserve. Three of these patients were first seen in the hospital during an episode of congestive heart failure. The other 2 were initially seen in the out-patient clinic. All had had repeated episodes of congestive heart failure. The initial method of study and formulation was the same for this group as for the larger consecutive series. In addition, these patients were subsequently followed in the out-patient clinic at weekly intervals for periods averaging 9 months. This continued observation afforded opportunity for concurrent rather than retrospective observations concerning the association between life experiences (including doctor-patient relationship)

and fluctuations in clinical course. Medical measures, such as digitalization, salt-poor diet[3], and diuretics were carried out in accordance with the usual clinical indications.

Results

Twenty-five Consecutive Cases of Congestive Heart Failure

Identification of Precipitating Factors

Precipitating factors could be identified in 23 of the 25 patients (fig. 1). In 19, or 76%, it was felt that emotional tension was the factor immediately responsible for increasing the work load beyond cardiac capacity. In 4, or 16%, organic factors were felt to be responsible. (These are listed in the upper half of table II.) In 2 cases it was impossible to isolate a single responsible factor, no single event or complication appeared to have exerted a predominant effect. (The findings on these 2 patients are listed in the lower half of table II.) Although it was found that all patients in this series had markedly diminished cardiac reserve from organic disease and had been living under severe, chronic emotional

[3] The cardiac 'salt-poor' diet used at the Cincinnati General Hospital contains not more than 0.9 g of sodium per day.

Table II. Precipitating factors in 6 of the 25 consecutive cases of congestive heart failure (also see table III)

Organic factors predominate (4 cases)

F.B. Pulmonary infarction
      Acute myocardial infarction
H.S. Severe acute bronchitis (Syphilitic
      heart disease)
M.B. Pulmonary infarction
S.J. Digitalis intoxication (Arteriosclerotic
      heart disease)

No specific precipitating factor identified (2 cases)

M.Y. Rheumatic heart disease
      Auricular fibrillation
      Chronic emotional tension
C.C. Arteriosclerotic heart disease
      Malnutrition
      Chronic emotional tension

---

strain, these factors alone were not felt to be adequate explanation for the precipitation of congestive failure in the majority of them. In 92 % an added stress of acute and overwhelming nature was found to have been superimposed on the chronic tension state and diseased cardiovascular system for precipitation of the acute episode. In the 19 cases in which this added stress was primarily emotional in origin, there were frequently concomitant complicating factors, such as coexistent diseases of other systems, malnutrition, or digitalis intoxication, which appeared to play contributory rather than immediately precipitating roles.

The following case résumé illustrates strikingly, and in some detail, the findings in one of these 19 patients:

Case 1[4] (fig. 2). F.Y., a 49-year old-single, white salesman, was admitted to the Cincinnati General Hospital on September 4, 1949, in severe congestive heart failure, with a diagnosis of rheumatic heart disease. He had been well until 8 weeks before admission, when he noted the onset of exertional dyspnea. Several days later 'I ran up eight flights of stairs to

prove to myself that I was all right'. That same evening he drank excessively and awoke the next morning gasping for breath and noted swelling of his feet and legs. During the ensuing 6 weeks he failed to contact a physician and treated himself 'with exercise and vitamin E'. Finally, 1 week before admission, because of the increasing severity of his symptoms, he went to a physician who diagnosed 'heart trouble' and cirrhosis of the liver. Hospitalization was advised; but he refused. He was treated with digitalis and daily mercurials, but failed to respond. Because of this he finally submitted to hospitalization. Although at first he refused to admit that he had ever had heart trouble in the past, he finally said that he had been told in 1930 that he had heart murmurs, and that he had been rejected from the Army in 1942 for the same reason. For the past 20 years, he had been a heavy consumer of alcohol.

Physical examination showed an acutely ill man with extreme dyspnea and orthopnea. The blood pressure was 135/40 mm Hg; the pulse rate, 96/min; and respiratory rate, 28/min. There was moderate cyanosis of the lips and nail beds. Moist rales were present over both lung fields and there was dullness with decreased breath sounds at the right lung base. The point of maximum cardiac impulse was in the sixth interspace, 2 cm inside of the anterior-axillary line. A systolic thrill was felt over the aortic area and there was a questionable diastolic thrill at the apex. On auscultation, a short systolic and a low blowing diastolic murmur were heard at the apex; there was an early short diastolic murmur and a loud, rough systolic murmur at the base which was transmitted to the neck. A2 was present. A diastolic gallop rhythm was heard at the apex, with occasional premature beats. The liver was tender and the edge was palpable 5 fingerbreadths below the right costal margin. Grade 3 pitting edema of the legs, ankles, and feet was present, and there was palmar erythema.

Fluoroscopic examination showed generalized cardiac enlargement with gross left ventricular enlargement, pulmonary congestion, and right pleural effusion. The electrocardiogram showed first degree A-V block and digitalis effect.

The patient was first seen by the investigator 12 h after admission, at which time he was

---

[4] Date of study, September, 1949.

severely dyspneic and required oxygen. In spite of this, when he was approached, he pulled off the oxygen mask, got out of bed, pounded on his chest, and exhibited his biceps as he flexed them (they were flaccid and atrophied).

He was visited on five successive days. The total time spent in the interviews was 3 h. Gradually, as he gave his story, it became evident that he was seriously depressed, felt hopeless, and had a strong fear of death.

The patient was born in Syracuse, N.Y. His father was an inspector in a steel plant in Syracuse, and one brother, 40 years old, is now superintendent of a steel plant in Utica. 'He (brother) has had a college education. He goes around teaching young men. He has

great responsibilities.' The patient stated that he had good parents. 'They never hit me, but I always wanted to be on the road.' He stayed home until he was 21 years old, but said that he started traveling sporadically at the age of 16. He went through the first year of high school and then stopped. 'I didn't like it, and I wanted to build myself up. I thought I should begin with the body. I gained 20 lb. by exercise and I walked 20 miles a day, took cold showers summer and winter, exercising morning and night. That will cure anything. My father exercised. He was a great athlete. I built myself up and I couldn't stop. I was a salesman for many different companies. I've always been a physical culture man. I've always been interested in Charles Atlas,

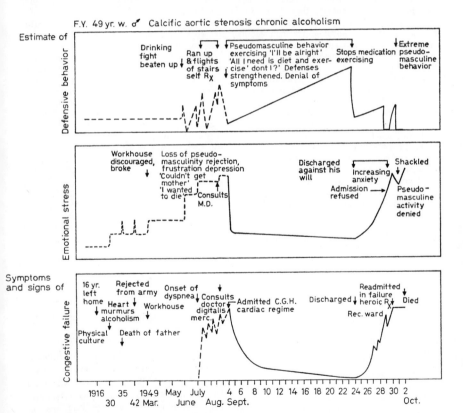

Fig. 2. Symptoms and signs of congestive failure, emotional stress, and defensive behavior in case 1.

Bernarr McFadden, and all the rest of them. I worked with them when I was 18 years old. I started drinking when I was 30 years old and have continued to the present. I've never married and have always been on the road. I used to shack up, but never much. I never had much desire for women, and now I'm impotent. I've always been interested in building myself up.'

He then talked about his many different jobs, repeatedly stating, 'I was a leader in it', or 'I was a great success at it'. 'When I lived in Niagara Falls, I used to walk back and forth to Buffalo in the same day, 50 miles. I felt wonderful. I was going to be a school teacher then.' He came to Cincinnati 3 years ago but would not give the reason for this. The patient denied any overt homosexuality but frequentlye mad reference to 'those guys'. 'I've done a lot of reading of psychiatry and I know it's because of their mothers.' He then told at length of a man who approached him when he was in a bar, but denied that he had anything to do with him.

The patient was sent to the workhouse for 19 days in March, 1949. He stated that he was going from house to house selling coupons and 'two old hens had me locked up. I had never been held by the police before. It was terrible. Then I began to worry about everything. About 3 months ago, I was drinking with a veteran. He invited me to his house. He started to give some beer to his little niece and I said, "You're not going to give any to her, are you?" He turned around and slammed me in the face and hit me over the head with the bottle. When I was down he kicked me in the face. I was lying there, covered with blood, but got up. I couldn't fight back, and he ran away. I was afraid the police were going to get me and I began to worry again. I couldn't get to my mother or brother and I had no money. I was selling, but I drank it all up. I was completely discouraged and didn't care if I lived or not; I was eating very poorly.'

'Three months ago was when I began to go to pieces and I wanted to die.' He then told of running up eight flights of stairs again shortly before the onset of his present illness 7 weeks before and of taking cold baths, standing before open windows exercising excessively morning and night. Throughout the conversations the patient constantly asked for reassurance. 'That's not too bad, is it?' 'That can be cured, can't it?' 'How about vitamin E for the heart? They have reported miraculous cures

of the girl in Canada.' 'I'll be all right, won't I?' He repeatedly recounted the story of his violent drinking bout at the onset of his present illness. 'I was O.K. the night before and I had run up eight flights of stairs. But when I woke up the next morning with a terrible hangover, I was all out of breath and my ankles were swollen. I thought it would pass off, and it did, because I exercised and I felt better. I continued to exercise until I couldn't any more. Then I went to a doctor, 1 week before coming here. I always thought it would get better. I've never been sick before. I couldn't work. It all began 3 months ago when I got knocked down. It was being knocked down that was so terrible. I've never got knocked down or arrested before; and then I was knocked down and I felt all gone.'

During his entire hospitalization he would jump up from his bed, beat his chest before the open window, take deep breaths, and make deep knee bends; all this time in severe congestive heart failure. He was allowed considerable freedom in his activities in spite of his severe failure, and his failure responded dramatically. He was discharged, probably too soon for his own extremely dependent needs, and remained compensated for only 2 days. He came back to the Receiving Ward, was given emergency treatment, and was sent out again. This time he was severely apprehensive and anxious. He returned the same evening and was readmitted because of severe failure. Throughout the final hospitalization his anxiety was extreme. On this admission he was in the care of different personnel who were unfamiliar with his record and shackled him in bed, thus blocking any possibility of his utilizing the pseudomasculine defenses. His condition became increasingly worse and he died 2 days after admission. The postmortem diagnosis was nodular calcific aortic stenosis, probably on a rheumatic basis.

The emotional stress extant at the onset and during this man's illness is readily apparent in the direct interview material. It is felt that the conflicting life situation exerted a noxious influence on the tenuous circulatory equilibrium in at least two ways. First, the intensification of his long-standing, pathologically exaggerated pseudomasculine defenses (in response to his growing feelings of helplessness) led to

excessive physical exertion and other in-
discretions, which greatly increased the
cardiac load. Second, the physiologic
changes incident to the anxiety and hostility engendered when he found himself
realistically forced to face his dependent
and passive needs further increased the demands on the already failing circulation.
With the breakdown of the 'illusion' afforded by denial, this individual was over-
whelmed and unable to cope satisfactorily
with the conflict over his basis intense passivity. Figure 2 illustrates graphically the
parallelism between the degrees of circulatory failure and emotional stress, and the
inverse relationship of these two phenomena to the 'effectiveness' of the pseudomasculine acting out.

The data on the remaining 18 patients
(cases 2 to 19) in the consecutive series in
whom emotional stress was felt to have been
responsible for the precipitation of congestive heart failure are summarized in the
appendix.

Nature of the Emotionally Stressful
Precipitating Events

The nature of the events identified as
precipitating emotional factors were, in
their general characteristics, remarkably
uniform in these 19 cases. They can be
readily grouped under two major headings
determined by the predominant effects or
feeling states evoked by them in the patient
(table III). (1) events leading predominantly
to feelings of rejection and loss of security;
(2) events leading predominantly to feelings
of frustration and rage.

Situations to which the patient responded with feelings of rejection and loss of
security occurred in some form in each of
the 19. In 12 patients these episodes occurred in close combination with other
(sometimes related) events which stirred up
additional, intense feelings of frustration
and rage. Such superimposed or concomitant events were often related to conflicts
with persons close to the individual, to
business reverses, loss of job, or other
factors.

Nature of the Interview

The nature of the interviews varied
greatly in relation to the timing of the first
contact with the patient. Nineteen patients
were initially seen within the first 48 h of
hospitalization when they were still seriously ill, in acute physical distress, and
experiencing realistic fears of death. All of
these patients related quickly to the doctor
in a trusting and help-seeking way, and
were willing and often spontaneously eager
to discuss their personal affairs and feelings.
Pertinent psychiatric data were obtained in
each of these cases. In 17 of these 19 patients, emotional precipitating factors were
identified, in 13 cases (75%) from the data
supplied by the patient alone. These 'early'
interviews are most aptly described as
'confessional' in nature in 17 of the patients;
highly charged life experiences and intimate
feelings were brought out as if the patient
were under internal pressure to 'get them
out in the open'. These sessions were followed by visible evidences of relief and
relaxation (both physiologic and psychologic). The experience with the 6 patients
initially seen after the first 48 h (when the
physical distress had been greatly reduced)
stands in marked contrast. All of this
group showed the more usual types of resistance to the interviews, although there
was no consciously intended difference in
the manner in which they were conducted.
None developed the exaggerated transference attitudes leading to confessional type
of behavior. In 2 a satisfactory or primarily
trusting relationship developed, while in 4
there was marked ambivalence and hesitancy throughout the series of visits. Only
one of these 6 patients brought out pertinent psychiatric material, and only 40% of
the precipitating events were discernible
from the patient's data alone.

Five Patients Selected for Long-Term Study

In the 5 patients who were selected for
more extended study, it was considered that
the importance of emotional factors out-

Table III. Precipitating factors in 25 consecutive cases of congestive heart failure (also see table II)

Emotional factors predominate (19 cases)		
Patients	Rejection and loss of security predominate	Frustration and rage predominate
C.M.	Desertion by relative	Threat of institutionalization
A.S.	Relatives refuse to care for her	Amputation of legs without patient's knowledge
C.B.	Sudden death of son	
C.L.	Desertion by one son and landlady Serious accident to other son	Threats of institutionalization
G.W.	Illness of mother Argument with wife	Severe business reverses
W.L.	Desertion by wife	Business reverses
F.K.	Sudden death of husband	
W.W.	Husband's death Rejection by relatives	Conflict with daughter-in-law
M.C.	Rejection by husband and son	Abduction of foster child
G.B.	Marriage of daughter Wife's leg amputation	Business failure
M.T.	Desertion by husband	Fight with nephew Daughter's drunkenness
B.K.	Rejection by children	Conflict with assistant
I.B.	Desertion by brother and sister-in-law	Conflict with brother about debts
J.H.	Rejection by employer	Loss of job (extreme regression)
L.F.	Rejection by husband	Fight with husband
G.F.	Rejection by employer	Loss of job
Geo. F.	Eviction from home of 18 years	
C.W.	Eviction from home of 17 years	
F.Y.	Loss of pseudomasculine defenses	Overwhelmed in fight

weighed the organic factors in precipitation of congestive failure in 4. Organic factors were considered the precipitating cause in 1 who had severe hypertensive cardiovascular disease and chronic glomerulonephritis, with recurrent episodes of failure related to acute exacerbations of nephritis. The nature of the emotional precipitating factors in this group were similar to those of the longer series.

Two of these patients were originally seen within the first 48 h of hospitalization.

They showed the characteristics of the larger series who were interviewed early by relating well to the physician, giving pertinent psychiatric material, and manifesting a confessional attitude in the early interviews.

The 3 patients who were seen later in hospitalization or in the out-patient department related more slowly, and pertinent psychiatric material was obtained only after many interviews. All eventually developed a strong and primarily dependent transference toward the physician, with the development and nature of the transference attitudes (degree of aggressiveness, passivity, sexual coloring, etc.) being related to the patient's basic personality structure and current emotional needs. Examples of the findings in 2 of these 5 patients are given in the following case presentations.

Case 20[5] (fig. 6). W.W. is a 31-year-old, feebleminded[6] Negro woman with hypertensive cardiovascular disease, paroxysmal auricular fibrillation and repeated episodes of acute congestive failure. Like so many others in this series, she had experienced severe deprivation throughout her life. Her father deserted her mother when she was an infant. The mother then gave the child to another woman to bring up while she worked, but kept in contact with her. The patient did not go to school. As 17, she became pregnant and developed grade 1 toxemia. At this time she was told that she had high blood pressure. When delivered, she put the child in a foster home and continued her wanderings. From 1944 to the present she has had yearly pregnancies, all out of wedlock, and all resulting in miscarriages or stillbirths. In April, 1948, she came to Cincinnati at the request of her mother, who lived there. The mother had heart trouble and wanted her daughter to nurse her. The patient was first seen in the Cincinnati General Hospital in August, 1948, again in grade I toxemia of pregnancy. At this time it was noted that she had hypertension, but there was no evidence of heart disease. She had a stillbirth in November, 1948. In December, 1948, her mother, who had recovered from her illness, married the patient's boy friend. 'My mama always gave me everything until she married him. Then she wouldn't give me a thing.' At this time her grandfather, of whom she had always been fond, died. She felt completely abandoned and said, 'Everyone near me is dying'. In January 1949, she noted onset of exertional dyspnea. When seen in the obstetrical out-patient clinic on February 11, 1949, she was in congestive failure and was referred to the cardiac clinic. She did not report to the cardiac clinic but was admitted to the hospital 2 weeks later with severe congestive failure. She responded well to digitalization and cardiac regimen and was discharged in 1 week, to be followed in the cardiac clinic, where she was seen at weekly intervals.

However, she did poorly and in spite of mercurial diuretics gained weight and remained in mild congestive failure. Her physician at this time openly expressed his hostility to her. On June 12, 1949, her stepfather and mother, with whom she was living, had a violent argument, followed by a fight in which the mother was knocked unconscious. The stepfather then raped the patient. On the following day, both mother and daughter were admitted to the hospital, the mother in a coma in which she died of a subdural hematoma 2 days later, the daughter in severe congestive failure. It was at this time that the observer's contact with the patient began. The patient again responded well to hospitalization, during which a strong dependent relationship developed. She talked freely, acting out various incidents in her life. During these descriptions, she would become excited, taking the parts of the various individuals involved, obviously reliving the experiences, wildly gesticulating and grimacing. Several days after hospitalization, she acted out for the observer much of the situation which occurred on the night before her admission. Like the other patients who had a therapeutic relationship with the physician, she did not have a recurrence of congestive failure during these highly-charged confessions.

The patient was discharged after approximately 1 month's hospitalization and was followed at weekly intervals in the clinic. Compensation was maintained throughout the period from July, 1949, through the third week in March, 1950. During the first few months of her clinic follow-up, mercurials were required twice weekly, but this was gradually decreased; she required no mercurials and showed no evidence of congestive failure for 6 months. During this time the patient was seen for 10 to 15 min once a week, and a social worker also saw her for the same amount of time. She utilized these visits for discussion and ventilation of her current problems. 'I'm going to court tomorrow. I don't like that proposition, but I'm going. I dreamed he got out of jail and after what he done to my mama. He said if I put him in jail and if he got out, he would jump me.' She went through court proceedings (which resulted in the conviction of her stepfather for manslaughter) and many other trying life situations without

---

[5] Date of study, June, 1949.
[6] I. Q. 53 (Wechsler-Bellevue).

any recurrence of failure. In November, 1949, she was admitted to the obstetrical service for observation because she was again pregnant. Venous pressure, circulation time, and PSP excretion were normal at this time, although fluoroscopic examination of the heart revealed marked left ventricular enlargement; electrocardiogram showed left ventricular hypertrophy. Therapeutic abortion was strongly advised, but the patient refused on religious grounds. On February 19 she had a stillbirth, but again there was no evidence of congestive failure. She was discharged 2 days later and was followed in the medical clinic, where she did well for the ensuing month. On March 22, 1950, the observer told her of his approaching departure. Her only statement was: 'Oh, father'.

She returned to the receiving ward two nights later in mild congestive failure, was

given Mercuhydrin and discharged, but returned in 2 days again in congestive failure in a state of extreme anxiety. When seen on March 29 she was in moderate congestive heart failure and was admitted to the ward service. Her response was poor and she remained in mild failure; she talked continually of her aloneness and of the fact that her physician was leaving her. 'I feel just as I felt before you started taking care of me.' (After discharge from the hospital she remained in chronic congestive failure despite clinic care, and it eventually became necessary to send her to the County Home and Chronic Disease Hospital.)

It is of interest to note that the patient was able to tolerate numerous difficult situations without any recurrence of congestive failure during the period in which a

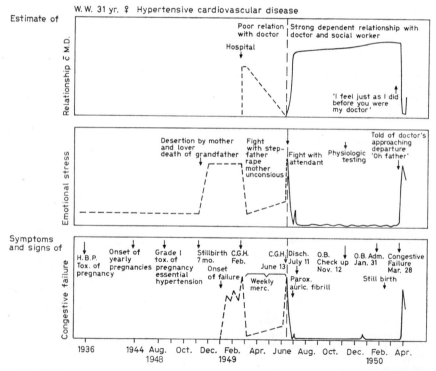

Fig. 3. Symptoms and signs of congestive failure, emotional stress, and relationship in therapy in case 20.

good therapeutic relationship was maintained. The threat of dissolution of this relationship, however, precipitated a recurrence of circulatory failure. Figure 3 graphically depicts the relationship between emotional stress and degree of congestive failure and the ameliorating effect of the doctor-patient relationship, through the relief of emotional stress, on the patient's course.

Case 21[7] (fig. 4). A.H., a 49-year-old Negro woman with a severe hysterical masochistic character neurosis, was found to have syphilitic aortitis in 1937 and hypertension in 1939, which was subsequently sustained. Her first bout of congestive failure occurred in October, 1948, during a period of severe conflict with her husband. Although she was able to work as a maid, she would develop dyspnea and orthopnea whenever her husband demanded intercourse. 'I married my second husband in 1932, but he just didn't pay any attention to me. He was always running around with other women. He had feelings only for himself. He didn't know I was sick. I stayed with my second husband until 7 months ago. I left him in April, 1949. My husband always wanted intercourse. He wanted it every night. I couldn't stand it. I told him I wanted to live. When he was around, there was a terrible load on my chest. I just couldn't stand it. I was afraid I'd die if I had intercourse. He was terrible; he fussed at me all the time for intercourse. I know a friend who died that way. When we were to have intercourse I would start gasping and I would say, I can't go on any further, and he would leave me, but he would be terribly mad. Then we'd try it the next night and I would get choked up so I'd tell him he would have to stop. He'd get mad again and he would argue all the time. I had to sit up. It was terrible. I got so upset I couldn't even talk. I lived with him for 17 years, and we fought for 17 years. We'd argue all the time. I'm sure he is trying to kill me.' Finally he left her in late April, 1949, by which time she had been in mild failure for 7 months without seeking medical attention.

The patient returned to the clinic in May, 1949, the last previous visit having been in 1945. At this time she was found to be in moderately severe congestive failure. She was digitalized, put on a salt-free diet, and given 2 ml Mercuhydrin i.m. weekly. Although her failure improved somewhat, she remained in mild decompensation. In August, 1949, one of us (W.N.C.) began to take care of her and continued to see her at weekly intervals until April, 1950. The precipitating factors, came out early in the interviews, but the personality structure, genetics, and dynamics became clear only after prolonged contact. An intensely dependent relationship was immediately established and was maintained throughout the period of study. One injection of Mercuhydrin was given after the first visit, but was not required subsequently as all signs of failure disappeared.

In late November, 1949, the patient was used for testing depressor drugs, a procedure which necessitated intravenous injections on repeated days and which was frequently accompanied by nausea and vomiting. The patient became quite anxious. Gradually it became clear that the patient was developing a strong pseudosexual transference to the investigator. She was admitted to the hospital at the end of November for study of a left renal cyst. While on salt-free diet and digitalis in the hospital, the interne told her she was to have a treatment and explained to her the procedure of retrograde pyelography. She became very alarmed, dyspneic, orthopneic, and developed acute pulmonary edema. The investigator saw her the following day when she was in obvious congestive failure. The transference anxiety was handled by direct explanation in an accepting but firm manner. She was given strong reassurance and was started on 2 ml Mercuhydrin daily.

Subsequently, she was able to tolerate the retrograde pyelogram and other tests with no difficulty. She was discharged after a week in the hospital again well compensated. The patient did well for the subsequent 4 months and returned to part-time work. However, on being informed of the observer's impending departure, she became anxious and developed increasing exertional dyspnea. One week later, when seen in the clinic, she was in mild congestive heart failure and talked constantly of the observer's leaving her.

Figure 4 depicts the relationships between clinical course, degree of emotional stress, and the therapeutic relationship.

Repetition in the transference relationship of the patient's basic sexual conflicts

[7] Date of study, August, 1949.

was accompanied by a recurrence of failure in the face of a carefully-controlled regimen. Resolution of this anxiety increased the patient's dependent security in the relationship and was accompanied by subsidence of the failure.

Discussion

Although it has always been considered that emotional stress may be a precipitating factor in congestive heart failure, in this series it was found with greater frequency than had previously been anticipated. It was felt that emotional factors played a primary role in the precipitation of congestive failure in 19 (76%) of the 25 consecutive cases studied. Each of them had, at the time of study, markedly limited cardiac reserve, and had been living under severe, chronic emotional strain. However, in each of these 19 patients the superimposition of an acute and overwhelming emotional experience was the factor immediately responsible for throwing him (or her) into cardiac decompensation.

It should be noted that similarly stressful experiences had been suffered by many of the patients earlier in life, at times when myocardial reserve was not yet so limited. At such times the stress was inadequate to break the circulatory equilibrium. However, with the progression of the heart disease and greater and greater loss of cardiac reserve such stressful life events assumed clinical importance in the maintenance of adequate circulatory equilibrium. These patients were found to be in a similarly precarious state of psychological or emotional equilibrium: there was little flexibility or reserve. All were from the poorest social and economic group, in which deprivation and lack of security is so commonly a prominent aspect of early life experiences and development. In addition, the life histories were characterized throughout by realistic lack of material and social security and stability. At the time of study, most of them were functioning in an environment and social milieu which had very limited capacity for affording real material and emotional support. Dependence upon tenuous relationships with relatively few key figures, upon symbols (such as familiar living quarters), and even upon illusions, is understandably exaggerated in such a setting.

In view of the social homogeneity of the patients studied, it is not surprising that a common denominator of sudden rejection and loss of security was found to run through the various emotional precipitating situations. It is interesting to note that when the relationship with the physician deteriorated or was withdrawn, congestive failure recurred in several instances. It is probable that a similar study of a series of patients from a more fortunate social and economic group might not lead to such pronounced emphasis on overt rejection and loss of security. (In other groups one might anticipate a greater variety of overt problems and from a dynamic viewpoint a greater breadth of problem areas involving several levels of psychosexual function.) It is not felt that the prominence of this factor in the series bears any specific relation to the problem of heart failure *per se*, but rather that it is related to the population studied. The important point is that life events specifically stressful for the patients with heart disease studied were found, with high frequency, to have precipitated congestive failure.

The semidirective technique of interviewing was chosen because the experimental design called for obtaining as much pertinent psychiatric material as was feasible in a comparatively brief period of time. There was no therapeutic intent in the contacts with patients in the consecutive series, although it was realized that all interviews would automatically assume such coloring. As it worked out, this phenomenon became a powerful catalyst to the investigative procedure in those patients who were seen when acutely ill and severely threatened by death. They seemed to reach out immediately and desperately for help and poured forth much highly-charged emotional material, as though making their last confession. It might be expected in patients whose circulation was already embarassed that further decompensation could result from the mobilization of such charged topics. Actually, it was evident from the clinical findings that this did not happen in any of the patients studied. Further, the confessional nature of the interviews seemed to exert a distinctly salutary effect in some.

Several factors seem to have contributed to the dramatic lowering of the usual psychological defenses with the resultant free confiding of material which, under other circumstances, would be highly guarded:

1. The overwhelming fear of death (attested to by the reality of the situation, the widespread occurrence of attitudes of hopelessness and depression, and the extensive attempts by nearly all of the patients on admission to use an exaggerated and blatantly illogical denial of symptoms as a defense against anxiety). This sort of interview occurred only in patients seen at a time of acute distress.

2. Individuals with lifelong histories of insecurity and deprivation had become ill in relation to loss of contact and relation-

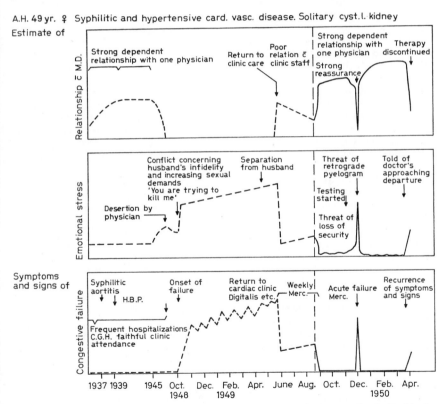

Fig. 4. Symptoms and signs of congestive failure, emotional stress, and relationship in therapy in case 21.

ship with key supporting figures. The avid reaching out to someone who represented potential help, support, and warmth, is quite understandable under such circumstances.

3. The combination of the first two factors apparently operated in such a way as to evoke warmth, sympathy, and helpful attitudes in the physician, so that more of an accepting and therapeutic 'set' developed than had been intended in the original design of the study. The interviewer responded to the situation by accepting the patient's transference needs for him to assume the role of a protecting and forgiving parent figure. It seems highly probable that this latter factor not only contributed to the further revealing of confidences by the patient, but that it also in large part accounts for the absence of deleterious effects. The 'confessional' interviews in essence seem to have been opportunities for the patient to share conflict experiences and feelings with another human being in a setting conducive to the relief of tension, although tension was simultaneously mobilized with the verbalizations. Any accumulation of tension almost certainly would have added to the physiologic strain and led to further circulatory embarrassment in these patients.

Our experience does indicate, however, that abrupt or unexplained withdrawal of the physician after such interviews have taken place may be taken by the patient as another rejection by a meaningful figure and thus precipitate recurrence of failure. This is quite evident in the group of 5 patients who were selected for long-term observation. In these patients, the clinical response appeared to be determined, in large part, by the degree and nature of the dependency on the physician. One patient who remained in chronic congestive failure was the most regressed of the group and so infantile that no meaningful relationship could be established with him. With a second patient (case 20), a more actively dependent relationship was established in which congestive failure was adequately

controlled for many months during difficult life situations but was again precipitated when she was threatened by the departure of the physician. The other 3 patients, all more emotionally mature, benefited by the dependent relationship in a more active way. These patients also remained compensated for many months, during which they were frequently able to express or act out some of their hostile feelings toward the physician. These episodes were worked through and, when resolved, seemed to result in a stronger relationship. Two of these patients died of other causes; the third (case 21) developed congestive failure when informed that the physician was leaving, but subsequently was able to establish a similar relationship with a new physician and again became compensated. Loss of the second physician led to another exacerbation of failure, which responded for a third time as soon as a good relationship had been established with a third physician.

The beneficial influence of the dependent relationship in all patients in the group – and more particularly the 5 long-term patients – makes the therapeutic importance of the doctor-patient relationship obvious. Its therapeutic effect appeared to be related primarily to the relief of anxiety and tension, achieved through satisfaction of the patients' strong dependent needs (which had been left totally unsaturated by the original precipitating events). In addition, continuation in the relationship offered opportunity for constructive and maturing emotional experience for some. The substitutive acceptance and support gained through the relationship seemed to allow the patient to function on a more adequate level both psychologically and physiologically (within the limits of the reserves of both systems). When these patients decompensated psychologically (either through breakdown of intrinsic defenses or through loss of the therapeutic relationship), they seemed also to decompensate physiologically by developing congestive heart failure.

Emotionally stressful situations were found with surprisingly high frequency to have acted as the 'straw that broke the camel's back' in precipitating episodes of congestive failure in this series of patients. In this regard it should be emphasized that although the 25 consecutive patients represent an unselected series of the population of the hospital at which the study was carried out, they do, nonetheless, represent a relatively homogeneous segment of society and practice. Because of this, and because of the special circumstances surrounding the experimental situation, the conclusions to be drawn from these results must be limited. These data are not drawn from a large or broad enough sampling of the total population to suggest or infer that the incidence reported here is necessarily representative of what may actually be obtained in a broad general experience. The findings do demonstrate that emotional stress may operate as a precipitating factor in the development of congestive heart failure in the patient with limited cardiac reserve, and that it may operate with much higher frequency than had previously been thought. The practical implication to be drawn is that these findings constitute strong indication for a consideration of, and search for, such factors in the diagnostic and therapeutic approach to the patient with congestive heart failure. It is particularly important to note that these patients were seriously ill, and all exhibited severe degrees of cardiac decompensation. It is in just such patients (those with severe physical difficulties) that there may be a tendency to minimize or ignore the possibility of an emotional component to the illness. We feel it is evident from the data presented that the extent of structural heart damage and cardiac decompensation do not necessarily serve as indications or clues to the *nature* of the forces responsible for the loss of circulatory equilibrium at a specific time. Experience with patients who were followed on a long-term basis is felt to point up the important role the doctor-patient relationship may play in the overall handling of this medical problem.

Summary

In a study of the precipitating events connected with episodes of congestive heart failure in 25 consecutive hospital admissions, emotional stress played a major role in 76 %. From a consideration of the patients' personality structures and their verbalizations, it was evident that these time-correlated life situations had strong emotional meaning. This unexpectedly high incidence of precipitating factors related to emotional stress may, in large part, be explained by the circumstances of the study, in which the patients were interviewed with a warm and helpful approach at a time when they were experiencing acute and overwhelming fear of death. This situation seemed to result in a dramatic lowering of psychological defenses. Material which otherwise would have been guarded was freely confided. This experience was associated with no deleterious effects to the patients; in some instances it seemed to have a beneficial influence on their physiologic status. It was observed that loss of security through rejection by some key figure upon whom the patient was dependent constituted an overwhelming threat for the patients in this series, and that this stress was common to the various life events responsible for the precipitation of failure in the group studied.

This was also observed in the longer studies, in which compensation was maintained as long as the patient-physician relationship was satisfactory; but as soon as this relationship was threatened, the patients again developed congestive heart failure.

Conclusion

Emotional stress is a frequent precipitating factor in the development of congestive heart failure in the patient with limited cardiac reserve.

Appendix

Case 2. C.M., a 72-year-old white woman, was diagnosed as having hypertensive and arteriosclerotic heart disease with auricular fibrillation; chronic cystitis, and congestive heart failure of 2 weeks' duration.

Background
This patient had long-standing, severe hypertension and marked arteriosclerosis. There had been previous episodes of congestive failure, but the recent attack had been preceded by several years of compensation. She had a background of severe deprivation, but had always maintained an independent status and said that she never wanted to be a bother to anyone. For the previous year she had been obliged to live with a relative because of her failing vision.

Precipitating Factor
The relative with whom the patient was living found herself unable to continue with this arrangement. A social worker visited the home and informed the patient that she would have to go to the 'County Home'. Immediately following this, she developed severe congestive heart failure.

Case 3. A.S., a 65-year-old Negro woman, was diagnosed as having arteriosclerotic heart disease with auricular fibrillation; arteriosclerosis obliterans, right leg; generalized arteriosclerosis; and congestive heart failure of 2 months' duration.

Background
The patient had been an extremely hard worker all her life and had always been independent, controlling, and demanding of those about her. For several years she had managed to remain self-sufficient despite the disability and pain attendant on severe obliterating arteriosclerosis of the right leg. During this period there had been no congestive failure.

Precipitating Factor
Amputation of the right leg without the patient's consent. She was not told that actual amputation was to be done. On recovering from anesthesia she was furious that the leg had been removed. At this time there was onset of the first attack of congestive heart failure. She repeatedly said, 'How come you put me in the hospital and let them take my leg off.' Following this she would become quite violent and would have an attack of severe dyspnea. 'And now I have to sit where they put me ...

It's bad just to sit down – it's terrible. I worry and fuss all the time. I start to do something, and then I find I can't do anything without help. I was always very independent. I did things for myself and my children ... I don't want to have to depend on others. I need a leg, and I ain't dead yet. My left leg began swelling after they took my right leg off. They didn't swell before that. I had lots of feeling of misery after they took the leg off.' The daughter with whom the patient lived also dated the onset to this event. She further described how the patient repeatedly would develop pulmonary edema whenever she became 'excited and upset' over the loss of her leg, and the fact that she was not forewarned of the procedure.

Case 4. C.B., a 66-year-old Negro man, was diagnosed as having chronic bronchial asthma, pulmonary emphysema; corpulmonale; chronic alcoholism; and chronic, progressive congestive heart failure of 1 year's duration.

Background
The patient reported that he had been separated from his wife for 15 years and that he had been living alone for this period without maintaining much, if any, direct contact with any of his 5 children. His life story was characterized by mild pseudomasculine denial of dependency and chronic alcoholism. Life relationships had been tenuous; his work record was sporadic. He was extremely reluctant to discuss his children, stating that they were all failures and that they did not 'figure' in his life situation. He was obviously depressed and talked repeatedly of his aloneness and the fact that there was no one to help him.

Precipitating Factor
The sudden death of a son (age 33) who had been living with the patient for many years. Although the patient had not mentioned the fact of his son's death or talked of his relationship with him, it was learned through social service contacts that there had been an extremely close relationship between them. They had been living together, and the patient had been quite dependent upon him. Following the son's death, mild congestive failure developed. On hospitalization, digitalis intoxication was also found to be present.

Case 5. C.L., a 72-year-old Negro woman, was diagnosed as having arteriosclerotic heart disease; alopecia areata; chronic cystitis; chronic pyelonephritis; chronic, mild congestive heart failure for 3 years, and acute exacerbation of 3 weeks' duration.

Background

The patient had always been an extremely controlling, domineering woman who had invested all her energies in an excessively possessive relationship with her children. Her own childhood had been extremely deprived, both materially and emotionally. 'I don't think we ever had the feeling of love in our home ... I love my children to death; and they love me. I've always tried to show all the affection to my children, because if a child grows up without love then he loves nobody and nobody loves him ... They all say if I die they don't want to live. They will have nothing to live for if I did, even though they are married.' She had attempted to live with her favorite son, but had moved out 9 months previously because she was jealous of the attention the son showed to his wife. Subsequent to this her son had visited her regularly until 3 weeks preceding admission to the hospital, which was the time the episode of congestive failure developed.

Precipitating Factors

An argument with her favorite son during which he rejected her totally and said he would never return to visit her again. In addition, the patient's landlady threatened to turn her out and force her into a chronic disease hospital. During the same week another son suffered a leg fracture in an accident. The daughter described the onset of failure as follows: 'There was a terrible argument 3 weeks ago. He said he wouldn't come back to see her again. She told him everything she thought of him – all about his wife and all of that. She had been fine until then, and then came the terrible argument, and she was sick and terrible short of breath. The next morning she said, "I'm terribly short of breath. I can't get my breath. It all happened last night." And she was unable to get up and go downstairs.'

Case 6. G.W., a 45-year-old Negro man, was diagnosed as having hypertensive cardiovascular disease and acute congestive heart failure of two weeks' duration with rapid progression during the 6 h immediately preceding hospitalization.

Background

The main theme of the patient's life story had been one of continual hard work, excessive ambition, perfectionism, and maintenance of an 'independent' front. His early life had been characterized by deprivation and strict, demanding parental attitudes (particularly on the father's part). The perfectionistic drives and needs for independence and success were felt to represent both a denial of his dependent strivings and a need to continually conform to the parental standards which had been set up in childhood. He had carried a responsible supervisory job with a taxi company for the 15 years previous. This had seemed to satisfy most of his ambition and strivings for prestige. His marriage was unsatisfactory and he had maintained close relationship with his mother and a sister who worked for the same taxi company. Although the sister was in a subordinate position to him, it was apparent that he had depended upon her for emotional support and advice in the management of his job. Some time before the present illness, his job had lost its gratifications and had become a source of worry instead. First, unionization had made the men, who formerly had accepted his supervision, rebellious and hostile. Second, the business began to fail, and 1 month prior to hospitalization the patient was faced with the prospect of his first failure.

Precipitating Factors

Failure of his business, followed by the serious illness of his mother, and the feeling that he had been deserted by his sister. At the time of the mother's illness and eviction from his apartment (2 weeks before hospitalization) mild congestive failure developed. The day before admission the patient had called his sister for advice and solace. He was told that she had left the city for a vacation. The symptoms of congestive heart failure developed within a few hours.

Case 7. W.L., a 59-year-old Negro man, was diagnosed as having arteriosclerotic heart disease; digitalis intoxication; and congestive heart failure, recurrent for the previous 3 years, persistently progressive for 6 months.

Background

This man's problems revolve about his unsatisfied wishes for security and dependence upon a maternal figure. He was one of 14 children born to an impoverished Southern Negro family. He had to leave home to work on the railroad when he was 10 years old. In his first marriage, his wife had little time for him since she was always busy bearing children. When he was 27 years old, she died, leaving him with 7 children to care for. After several years, he deserted his home and children to live with his mother. After his mother's death, he moved to Cincinnati and remarried, still seeking a satisfactory and secure relationship with a woman. About 5 to 6 years prior to the present illness his second wife began to consort with other men and to neglect their home. There were numerous arguments between them, but prior to the present illness there had been no separation, and the patient, despite his anger, never could bring himself to initiate such a step. He had been suffering recurrent episodes of congestive heart failure for the past 3 years.

Precipitating Factor

In February, 1949, the patient's wife deserted him and moved to another city. She told a friend that she didn't care if the patient lived or died. Within the next few weeks congestive failure recurred and persisted, despite medical treatment, until his admission to the hospital 6 months later in August, 1949. At this time, his course was complicated by digitalis intoxication. (During the early part of his hospital stay he developed a delirium in which the intense conflict in relation to his wife was reflected in paranoid delusions, she appeared as the central persecuting figure in these delusions, with murderous intentions toward him.)

Case 8.
F.K., an 83-year-old white woman, was diagnosed as having arteriosclerotic heart disease with auricular fibrillation, and acute congestive heart failure of 3 hours' duration.

Background

This 83-year-old woman had led a relatively uneventful life. One of her 4 children had died, and the other 3 had married and been out of the home for many years. She and her husband had been living out their old age alone. Prior to the present illness there had been no congestive failure, although physical examination had revealed left ventricular enlargement and auricular fibrillation. Her husband had been blind for 7 years and, according to the family, had become increasingly irascible, violent, and demanding of attention. For the 5 months preceding the patient's illness, he had been totally bedridden and had manifested outbreaks of demanding behavior and violent temper tantrums of psychotic proportions.

Precipitating Factor

The sudden and unexpected death of her husband. Immediately following his death, the patient seemed to show little grief: her son reported that she 'shed a few tears but held the rest in.' Six hours later, acute left ventricular failure developed and she was brought to the hospital.

Case 9.
W.W., a 57-year-old Negro woman, presented a medical diagnosis of hypertensive and arteriosclerotic cardiovascular disease; arteriolonephrosclerosis; congestive heart failure, chronic, with frequent acute exacerbations for the preceding 2 years.

Background

The patient was one of many children from a poor Southern Negro family. She had found some security and stability as an adult in her marriage and family life. Although her husband had as a young man been a nomadic person, he had always maintained contact with the patient and she had always been very attached to him. She had worked extremely hard and long in order to help him financially and keep the family together. There was also a close mutual attachment with the elder of her 2 sons. She expressed the feeling that he was the only person who mattered to her following the death of her husband in October, 1942. This favorite son had married in 1940 but had lived with his wife at his parents' home. Although he had moved to a place of his own shortly after his father's death, he and his wife had been forced within a few months to return to his mother's apartment. He felt that there was a great deal of competitive enmity and strain between the two women. Congestive heart failure had first developed in 1947 and had persisted in chronic form (with occasional acute exacerbations) until the time of study in August, 1949.

Precipitating Factors

Conflict with the daughter-in-law over the favorite son. The patient resented her son's attachment to his wife and was extremely hostile to her but, at the same time, realistically dependent upon her. She sensed that too frank a display of hostility would lead to an open break and loss of her son. The onset of congestive failure followed a 3 to 4 month period in which the daughter-in-law had been ill and the patient had been obliged to care for her and cater to her wishes. Subsequent acute attacks of congestive failure had followed arguments with the daughter-in-law, and the son had noticed that during periods of tension the patient would break with her medical regimen, eat large quantities of salt, and neglect to take her digitalis.

Case 10. M.C., a 67-year-old white woman, was diagnosed as having arteriosclerotic heart disease; chronic auricular fibrillation; generalized arteriosclerosis; portal cirrhosis; esophageal varices; nontoxic nodular goiter; cellulitis, right leg; and chronic congestive heart failure for the previous 2 years, with the development of an acute episode three weeks previously.

Background

This patient, the oldest of 6 siblings, had developed a pattern of hard work and caring for others early in her life. Her first marriage had failed and had been followed 9 years later by a second unsatisfactory, but permanent marriage to an irresponsible alcoholic. Her total adjustment had remained fairly satisfactory as long as she had been able to work productively and carry the responsibility for rearing a number of small children. Although she had been unable to have children of her own, she had cared for a series of 'adopted' and foster children. Following the failure of a family business venture in 1937, her relationship with her husband had deteriorated markedly, from that time on he had worked only sporadically as a laborer and had been an unreliable source of support. Following the disappointment of the business failure, the patient had discontinued work and had devoted all of her energies to the care of the children. Only one of them, a boy, remained permanently in her care and was 23 years old at the time of this study. In recent years, he and the husband had been rebelling more

openly against the patient's possessive demands. The 'son' particularly resented the fact that he was expected to help with the care of the infants whom the patient was still bringing into her home. She had been in chronic congestive failure for 2 years preceding the present hospital admission.

Precipitating Factor

Three weeks prior to the patient's admission, the unmarried mother of an infant that the patient had taken to raise changed her mind and decided that she wanted the baby back. The mother, knowing the patient's temperament, had sneaked into the apartment and 'stolen' the child. When the loss was discovered, the patient flew into a rage and developed an exacerbation of her failure, which eventually required that she be hospitalized. This incident was superimposed upon the chronic strain of the gradual deterioration of her relationship with her husband and 'son', and upon multiple organic predisposing and contributory influences, such as malnutrition, low grade infection, and advanced arteriosclerotic heart disease.

Case 11. G.B., a 71-year-old white man, was diagnosed as having rheumatic heart disease, inactive, with mitral stenosis and insufficiency; generalized arteriosclerosis; and chronic congestive heart failure for 9 years, with increasingly frequent episodes of acute decompensation for the preceding 2 to 3 years.

Background

The patient, who had been orphaned as a child in Germany, had been raised by strict and demanding grandparents. He had worked his way through architecture and engineering school and, following his arrival in the United States in 1909, his story was that of a typical, highly successful, self-made man. In 1935 he suffered severe business reverses: the story from then on is one of progressive loss of prestige and money, with desperate attempts at restoring his lost self-esteem through the old pattern of hard work and self-discipline. He entered a small restaurant business which had been established by his wife. Following the failure of this venture, he bought a small candy store. This was never successful, and the patient leaned heavily upon his wife and daughter for its operation. At the age of 65 he was 'managing' the store, and at the outbreak of World War II took an additional job as a night worker in a war plant. Congestive heart failure first appeared in 1940. In 1946 his daughter married, leaving only his wife to help at the store. In 1948 the wife developed diabetic gangrene and amputation of her leg was performed. The patient now had to care for her. The business was 'in the red' and he was able to keep the store open only by accepting contributions from relatives. However, he refused to give up. 'She (wife) has been progressively useless around the place and I have had to bear more and more of the burdens of the work. Everything has been terrible. I stand outside so I can breathe. I can't sleep at night ... I'm all gone, but I want to stay here with my little store in spite of the fact that everything has gone to pieces.'

Precipitating Factor
The combination of circumstances described above was accompanied by gradual increase in the severity of the congestive failure, finally necessitating hospitalization at the time of study (September, 1949).

Case 12. M.T., a 54-year-old white woman, was diagnosed as having hypertensive and arteriosclerotic heart disease, and congestive heart failure of 5 months' duration.

Background
The most outstanding characteristic of this patient's personality was her increasing intolerance for frustration. For years preceding this study she had been building up an increasing tension in connection with a progressive deterioration of her relationship with her second husband and her children. She had experienced two episodes of acute congestive failure in the preceding 5 months. 'My nerves get so bad, they overpower my heart. Just anything makes me nervous ... At times I get so nervous I don't want anyone around. I get so aggravated with my husband ... I've had lots of breathing attacks ... Before I have the attack I always have a nervous spell. I get cross. Nothing goes right. My husband says to me: "Well, I'm glad it's time for me to go to work. You're terrible to live with." And he walks out!' In the few months immediately preceding the present attack the patient had been experiencing marked conflict with a nephew who was living in her home but who

refused to conform to her wishes. In addition, her 29-year-old daughter had been an ever-increasing source of worry and aggravation.

Precipitating Factor
A fight with the daughter concerning drinking. 'She's 29 years old. She married a man who is 63. She is so mean. She's hotheaded. She was in the WACS. She drinks all the time and there is nothing that makes me so nervous. I just can't stand it. I tried to bring her up well, but she has taken to drink ... much worse in the past year; and that's why I'm worse in the past year. On Saturday night – that was three nights ago – we were playing Pinochle and she started to drink. I got so upset I got up and left. Her drinking upsets me more than anything else and that's what brought on this attack.'

Case 13. B.K., a 65-year-old white woman, was diagnosed as having hypertensive cardiovascular disease; obesity; congestive heart failure, mildly progressive for 1 week preceding admission; and acute pulmonary edema of 8 hours' duration.

Background
Patient was the youngest of 13 children and had been raised by a strict, demanding mother with whom she had had a poor and insecure relationship. Fifteen years preceding admission, her husband had died. This left the patient to her own resources for support, since her children were married and were not in a position to help her. She had managed by working as a cook in a home for the aged. She had always felt a great need to do things to perfection, and particularly to be in control and receive full credit for the kitchen work. For the preceding 3 years there had been increasing conflict with a younger woman who worked as her assistant and was becoming a threat to her authority and prestige. 'I work with a girl who is a nervous wreck. She makes my life miserable. I can't stand her. She is my assistant. I've worked with her for 3 years. She gets worse and worse. I just walk away; I can't say anything back. That's my trouble. If I could get it out, it would be all right; but I just keep it inside and get more and more nervous. She is married. Her husband is an orderly. They fight all the time. She makes me nervous, shouts at me, tries to argue, gets me all nerved up. Don't tell anyone about this. If you did I'd lose my job.'

Precipitating Factor

The return of her assistant from a vacation. The patient described with a good deal of guilt how she had enjoyed the 2 weeks' respite from her stormy contacts with this woman. During that period, however, she had suffered nightmares from which she would awaken 'screaming for help'. 'The assistant cook came back on the night I was brought here.'

Case 14. I.B., a 36-year-old white man, was diagnosed as having inactive rheumatic heart disease, with mitral stenosis and insufficiency; tricuspid insufficiency; auricular fibrillation; multiple arterial emboli; bronchopneumonia; azotemia; amputation of the right leg; progressive congestive heart failure of 15 weeks' duration (previous episode of congestive failure 3 years ago).

Background

The patient had always shown an excessive need to deny symptoms, to excel, to work extremely hard, and to maintain a strong 'masculine' front. He had suffered an initial attack of rheumatic fever at the age of 24, but continued to work effectively following recovery. He nursed his father through a long illness. 'He finally died because the water flooded his heart out.' His marriage was unsatisfactory from the start, but in the earlier years the patient's work and children had filled in the gaps, and there had been little overt friction. Five years before the time of study, his wife had left him and taken their 3 children with her. Two years later, she deserted the children, and the patient had to take them back into his home. It was at this time that the first episode of congestive failure occurred. Following this, he was advised to move in with his brother and sister-in-law and their 10 children. Gradually, his brother, who was irresponsible, began to run up large debts, and the patient (fearing for his own reputation and job) assumed responsibility for those debts and for the support of the brother's large family as well as his own. In addition, the brother had become ill during the past year and had to be hospitalized. The sister-in-law would frequently leave home to visit her husband, leaving the patient with the physical management of the household as well. 'My brother is very sick. He'll be on crutches for a year. He was a horse trainer, but didn't make any money. I was supporting him and his family as well as my own. Now everything has fallen on me. I can't work and am in the hospital. I'm broke. I haven't worked for 15 weeks. I had to stay home and take care of those brats while my sister-in-law went to see my brother.'

Precipitating Factor

Immediately prior to the onset of congestive failure the brother's creditors visited the patient at his place of employment and demanded that the ever-mounting debts be settled. The patient worried a good deal and attempted to make plans to settle the accounts if possible. He feared that his employers would think the debts were his own personal ones and that they might then fire him. He continued to work despite the onset of increasing dyspnea and ankle edema. Routine treatment by a local physician failed to arrest the progress of these symptoms. 'I felt there was no hope. My father got dropsy just like me, and he died.' During this time, the sister-in-law deserted the home leaving the care of the 10 children to him. It was in this setting that his symptoms became extremely severe and he was admitted.

Case 15. J.H., a 48-year-old Negro man, was diagnosed as having arteriosclerotic heart disease; generalized arteriosclerosis; and chronic recurrent congestive heart failure of 8 months' duration. The patient had suffered a myocardial infarction a year before the present hospital admission.

Background

The patient, the youngest of '14 head', had been mother's favorite and had remained at home until the age of 25. He had had a short-lived common-law marriage but had deserted his wife and children after a few years. 'After I lost my mother, I didn't get back home ... I left my wife 17 years ago; I have no friends. People did not help me out. Mother died 17 years ago at the same time that I left my wife.' From that time until he suffered a myocardial infarction in 1948 the patient had led a no-madic day-to-day existence. Following the myocardial infarction, his employer, who had previously been indulgent, became less supportive and finally fired him. He adjusted poorly and within 4 months developed congestive failure. There followed a series of readmissions to the hospital. On each admission he would show overt regressive behavior.

As soon as compensation would be achieved, he would be discharged, only to return again within a few weeks or months with massive edema and dyspnea. Between admissions he would fail to take his digitalis and would not report to the clinic for mercurial injections.

Precipitating Factor
It became clear that the protective atmosphere of the hospital was so gratifying to this overtly dependent individual that he was actually having repeated attacks of failure, which were self-induced through conscious neglect. After the pattern became clear, the patient was transferred to the Chronic Disease Hospital. This he readily accepted and congestive failure did not recur after his admission to the more permanent institution during the period of observation.

Case 16. L.F., a 30-year-old Negro woman, was diagnosed as having hypertensive cardiovascular disease; chronic progressive congestive heart failure of 6 months' duration with acute progression in the 2 weeks preceding admission and paroxysmal dyspnea of 12 hours' duration.

Background
The patient had been raised by strict foster parents, her own parents having died during the first year of her life. She married at the age of 16 to get away from her foster mother. Her marriage had turned out to be insecure and unsatisfying as she felt that her husband was unfaithful and inattentive. She had always been an extremely volatile person emotionally and had been a chronic alcoholic for many years. In recent months she had felt doubly frustrated by her husband, who had begun to walk away from her when she would lose her temper. 'I always get mad and shake all over. Then I get an attack. Sometimes when I get mad I want to throw something or hit somebody. If I can't, then I cry and I wheeze all up and I get an attack. I get mad at my husband when he won't do what I want. When I get mad I can't talk. I shout so loud they can hear me for 3 miles. My husband shuts all the doors and the windows so the neighbors won't know our affairs. He mostly walks out when I get mad, and that makes me madder. I always want sexual intercourse 2 times a night. It doesn't make me get out of breath. My husband says, "You're sick", but I say I'm not

sick down there. He doesn't want it much, only once a week; I tell him he goes out with other women. I get mad when he doesn't come home. I peek out the windows, and I get so mad I choke all up.'

Precipitating Factor
Increasing tension in relation to the husband. The night before admission the patient had flown into a rage against her husband and then developed the attack of acute dyspnea which necessitated hospitalization.

Case 17. G.F., a 70-year-old white man, was diagnosed as having arteriosclerotic heart disease with auricular fibrillation; benign prostatic hypertrophy; malnutrition; and congestive heart failure: acute episode 1 year previously, chronic failure for past 6 months, with acute exacerbation of 3 weeks' duration preceding current admission.

Background
The patient was born and raised in Germany by strict, demanding, and rigid parents. His father had been a butcher; the patient always felt that his father had been excessively demanding of him and yet had given little or nothing in return. The patient did not marry. At the age of 27 he had come to the USA, where he worked at various jobs, never finding security or realizing any productivity. He had made no lasting relationships until 12 years previously when he had taken a job as gardener and caretaker for a wealthy butcher and his wife. His relationship to the butcher and his wife reproduced in many ways his earlier life relationships to his parents. He felt that they were too demanding and too dependent upon him. He felt closer to the wife than to the husband, just as he had felt closer to his mother than to his father. Many times he had wanted to leave, but each time they would plead with him to stay. Finally, a year before the present study, the patient had quit his job and taken a room in a men's hotel. He left because he felt that his employers were stealing his tools and using many of his possessions without permission.

Precipitating Factor
Dissolution of his relationship and home with his employers. The first episode of failure followed this incident. The episode 3 weeks prior to admission was preceded by the death

of his former employer. The patient became very excited as he spoke of his determination to get his tools back now that the employer had died. 'They all had long fingers. Everything disappeared, so finally I left. I get all upside down when I get so excited. I can't stand it. It's just like lightning strikes you.'

Case 18. G.F., a 73-year-old white man, was diagnosed as having hypertensive cardiovascular disease with auricular fibrillation; Adams-Stokes syndrome; and chronic congestive heart failure with recurrent attacks of paroxysmal dyspnea of 1 year's duration.

Background

The patient had lost both parents at the age of 4 and had been raised then by an uncle 'who despised me and treated me like an animal'. He finally left the uncle's home and wandered the country working at various laboring and construction jobs. He had married 37 years previously during the course of his travels; there were no children. For years he and his wife had led a nomadic type of existence, but 18 years ago they had settled down in an apartment in Cincinnati. Although the patient had a need to impress the examiner with his abilities and the importance of his work, his wife reported that his jobs had always been unimpressive and that they had never managed to accumulate much in the way of savings or attain any degree of security. Five years prior to the present study, he had begun to suffer from attacks of Adams-Stokes syncope. This necessitated his discontinuing work. Since that time he and his wife had been 'ailing' and spent all of their time together in the small apartment which they were struggling to hold on to by working as caretakers of the building.

Precipitating Factor

Threatened eviction from his apartment. 'Yes, that is the time I got sick. That caused it ... We are both old and failing, and then finally we ran that place so that we could stay there. We'd lived there for 18 years. It was hell in the first degree for her to keep taking care of me and us trying to make a go of it together. Then they tried to force me out; and that's when I got sick. But I ain't beholdin' to nobody. I don't owe nobody a nickel. I'd die right now if I could. I have no desire to go on living. I have nothing to live for.'

Case 19. C.W., a 69-year-old white man, was diagnosed as having hypertensive cardiovascular disease with auricular fibrillation; generalized arteriosclerosis; and chronic, progressive congestive heart failure of 3 month's duration.

Background

The patient, with a background of dependency and chronic alcoholism, was, prior to onset of congestive failure, living out his years in the care of an unmarried daughter. His life had been colorless and routine. His wife had died 15 years previously and the daughter had remained unmarried in order to make a home for him. In 1944 (5 years prior to the present study), he had had a brief, acute psychotic episode which, on the basis of diagnostic study at that time, was felt to be due to vascular brain disease. He had not worked since that time and had adjusted fairly well to a simple, uncomplicated life which centered in and around his apartment and his daughter.

Precipitating Factor

Forcible eviction from the apartment in which he had been living for 12 years. 'The landlord had become nasty and mean, did everything against us he could. I think because I lived there long I was terribly upset. It was impossible to find a new place. I ain't got no home.'

References

1. DUNCAN, C. H.; STEVENSON, I. P., and RIPLEY, H. S.: Life situations, emotions, and paroxysmal auricular arrhythmias. Psychosom. Med. 12: 23 (1950).
2. GROLLMAN, A.: The effect of psychic disturbances on the cardiac output, blood pressure and oxygen consumption in man. Amer. J. Physiol. 89: 584 (1929).
3. HARRISON, T. R.: Failure of the circulation, 2nd ed., p. 123 (Williams and Wilkins, Baltimore 1939).
4. HICKAM, J. B.; CARGILL, W. H., and GOLDEN, A.: Cardiovascular reactions to emotional stimuli. Effect on cardiac output, A.V. oxygen difference, arterial pressure and peripheral resistance. J. clin. Invest. 27: 290 (1948).
5. KATZ, L.; WINTON, S. S., and MEGILOW, R. S.: Psychosomatic aspects of cardiac

arrhythmias. A physiological dynamic approach. Ann. intern. Med. *27:* 261 (1947).

6. STEAD, E. A., Jr.; WARREN, J. V.; MERRILL, A. J., and BRANNON, E. S.: The cardiac output in male subjects as measured by the technique of right atrial catheterization, normal values with observations on the effects of anxiety and tilting. J. clin. Invest. *24:* 326 (1945).

7. STEVENSON, I. P.; DUNCAN, C. D., and WOLFF, H.: Circulatory dynamics before and after exercise in subjects with and without structural heart disease during anxiety and relaxation. J. clin. Invest. *28:* 1534 (1949).

8. WENDKOS, M. H.: The influence of autonomic imbalance on the human electrocardiogram. I. Unstable T waves in precordial leads from emotionally unstable persons without organic heart disease. Amer. Heart J. *28:* 549 (1944).

9. WHITE, P.: Heart disease, 3rd ed., p. 753 (Macmillan, New York 1945).

10. WOLF, G. A. and WOLFF, H. G.: Studies on the nature of certain symptoms associated with cardiac vascular disorders. Psychosom. Med. *8:* 239 (1946).

Some Experimental Observations on Gastrointestinal Lesions in Behaviorally Conditioned Monkeys[1]

R. W. PORTER, J. V. BRADY, D. CONRAD, J. W. MASON, R. GALAMBOS and D. McK. RIOCH

Retrospective comment by Dr. H. Weiner. The work reported in this paper was the outcome of two trends in research on the pathogenesis of peptic ulcer: (1) Clinical observation that the onset of peptic ulcer begins in specific environmental situations which are 'stressful' to the predisposed individual, (2) Experimental observations in animals that the conflict between the need to obtain food and water (in a rat deprived of them), and the need to avoid electric shock, seemed to produce gastric erosions [SAWREY et al.]. Similar lesions could be produced merely by immobilizing a rat [SELYE].

One of the remarkable experimental findings of PORTER and coworkers (which is the subject of this reprint), was that only the 'executive' monkeys developed the gastrointestinal lesions. In a study reported at about the same time (1958), BRADY et al. found gastric and duodenal ulcers at the autopsy of monkeys which had performed for many days a lever-pressing response to avoid shock to himself and another monkey. This other monkey was not trained to perform the response and never developed an ulcer.

In 1962 POLISH et al. working in the same laboratory as PORTER and BRADY, employed similar schedules of avoidance conditioning. Two of 9 monkeys were found to have duodenal ulcers, the remaining seven had no gastroduodenal lesions. In 1964, FOLTZ and MILLETT reported that they could not reproduce PORTER's and BRADY's findings. But they did not examine the upper GI tract at autopsy. Rather, in their 6 monkeys, they examined the stool for blood daily, and found none. A laparatomy was performed on one monkey and no lesion could be palpated. It has been suggested that the differences in results reported from the two laboratories could be explained on the basis of species differences. It seems that at least two pairs of monkeys in PORTER's experiment were *Macaca iris*. While FOLTZ and MILLET used *M. mulatta*.

On balance the data suggest that gastric and duodenal lesions can be produced by avoidance conditioning. The temporal patterning of the avoidance task is most important if lesions are to be produced. Additional factors, such as strain and other individual differences (some of which remain unknown) probably also play a role in the pathogenesis of ulcers in monkeys. The central nervous mechanisms which mediate the effects of such conditioning remain to be worked out in full.

A high incidence of gastrointestinal disease in a group of monkeys undergoing psychological conditioning studies has been observed in our laboratories. As the underlying disease processes were not those usually encountered in a monkey population under laboratory conditions, further inquiry into the possible etiological factors contributing to this occurrence seemed indicated. For the most part, the experimental procedures undertaken with these animals were directed toward an analysis of various aspects of emotional behavior, although the program differed somewhat for each animal during the initial observations. These somewhat fortuitous findings, however, did appear to justify a more detailed and sys-

[1] From the Division of Neuropsychiatry, Walter Reed Army Institute of Research, Walter Reed Army Medical Center, Washington 12, D.C.

tematic analysis of the possible psychosomatic relationships discernible under such experimental conditions.

The present report first describes the observations on the initial series of 19 rhesus monkeys, to include a descriptive analysis of both the various behavioral procedures used with these animals, and the somatic pathology which developed during the course of these behavioral experiments. Secondly, the initial results of a more systematic follow-up study with an additional series of 4 rhesus monkeys utilizing a single behavioral procedure with suitable controls will be described along with the correlated gastrointestinal findings in these animals.

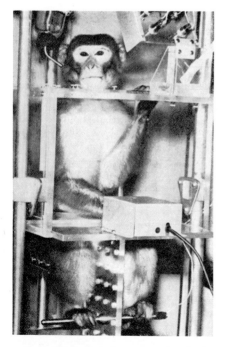

Fig. 1. Illustration shows a monkey in the chair-type restraining device used in these studies.

Experiments with Intermixed Programs

General Procedure

Nineteen rhesus monkeys of the initial series in this study were gently restrained in plastic chairs, as illustrated in figure 1, providing for freedom of all limbs, self-feeding facilities, and collection of excreta for hormonal determinations [21]. In addition, the chairs were equipped with attachments for presentation of auditory and visual stimuli, automatic delivery of sugar-pellet rewards and brief electric shocks, and a lever-operated microswitch within easy reach of the monkey. All animals were trained to press the lever in this situation for a food reward, to avoid an electric shock, or to adjust to some combination of these positive and negative events. Both the experimental program and the length of time in the chair differed in greater or lesser degree for each animal, as indicated in the tables I and II. Some monkeys were removed from and returned to the chair several times during the total experimental period (column 1, tables I and II). All animals were kept on their usual diet of fresh fruit and vegetables and biscuit-type monkey food (Dietrich & Cambrill Co.), although the time of the daily feeding varied in accordance with the experimental program. Upon termination of the behavioral studies, all animals were sacrificed and a complete gross and microscopic *post mortem* examination was performed.

Lever Pressing for Food Reward

All but 1 animal in the first series were trained to press the lever for sugar-pellet rewards. The monkeys were deprived of food for 24 h or more and then initially permitted to obtain one 45 mg glucose tablet every time they pressed the lever and closed the microswitch (continuous reinforcement or CRF). Within a few sessions, however, all animals were shifted to one of two reward schedules which permitted delivery of the sugar pellet for a lever response only on a 'partial reinforcement' basis. On one of these schedules (variable interval reinforcement or VI), a sugar pellet was delivered to the monkey for a lever response only after varying intervals of time (average, 60 sec) had elapsed since delivery of the last pellet reward. On the other positive reward schedule (fixed ratio reinforcement or FR), a sugar pellet was delivered to the monkey for a lever response only after a fixed number of bar presses (i.e., 100) had been made since delivery of the last sugar-pellet reward. Both these reinforcement schedules produce stable but characteristically different response patterns, which provide baselines for the behavioral procedures described below [3, 8, 32, 33].

Conditioned 'Anxiety' Procedure

All the monkeys studied in this emotional conditioning situation were first trained in lever pressing for sugar-pellet rewards on the variable interval reinforcement schedule described above. Then, the conditioned 'anxiety' response was superimposed upon the stable lever-pressing habit according to a procedure previously described in some detail [3]. Briefly, the animals received a series of conditioning trials, each consisting of the presentation of a clicking noise for 5 min terminated with a brief painful electric shock (5–8 mA, 60 cycles AC, for 0.5 sec) to the feet during the sugar-rewarded lever-pressing sessions. After a few pairings of clicker and shock in this fashion, the anticipatory 'fear' or 'anxiety' response appears as a disruption of the stable lever-pressing pattern accompanied by alternating immobility and intense locomotor activity, trembling, piloerection, and frequently urination and defecation in response to presentation of the clicker. With continued training on this procedure, the animals developed a stable pattern of responding during experimental sessions of up to several hours with 5-min presentations of the clicker interspersed with 10-min periods of no clicker. During the no clicker periods, the monkeys maintained a steady lever-pressing rate for the variable-interval sugar-pellet reward and showed a marked suppression of such responding during the clicker cycles, even though the lever responses would have produced sugar pellets on the same schedule.

Table I. Individual behavioral conditioning programs and lesions observed

Monkey	Days in chair	Total experimental days	Food reward hours	Conditioning anxiety 15-min trials	Conditioning punishment 5-min trials	Conditioning avoidance hours	Combined conditioning procedure 6–8-hour sessions Total	Night sessions	Pathology
M 3	37	30	2	–	–	2	28	25	Gastric hemorrhage and erosion
M 32	9	9	9	–	–	–	–	–	
	54	32	7	7	–	3	25	6	Duodenal ulcer
M 34	65	53	12	–	–	13	26	26	Gastric hemorrhage and erosion
M 41	14	10	–	–	–	2	8	4	Intussusception
M 1	36	15	12	–	–	8	–	–	
	19	4	4	–	–	–	–	–	Chronic colitis
M 48	30	12	5	–	3	7	–	–	Perforated duodenal ulcer,
	7	3	1	–	3	3	–	–	gastric hemorrhage
	35	22	13	–	41	21	–	–	
M 5	59	44	28	–	76	13	–	–	Gastric erosion
M 20	11	9	–	–	–	9	–	–	Normal
M 31	67	5	5	–	–	–	–	–	Normal

Conditioned 'Punishment' Procedure

In this emotional conditioning situation, too, all monkeys were initially trained in lever pressing for sugar-pellet rewards on a variable-interval reinforcement schedule. Then, the conditioned 'punishment' procedure was superimposed upon the stable lever-pressing behavior in a manner similar to that described above for the 'anxiety' procedure. In this situation, however, the pain-shock was administered concurrently with a lever response in the presence of the warning stimulus (a tone or light) and only if the monkey pressed the bar during this 5-min period [16]. In this instance, then, lever pressing was actually 'punished' in the presence of the warning stimulus, whereas in the 'anxiety' situation, the pain-shock was administered, independently of the lever response, upon termination of the clicker. As a consequence of this 'punishment' procedure, suppression of bar pressing during presentation of the light or tone and maintenance of response rates in its absence is also seen to develop as a stable behavior pattern. For the most part, however, the autonomic concomitants of the conditioned 'anxiety' response described above do not develop as stable components of the 'punishment' situation.

Conditioned 'Avoidance' Procedure

In this related but somewhat different emotional conditioning situation, the monkeys were trained to press the lever to avoid an electric shock to the feet according to a procedure previously described [30]. Brief shocks (5 mA, 60 cycle AC for 0.5 sec) were delivered to the animal's feet at fixed intervals (20 sec) unless the monkey pressed the lever within the 20-sec interval to delay the shock for another 20 sec. Under these conditions, which were obtained whenever a flashing red light was presented, the monkeys rapidly learned to press the lever considerably faster than once every 20 sec, and the stable maintenance of bar-pressing rates approximating 15–20 responses/min effectively avoided all but a few shocks during sessions of several hours or more in duration.

Combined Conditioning Procedures

With some of the animals, as indicated in table I, multiple programs consisting of several reinforcement schedules and emotional conditioning procedures were combined in fixed temporal sequences [9]. In one of these multiple programs, for example, the flashing red light was presented for 15 min, during which time the 'avoidance' contingency described above was in effect; this was followed by a 15-min period during which no stimulus was presented and lever responses did nothing; then, a green light was presented for 15 min and the monkey could obtain sugar pellets on a 100 to 1 fixed ratio schedule; finally, another 15-min period with no stimulus followed before the entire cycle was repeated. Another multiple program utilized with some of the animals combined alternating cycles of the 'avoidance' and 'punishment' procedures superimposed upon a baseline of lever pressing for sugar pellets on a variable-interval schedule of reinforcement. Typically, experimental sessions on the repeated cycles of these multiple programs approximated 6 to 8 h in length, and, for several of the monkeys, sessions were run during the night.

Intracerebral Self-Stimulation Procedure

With 6 of the monkeys in this initial series, as indicated in table II, electrodes were permanently implanted in several different brain loci (principally 'limbic system' structures) according to a procedure previously developed [29]. The electrodes used were bipolar and were secured to a socket on the calvarium from which leads could be taken for stimulation or recording purposes. In this phase of the study, the monkeys were trained to press the lever to obtain a brief electrical-stimulus reward through these electrodes, as originally described by OLDS and MILNER in rats [24] and were placed on different schedules of reinforcement (continuous, variable interval, and fixed ratio) as previously described [2, 31]. The electrical stimulus consisted of a biphasic pulse at a frequency of 100 cps for a train duration of 0.5 sec [19]. The current intensity varied for different animals from 5 to 60 'peak' mA (6–72 V), although the usual 'rewarding' value approximated 20–25 mA (20–30 V).

The procedure followed with these animals involved several 45-min self-stimulation periods, as indicated for each animal in table II. The electrode placements differed for each animal, and the degree to which the electrical

Table II. Behavior programs including self-stimulation

Monkey	Days in chair	Total experimental days	Food reward hours	Conditioning anxiety 15-min trials	Conditioning avoidance hours	Intracerebral self-stimulation[1,2], 45-min periods										Pathology
						Total days	MFB	Amy	Hip	CN	Ant Thal	Hyp	MRF	Sep	GP	
M 30	117	22	2	–	–	20	13±	28+	10+	5±	–	–	–	–	–	Duodenal ulcer
M 36	52	32	8	11	–	21	41+	6–	1–	2–	20+	1–	1–	3–	–	Duodenal ulcer, chronic colitis
R 6	14	12	12	13	–	–	–	–	–	–	–	–	–	–	–	Scarred duodenal pyloric obstruction
	8	7	–	–	–	7	2+	–	2–	–	–	1+	2+	4±	–	
	47	41	6	9	3	25	12+	2–	37±	–	2±	66+	11+	4±	–	
M 21	69	45	12	22	–	4	–	–	–	–	–	–	–	–	4+	Normal
	17	15	10	5	–	7	–	–	–	–	–	–	–	–	7+	
	29	24	16	–	–	15	–	–	–	–	–	–	–	–	16+	
M 53	60	40	24	28	–	16	12+	–	–	–	–	–	–	20–	–	Perforated duodenal ulcer
M 50	44	34	16	42	6	4	–	3±	–	–	–	–	–	1±	–	Normal
	5	4	–	–	–	4	–	2±	2±	–	–	–	–	1±	–	

[1] Intracerebral self-stimulation sites: MFB = median forebrain bundle at preoptic level; Amy = amygdala; Hip = hippocampus; CN = caudate nucleus; Ant Thal = anterior thalamic nucleus; Hyp = hypothalamus; MRF = mesencephalic reticular formation; Sep = septal nucleus; GP = globus pallidus.

[2] + indicates over 1,000 responses; ± indicates 500–1,000 responses/45 min period; – indicates less than 500 responses.

stimulus provided a rewarding effect varied considerably with different placements. In many locations, the high response rates maintained by the animals indicated a highly rewarding effect, while in others, the rather obvious aversive effects of stimulation suppressed the lever-pressing rate. Table II shows the number of days on which self-stimulation sessions were conducted for each of these animals (first column under intracerebral self-stimulation) and the rate of responding for the brain-stimulus reward is roughly indicated as follows: +, greater than 1,000 responses per 45-min period; ±, 500–1,000 responses per 45-min period; and –, less than 500 responses per 45-min period. Histological verification of the electrode placements in each animal upon completion of the study revealed that self-stimulation of the monkeys' brains had included the following locations: median forebrain bundle at the preoptic level (MFB), amygdala (Amy), hippocampus (Hip), caudate nucleus (CN), anterior thalamic nucleus (Ant Thal), hypothalamus (Hyp), mesencephalic reticular formation (MRF), septal nucleus (Sep), and the globus pallidus (GP).

Control Restraint Procedure

A series of 5 additional monkeys were confined in the primate chair-restraining device, as described above, without any additional behavior conditioning or intracranial stimulation. These animals remained in the chair environment with nothing else being done to them for 5 to 6 weeks and appeared normal in every respect throughout the entire period. No *post mortem* examination has as yet been completed on these monkeys, however, since they were not sacrificed.

Gastrointestinal Findings

Eleven of the 19 monkeys subjected to these various combinations of behavioral conditioning procedures died or became moribund and had to be sacrificed after 2–17 weeks of experimental study. With but few exceptions, these animals appeared quite normal during the experimental period and gave no external indication of ill health until 12 to 72 h before their death. As soon as any gross abnormality was noted, the monkeys were removed from their chairs and returned to cages. Only 1

animal (R 6) seemed to recover but succumbed at a later date when experimental studies were resumed. Complete *post mortem* examinations were performed on the 11 animals. Four additional animals were sacrificed for other reasons and no pathological findings were observed. The remaining 4 monkeys were studied for periods of 1 to 4 weeks and are still alive and well.

In each of the eleven animals, the most prominent pathological findings were located somewhere in the gastrointestinal tract. Among the findings were hemorrhage and/or erosion of the stomach, chronic ulceration of the duodenum, enteric intussusception, and chronic colitis. Two animals showed more than one of these lesions (M 36, 48). Complications of these disease processes accounted for the death of the monkeys in many instances.

Gastric Hemorrhage and Erosion

In 4 (M 3, 34, 48, 5) of the 11 monkeys exhibiting gastrointestinal disorder, extensive hemorrhages and/or erosive lesions of the

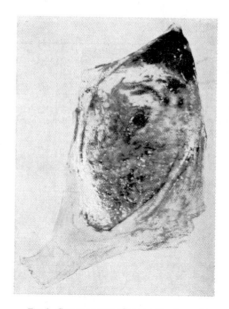

Fig. 2. Gross aspect of stomach of monkey M 3 subjected to intensive combined conditioning procedures showing hemorrhage and erosion of mucosa.

stomach were noted (fig. 2). In each, the stomach was markedly dilated, atonic, and those showing mural hemorrhage contained 50–100 ml of blood. The wall was quite thin, and the normal rugal pattern was lost. Large areas of hemorrhage in the wall were obvious on inspection of 3 of the gross specimens (M 3, 34, 48). Microscopic examination showed the hemorrhage to be confined largely to the submucosal layer, although in some regions it extended into the mucosa as well. Few areas of hemosiderin deposition could be found. An area of erosion (3 to 6 mm in diameter) was encountered on the posterior surface of the fundus in 2 (M 3, 5), and on the greater curvature in the third (M 34). All 3 were in areas not involved by hemorrhage. There was one incident of perforation in the 3 specimens (M 5). These craters were well circumscribed, and in the nonperforated ones, there was complete loss of mucosal substance through superficial muscularis mucosae into the submucosa. There was little indication of tissue reaction to this erosive process in any of the three.

Duodenal Ulceration

Five examples of well-developed duodenal ulceration (M 32, 48, 30, 36, 53) were noted. All were situated in the proximal portion of the duodenum within 3 cm of the pyloric-duodenal junction (fig. 3). Two of the lesions were anterior in position (M 48, 30), while the remaining three were on the posterior side of the intestinal wall. Perforation of the duodenum in 2 animals (M 48, 53) was readily apparent on removing the viscera. Approximately 20 to 30 ml of serous fluid containing intestinal contents was encountered in the peritoneal cavity of these animals. Acute inflammation of the serosa was obvious on gross and microscopic examination.

The diameter of the craters was relatively constant (4 to 5 mm). In all cases the erosion had progressed at least through the submucosa into the muscular layer. The base of the ulcer was composed of granulation tissue in most cases. The circumferential tissue was characterized by some edema, lymphocytic infiltration, and undermining of the mucosal edge.

Post mortem study of an additional animal (R 6) revealed a stellate-shaped cicatrix on the posterior aspect of the proximal duodenum. The lumen of the intestine was markedly attenuated at this point, and the stomach was distended with undigested food. Microscopic examination showed the connective tissue scar to have replaced the mucosa and subcosa and to have involved the inner muscular layer as well.

Intussusception

Monkey M 41 died after failing to eat and vomiting intermittently for 3 days. Autopsy showed an intussusception in the distal ileum with obstruction of the small bowel proximal to this point. The intussusceptum had advanced 8 cm and was markedly discolored with areas of frank hemorrhage in its wall. A specific cause of this occurrence was not readily apparent.

Chronic Colitis

Two well-developed instances of colitis were seen in animals M 1 and M 36. Both these monkeys had obvious signs of inanition. One of these, for which a pre-experimental weight was available, showed a 25% weight reduction. Both had diarrhea and melena intermittently during the 2 weeks prior to the termination of the experiment, which did not respond to antibiotic therapy. Repeated stool specimens examined in each case were negative for parasites. Gross abnormality was obvious on inspection of the mucosal surface of the colon, consisting of areas of hemorrhage and punctate ulceration. The thickness of the wall was greatly increased in the involved areas. In 1 case (M 1), an area of the rectosigmoid colon was so thick that it would not lie flat after the colon was longitudinally opened (fig. 4). This animal showed an additional segmental involvement of the cecum and ascending colon, as well. The rectosigmoid colon was the only area afflicted in the second monkey. The terminal ileum was not involved in either case.

Microscopic examination showed disorganization of the mucosa in all involved regions with degeneration of the glands. Small areas of erosion of the mucosa with very ragged edges were found. The submucosa was characterized by marked thickening, due to the presence of excessive fibrous connective tissue. The muscularis was thickened from edema. Lymphocytic infiltration and hemosiderin deposits were present in both mucosal and submucosal layers, most prominent around blood vessels. Thrombi were occasionally noted in the latter. Microscopic search for parasites was unrewarding.

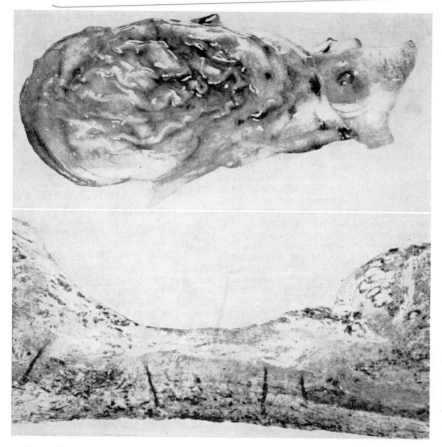

Fig.3. Gross (top) and microscopic (bottom) illustration of duodenal ulcer in monkey M 32 subjected to chronic behavior conditioning procedures.

Experiments with Avoidance Behavior

Despite a careful analysis of both the behavioral and physiological findings on this initial series of 19 monkeys, it proved difficult to isolate the psychological factors presumed to be responsible for these somatic observations. Consequently, a more systematic investigation of the individual behavioral conditioning procedures was undertaken under suitably controlled conditions in an effort to provide more definitive

data on the factors contributing to this occurrence. Since the conditioned avoidance procedure was found to be common to many of the animals in the initial series described above, this was the first behavioral program selected for analysis.

General Procedure

Four monkeys, restrained in chairs as above, were divided into pairs and conditioned according to a 'yoked-chair' avoidance procedure. The animals selected for each pair were similar in species (*Macaca iris*), size, weight (10–11 lb.), and sex (female), and had no known experimental history. Following an initial adaptation period of 5 days in the chair, each pair of monkeys was trained according to a variation in the avoidance procedure described above which permitted only 1 animal of each pair (the experimental monkey) to delay the shock for both itself and its partner (control monkey) by pressing the bar. In this way, only the experimental monkey of each pair learned and continued to perform the lever-pressing avoidance responses (the 'psychological stress' factor), although both animals were subjected to precisely the same number and temporal distribution of electric shocks (the 'physical trauma' factor). Each pair of monkeys received 6-hour sessions on this 'yoked-chair' avoidance procedure (4 to 10 a.m. and 4 to 10 p.m.) alternating with 6-hour 'off periods' (no shocks), 24 h each day, for periods of up to several weeks. A red light was illuminated in plain view of both animals during the 6-hour 'avoidance' periods, and was turned out during the 6-hour 'off' periods. Programing of the experimental procedure and recording of the animal's behavior were accomplished automatically by timers, magnetic counters, cumulative work recorders, and associated relay circuits. Lever

response and shocks were recorded continuously for all animals, and separate counts were maintained for the 'avoidance' periods and for the 'off' periods. Animals were fed their usual diet during the daytime 'off' period between 10 and 11 a.m. Throughout the entire experiment, urine was collected continuously from all animals in 24- or 48-hour samples for 17-hydroxycorticosteroid determinations. In addition, both before and intermittently during the course of the experiments feces were examined for blood and parasites.

Avoidance Conditioning

Initial training of the avoidance behavior was accomplished during 2 preliminary daily sessions of 2 to 4 h in duration. The training procedure involved the use of a short 5-second interval between shocks in the absence of a lever response (the 'shock-shock' or 'S-S' interval) and a 20-second interval between lever responses and shocks (the 'response-shock' or 'R-S' interval). At the outset, a lever response by either animal of a given pair delayed the shock for both animals and no further 'shaping' of the behavior was attempted. Within the first preliminary sessions, however, 1 monkey of each pair was observed to develop avoidance lever-pressing before its

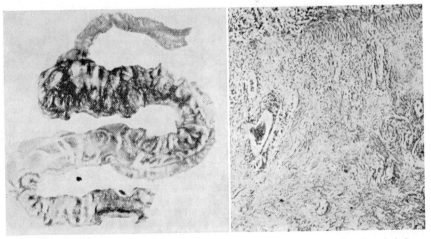

Fig.4. Photograph of gross aspect (left) of colon from monkey M 1 showing chronic inflammatory changes. The photomicrograph (right) was made at the level of the markedly thickened rectosigmoid colon.

partner and was selected as the experimental animal. At this point in the preliminary training procedure, both the 'shock-shock' and the 'response-shock' intervals were set at 20 sec and the control monkey's lever was made ineffective with respect to avoiding shocks for the remainder of the experiment.

Within a few hours after the initiation of the alternating 6-hour sessions, the experimental animals of each pair had developed stable avoidance lever-pressing rates which showed little change throughout the course of the experiment. Responses during the 6-hour 'off' periods in the absence of the red light rapidly dropped to a low level and remained there throughout the experiment. Since the lever-pressing rates for the experimental animals during the 6-hour 'avoidance' periods approximated 15 to 20 responses/min, the behavior effectively prevented all but an occasional shock for both animals. The shock rates never exceeded 2/h during the 6-hour 'avoidance' periods, and typically averaged less than 1 per hour. For the most part, only somewhat variable 'operant levels' of lever pressing were maintained by the control animals of each pair, although 1 of these animals did appear to develop what might be termed a 'superstitious-avoidance' rate during the course of the 3-week alternating procedure. From an initial rate not exceeding 1 response per hour during the first few days on the procedure, this control monkey gradually increased its output to 2 responses/min by the tenth day, and ultimately reached a peak of 5 responses/min on the twentieth day. During the succeeding 5-day period, however, its rate again gradually declined to relatively high levels of considerably less than 1 response/min. Throughout this entire period, the experimental animal of this pair maintained a lever-pressing response rate of almost 20 responses/min.

Gastrointestinal Findings

The experiment was terminated in each case by the death of the experimental monkey of each pair. The control animals were sacrificed immediately by the intravenous injection of sodium pentobarbital (5 ml) and complete autopsies were done on all animals.

In the first experiment there was little indication of the impending fatal outcome of the avoidance animals. The day before death this monkey failed to eat but continued to respond effectively. It was found dead on the morning of the twenty-third day during one of the 6-hour 'avoidance' periods. There was no weight loss during this period in either animal of the pair. *Post mortem* studies were done within a few hours after the death of the experimental animal. On opening the abdominal cavity approximately 25 ml of fluid containing food particles escaped. Areas of acute inflammation of the mesentery were apparent. A perforation of the wall of the duodenum was found on its anterior side just above the level of the ampulla of Vater. Inspection of the mucosal surface revealed an erosive lesion measuring 5 mm in diameter surrounded by an area of erythema. Microscopically, this lesion was indistinguishable from those ulcers previously discussed. Evidence of both acute and chronic inflammation was present in the sides of the crater. No additional gastrointestinal findings or evidence of parasitic infestation were noted. The control animal showed no abnormality of the gastrointestinal tract.

The avoidance animal of the second pair was removed from the experimental situation when he was no longer able to avoid shocks efficiently and died several hours later. This occurred on the twenty-fifth day after the beginning of the experiment. During the 3 days prior to this, the monkey ate poorly and vomited on one occasion. There was no change in body weight in either animal from their pre-experimental values. The principal pathology found in the experimental animal was located in the upper gastrointestinal tract. An erosion was noted in the duodenum 1 cm below the pylorus. It measured 4 mm in diameter and was situated on the posterior side. The duodenal wall was not perforated, in fact microscopic examination showed the ulcer to have penetrated only to the muscularis. There was acute inflammation and edema surrounding the area which conceivably might have caused partial obstruction of the intestinal lumen. This was suggested by marked distention of the stomach with undigested food. Streaks of hemorrhage were grossly visible in the wall of the stomach. Again, examination of the control animal revealed no gastrointestinal abnormalities.

Measurement of the urinary excretion of total 17-hydroxycorticosteroids (17-OH-CS) at selected stages during the experiment revealed slight increases in 24-hour 17-OH-CS output in both monkeys of each pair during the initial phases of avoidance conditioning. Otherwise the samples tested in subsequent phases of the experiments showed no evidence of increased adrenal cortical activity as judged by the 24-hour 17-OH-CS excretion. Fluctuations outside the normal range which may have occurred within individual 6-hour avoidance or rest periods cannot, however, be excluded by the data on 24-hour urine portions.

Discussion

The results of these experiments indicate quite clearly that the incidence of gastrointestinal disease is significantly greater in a population of rhesus monkeys subjected to chronic behavioral conditioning than in laboratory monkeys not so conditioned. The complexity of the behavioral conditioning procedures makes it difficult to isolate and analyze the specific psychological factors contributing to the etiology of these somatic changes. Although there would appear to be little doubt that certain aspects of the behavioral situations under study have figured prominently in the development of the gastrointestinal findings, the precise nature of these 'psychosomatic' relationships must continue to be speculative with only the present data at hand. Careful consideration of the possibilities suggested by such observations, however, may well provide the basis for a more definitive experimental analysis.

The first and most obvious consideration is the confining environment of the primate restraining chair itself as a common factor in all the experiments comprising this report. Previous reports [4, 10] have shown that short periods of restraint can be physiologically stressful in several species, at least during the early phases of such experiments. In monkeys, however, gradually decreasing adrenal cortical responses appear to accompany repeated restraint sessions. MASON, HARWOOD, and ROSENTHAL have reported the result of a study on monkeys dealing directly with the effect of continued restraint upon adrenal cortical function in the same primate chair used in the present experiments [22]. During the first 1 to 3 days in the chair, the animals showed an increased urinary excretion of 17-OH steroids. No further rises in adrenal cortical steroid levels were observed after this initial period, however, and a fairly stable baseline of hormone output was maintained for periods up to 4 or 5 weeks in a group of 5 monkeys without symptomatic evidence of disease. Although it is clear from these findings on control animals that restraint alone probably does not constitute the critical precipitating factor in the manifest somatic disorders observed in the experimental animals of the present series, the possible predisposing role of the primate chair cannot be easily dismissed.

With the initial series of the animals in the present study on combined conditioning procedures, the pathological changes appear to correlate more highly with the intensity of the behavioral program as a whole than with any of the specific conditioning techniques under investigation. Despite a careful analysis of the experimental histories of these animals trained with combined programs, it has been difficult to isolate any single behavioral procedure or group of specific procedures to which the gastrointestinal findings could be selectively related. Broadly considered, the more general relationship to program intensity appears to hold for both the site and nature of the observed lesions. Of the 5 monkeys subjected to intensive conditioning schedules (combined conditioning procedures or alternating avoidance-punishment), 4 show lesions of an acute nature, and three of the four were located in the stomach. For the most part, the monkeys on these programs participated in daily experimental sessions of several hours or more in duration, and in some instances these sessions lasted throughout the night. No animal subjected to these procedures for 5 days or longer has survived. Furthermore, it seems unlikely that this lethal outcome can be attributed to the physical trauma of the electric shocks employed. Although no specific control observations for this factor were included in the initial series, extended prior training on the individual 'avoidance' and 'punishment' components of these programs invariably reduced the incidence of actual electric shocks to a level well below that involved in many other procedures which have as yet shown no untoward somatic effects. This suggests that the environmental contingencies requiring constant attention to and rapid discrimination of continuously changing visual and auditory stimuli constitute potentially stressful etiologic factors. Unfortunately, it is impossible to elucidate specifically the apparent relationship of these operational contingencies to the more popular but ill-defined 'psychosomatic' concepts of 'anxiety', as an anticipatory phenomenological factor, or the even less meaningful 'mental fatigue'. But the possible contributing role of sleep deprivation and actual physical decrements as a consequence of these rather intense procedures cannot be overlooked, even though no overt signs of such disturbances were readily discernible.

The occurrence of acute ulcerations and hemorrhage in the stomach following systemic stress and intracranial disturbances is well documented both clinically and experimentally [5, 6, 11, 18, 25, 28, 37]. Although the pathogenesis of such gastrointestinal pathology is far from being well understood, it has been presumed to develop as a consequence of physiological exhaustion of the organism's somatic defense mechanisms in the face of overwhelmingly stressful stimuli. The question of adrenal cortical participation in this process has been discussed from both the clinical and experimental standpoint [7, 14, 28]. Lesions of the hypothalamus and related structures frequently, although not invariably [6, 20] appear to predispose to such an imbalance between autonomic and hormonal factors, presumably by interfering with the appropriate neural response to stressful stimuli. It is also of some interest that multiple gastric ulcers have been produced in rats subjected to a 'food approach – shock avoidance' conflict situation for periods of

3 or 4 weeks [26, 27, 38]. With the exception of a 1-hour break and feeding period every 2 days, these animals lived continuously in a situation which required that they take a shock by crossing an electrified grid in order to get a pellet of food. Despite these important experimental contributions, however, the precise relationships between such presumably 'psychological' factors and specific somatic disease processes remain to be experimentally defined.

The finding of an enteric intussuception in these intensive conditioning experiments seems worthy of comment. The etiology of this condition in man is not demonstrable in a majority of the cases [34]. WATTS and FULTON reported this phenomenon in monkeys following ablation of the premotor cortex, and they also induced intestinal hypomotility and intussusception by electrical stimulation of this same brain region [36]. They explained this apparent paradox on the grounds that the premotor area of the frontal cortex could be assumed to exert both stimulatory and inhibitory influences on intestinal mobility. Although it is tempting to speculate about the etiologic role of behaviorally induced increases in autonomic activity in producing the case reported in the present series, it must be recognized that the validity of such a conclusion could hardly be justified on the basis of the available evidence. It is recognized that intussusception may occur as an agonal event in monkeys, but preterminal cases can usually be distinguished, especially if signs of obstruction are present.

In the more protracted experiments, the lesions were largely confined to the intestine and were more chronic in nature. The lesions observed were ulceration of the duodenum and inflammation of the colon. For the most part, the experimental programs with these animals were limited to sessions not exceeding 1 or 2 h in duration each day, and with but one exception, did not include combined conditioning procedures in a single experimental session. The probability of somatic fatigue, then, as a contributing etiologic factor appears much lower in these chronic lesions than in the more intensive programs discussed previously. Clearly more serious consideration must be given to psychological aspects with consequent involvement or stimulation of related neural events in assessing the critical antecedents of these more chronic lesions.

Duodenal ulceration has been induced experimentally by others in a variety of ways. Most of these investigations have altered gastric function either directly or indirectly through the influence of peripheral neural or humoral mechanisms or through systemically administered agents [17]. The importance of neural mechanisms in this regard has been reviewed by WENER [39]. Focal lesions of the stomach and duodenum have also been induced by chronic electrical stimulation of the brain. FRENCH and his coworkers stimulated the hypothalamus several times a day for 30 to 74 days, and observed a high incidence of mucosal abnormalities with erosion as a prominent feature [12]. It is noteworthy that these animals were otherwise in good health, and were in no way subjected to physical stress. In the present experiments, a focal duodenal lesion was induced by various conditioning procedures designed either to stimulate the brain directly or to produce psychological stress over a protracted period. Four monkeys which had received stimulation in the median forebrain bundle at the preoptic or rostral hypothalamic level, in addition to some behavior conditioning, developed duodenal ulceration. However, as other areas were stimulated as well no definite conclusions can be drawn as to the specificity of the stimulation site. It is interesting to note though, that a fifth animal which received extensive stimulation in the globus pallidus but none in this median forebrain bundle area failed to develop gastrointestinal abnormality. The duodenal lesions produced in this series of experiments were similar regardless of the conditioning schedule used, and are of special interest because of the evidence of chronicity which they exhibited.

With respect to the behavioral proce-

dures presumed to bear some relationship to the development of duodenal ulceration in the present study, perhaps the results of the second phase of the investigation with the conditioned avoidance procedure alone is most revealing. In addition to the prevalence of this procedure as a component of several of the combined programs studied in the initial series of animals, this procedure was selected for more detailed analysis in the second phase of the present investigation because of many apparently interesting psychological characteristics. The avoidance-conditioning procedure, as described above, provides a means of facing the animal with a continuous threat of punishment over a prolonged, though somewhat intermittent period of time. It is possible for the monkey to prevent the shocks only by virtually constant participation in the experimental situation during the avoidance periods, although the rather low incidence of shocks *per se* (all of which could have been prevented) appears to contribute insignificantly to the somatic pathology which is seen to develop. Thus the control animal of each pair received all the shocks which were not avoided by the experimental animal and in the same distribution over time. However, neither control monkey showed any indication of behavioral disturbance throughout the course of the experiment and neither developed gastrointestinal disease.

Although both the experiments in the second phase of the present investigation were surprisingly similar in their course and terminal result, a definitive statement relevant to the true incidence of duodenal ulceration as a consequence of such continued avoidance behavior can be seen to require more extensive experimental analysis. Follow-up studies, presently in progress, strongly suggest that such factors as the selection criteria for experimental and control animals, relative degrees of 'social contact' or isolation during the course of the experiment, the schedule of 'avoidance' and 'rest' periods, and even constitutional factors, may play a critical role in determining the relationship between such 'behavioral stress' and consequent somatic pathology.

Unfortunately, these studies provide as yet little or no indication of the physiological mechanisms concerned in the mediation of the chronic avoidance behavior effect on gastrointestinal function. Whether the adrenal corticosteroids play a role in the pathogenesis of the duodenal ulceration in these experiments, as the work of GRAY and associates [13] suggests, cannot be adequately assessed on the basis of the present data. Although the 24-hour urinary 17-OH corticosteroid determinations were essentially within normal limits, more recent studies indicate that the excretion of these hormones is significantly elevated during the 6-hour avoidance session and falls to a subnormal level during rest periods.

The observation of chronic colitis in 2 of these animals is difficult to assess from an etiologic standpoint. Such chronic lesions have never been observed in monkeys used in other programs in the laboratory. The most obvious cause which must be given careful consideration is specific parasitic infestation, even though all attempts to isolate a pathogenic organism were unsuccessful. The most common parasite encountered in monkeys under our laboratory conditions is *Strongyloides*. Animals known to be infected with this and other organisms have been examined but no evidence of chronic inflammation of the colon was found. The pathological findings of submucosal fibrosis, mucosal ulceration, and chronic inflammatory reaction are features characteristically seen in chronic amebic and bacillary dysentery and nonspecific ulcerative colitis in man. Final differentiation of these conditions is based on identification of a responsible organism when present [1]. The etiology of nonspecific inflammation of the colon is problematical and has recently been reviewed by WARREN and BERK [35]. The role of behavioral or 'emotional-stress' factors in its pathogenesis or in determining its course have been considered important by several investigators

[15, 23]. The relevance of the present observations to this problem can be determined only by further study.

The proper evaluation of results obtained in any study of 'psychosomatic' relationships with animals is difficult and extrapolation to similar problems in man is hazardous. The present study seems significant, however, in that disease processes which are not known to occur spontaneously in monkeys and which exhibit many features characteristic of human disease, have been observed in behaviorally stressful experimental situations. Further analysis of the limits of reproducibility and exploration of the defining variables determining the observed relationships in this experimental setting promises to provide a valuable method for exploring the intermediary pathophysiologic processes involved in the pathogenesis of such disease processes and for evaluating the efficacy of various preventive and therapeutic measures.

Summary

Eleven of 19 monkeys used in chronic psychological-conditioning experiments developed gastrointestinal disease. Although the program for each animal was different, for the most part experiments were directed toward a study of emotional behavior. Among the lesions found were gastric hemorrhage and erosion, duodenal ulceration, enteric intussusception, and chronic colitis. In a controlled study of a single behavioral procedure (avoidance behavior), 2 experimental monkeys developed duodenal ulceration while the 2 control animals showed no abnormality. The possible etiologic factors responsible for this occurrence and their significance from the standpoint of investigating the pathogenesis of 'psychosomatic' disease have been discussed.

References

1. ANDERSON, W. A. D.: Pathology (ed. 3), p. 770 (Mosby, St. Louis 1957).
2. BRADY, J. V.: Temporal and emotional factors related to electrical self-stimulation of the limbic system, in Reticular formation of the brain, p. 689 (Little, Boston 1958).
3. BRADY, J. V. and HUNT, H. F.: An experimental approach to the analysis of emotional behavior. J. Psychol. 40: 313 (1955).
4. COLFER, H. F.; DE GROOT, J., and HARRIS, G. W.: Pituitary gland and blood lymphocytes. J. Physiol. 111: 328 (1950).
5. CUSHING, H.: Peptic ulcers and the interbrain. Surg. Gynec. Obstet. 55: 1 (1932).
6. DAVIS, R. A.; WETZEL, N., and DAVIS, L.: Acute upper alimentary tract ulceration and hemorrhage following neurosurgical operations. Surg. Gynec. Obstet. 100: 51 (1955).
7. DRAGSTEDT, I. R. et al.: Stress and duodenal ulcer. Ann. Surg. 144: 450 (1956).
8. FERSTER, C. B.: The use of the free operant in the analysis of behavior. Psychol. Bull. 5: 264 (1953).
9. FERSTER, C. B. and SKINNER, B. F.: Schedules of reinforcement (Appleton, New York 1957).
10. FORTIER, C.: Dual control of adrenocorticotrophin release. Endocrinology 49: 782 (1951).
11. FRENCH, J. D. et al.: Gastrointestinal hemorrhage and ulceration associated with intracranial lesions. Surgery 32: 395 (1952).
12. FRENCH, J. D. et al.: Experimental observations on 'psychosomatic' mechanisms. Arch. Neurol., Chicago 72: 267 (1954).
13. GRAY, S. J. et al.: Chronic stress and peptic ulcer. J. amer. med. Ass. 147: 1529 (1951).
14. GRAY, S. J. et al.: Adrenal influences upon the stomach and the gastric response to stress; in SELYE and HEUSER Fifth annual report on stress (New York 1955).
15. GROEN, J.: Psychogenesis and psychotherapy of ulcerative colitis. Psychosom. Med. 9: 151 (1947).
16. HUNT, H. F. and BRADY, J. V.: Some effects of punishment and intercurrent anxiety on a simple operant. J. comp. physiol. Psychol. 48: 305 (1955).
17. IVY, A. C.; GROSSMAN, M. I., and BACHRACH, W. H.: Peptic ulcer, p. 258 (Blakiston, New York 1950).
18. KELLER, A. D.: Ulceration in digestive tract of dog following intracranial procedures: Preliminary study. Arch. Path. 21: 127 (1936).
19. LILLY, J. C. et al.: Brief non-injurious electric waveform for stimulation of the brain. Science 121: 468 (1955).
20. MARTIN, J. and SCHNEDORF, J. G.: The absence of changes in gastric activity and of gastrointestinal ulceration following hypothalamic lesions in the monkey and also in the cat. Amer. J. Physiol. 122: 81 (1938).
21. MASON, J. W.: A restraining chair for the experimental study of primates. J. appl. Physiol. 12: 130 (1958).
22. MASON, J. W.; HARWOOD, C. T., and ROSENTHAL, N. R.: The influence of some environmental factors on plasma and urinary 17-hydroxycorticosteroid levels in the rhesus monkey. Amer. J. Physiol. 190: 429 (1957).
23. MURRAY, C. D.: Psychogenic factors in the etiology of ulcerative colitis and bloody diarrhea. Amer. J. med. Sci. 180: 239 (1930).
24. OLDS, J. and MILNER, P.: Positive reinforcement produced by electrical stimulation of septal area and other regions of the rat brain. J. comp. physiol. Psychol. 47: 419 (1954).
25. ROKITANSKY, C.: A manual of pathological anatomy, vol. 2, p. 40 (Blanchard &Lea, Philadelphia 1855).
26. SAWREY, W. L.; CONGER, J. J., and TURRELL, E. S.: An experimental investigation of the role of psychological factors in the production of gastric ulcers in rats. J. comp. physiol. Psychol. 49: 457 (1956).
27. SAWREY, W. L. and WEISZ, J. D.: An experimental method of producing gastric ulcers. J. comp. physiol. Psychol. 49: 269 (1956).
28. SELYE, H.: A syndrome produced by diverse nocuous agents. Nature, Lond. 138: 32 (1936).
29. SHEATZ, G. C.: Personal communication (1957).
30. SIDMAN, M.: Avoidance conditioning with brief shocks and no exteroceptive warning signal. Science 118: 157 (1953).

31. SIDMAN, M. et al.: Reward schedules and behavior maintained by intracranial self-stimulation. Science 122: 830 (1955).
32. SKINNER, B. F.: Some contributions of an experimental analysis of behavior to psychology as a whole. Amer. Psychol. 8: 69 (1953).
33. SKINNER, B. F.: The experimental analysis of behavior. Amer. Sci. 48: 343 (1957).
34. TUMEN, H. J.: in BOCKUS Gastroenterology, vol. 2, p. 308 (Saunders, Philadelphia 1944).
35. WARREN, I. A. and BERK, J. E.: The etiology of chronic non-specific ulcerative colitis. Gastroenterology 33: 395 (1957).
36. WATTS, J. W. and FULTON, J. F.: Intussusception – The relation of the cerebral cortex to intestinal motility in the monkey. New Engl. J. Med. 210: 883 (1934).
37. WATTS, J. W. and FULTON, J. F.: The effect of lesions of the hypothalamus upon the gastrointestinal tract and heart of monkeys. Ann. Surg. 101: 363 (1935).
38. WEISZ, J. D.: The etiology of experimental gastric ulceration. Psychosom. Med. 19: 61 (1957).
39. WENER, J. and HOFF, H. E.: The neurohumoral aspects of peptic ulcer formation. Canad. med. Ass. J. 59: 115 (1948).

Autonomic Response Specificity[1]

An Experimental Study

J. I. LACEY, DOROTHY E. BATEMAN and RUTH VANLEHN

Retrospective comment by Dr. W. Bridger. This paper by JOHN LACEY and his co-workers is a landmark in the development of both psychophysiology and experimental approaches to psychosomatic medicine. The results of this experiment shifted the emphasis away from the concept of emotional specificity and towards the role of individual differences in autonomic responsivity in an attempt to explain predispositions toward specific psychosomatic symptoms. Since its publication, more and more researchers have left the problem of the symbolic meaning of psychosomatic symptoms to the theoreticians and have entered the exciting area of psychophysiology. The experimental psychophysiological approach that JOHN LACEY pioneered has become a dominant model in the search for predisposing factors in psychosomatic disease and has acted as the main impetus in the expanding field of developmental psychophysiology.

However, this paper has perhaps an even more important aspect. LACEY would not have been able to describe response specificity if he had not made a notable advance in the measurement of autonomic function. This, and LACEY's subsequent papers, became models for both rigorous experimental design and statistical sophistication. In this paper, the autonomic lability score is first described and applied to the law of initial values. It has become a widely used and also somewhat controversial technique in the analysis of psychophysiological data. Thus, in one experiment LACEY provided an experimental model for understanding predispositions to psychosomatic illness and also developed a methodology that has had a lasting influence on experimental psychophysiology.

This report presents the detailed results of a study that has been partially described in an earlier preliminary paper [10]. It is the fourth paper in a series devoted to the problem of differential emphasis in somatic response to stress. To date, our findings in this area are contrary to those which would be expected on the basis of the usual interpretation of CANNON's researches on the functioning of the autonomic nervous system [3, 4]. They are more in accord with the clinical phenomenon of specific symptom selection in psychosomatic neuroses. The autonomic nervous system does indeed respond to experimentally imposed stress 'as a whole' in the sense that all autonomically innervated structures seem to be activated, usually in the direction of apparent sympathetic predominance. But it does not respond 'as a whole' in the sense that all autonomically innervated structures exhibit equal increments or decrements of function. Striking intra-individual differences in the degree of activation of different physiological functions are found when the different reactions are expressed in equivalent units [7, 8].

Our previous studies have dealt with but one stress in each experiment; the reliability of the patterns of response obtained upon

[1] From The Fels Research Institute, Antioch College, Yellow Springs, Ohio.

retest have then been determined. The next requisite step appears to be to determine whether there is a tendency for individuals to respond with the *same* physiological pattern in a series of different stresses. Such a study constitutes an extension to 'normal' individuals of the principle of symptom specificity, as recently formalized by MAL-MO and his collaborators [11, 12]. They declare: 'This principle states that in psychiatric patients presenting a somatic complaint, the particular physiological mechanism of that complaint is specifically susceptible to activation by stressful experience [12].' In accordance with this hypothesis, MALMO and his collaborators find that psychiatric patients with somatic complaints referable, for example, to the neuromuscular system are more sharply differentiated from other groups by muscle potential reactions than by heart rate reactions to painful stimulation [11].

It is not known whether such a principle holds only for those who have already developed a frank psychosomatic disorder. In fact, the principle requires reformulation if the general concept of specificity of response is to be applied to 'normal' individuals. The reformulated hypothesis is designated as 'the principle of *relative response specificity*' and is defined as follows: For a given set of autonomic functions, individuals tend to respond with a pattern of autonomic activation in which maximal activation will be shown by the same physiological function, whatever the stress.

We choose the term 'response specificity' rather than 'symptom specificity' to avoid the premature inplication that the pattern of response secured in a 'normal' individual is predictive of the area of symptom production if psychosomatic neurosis should develop later. The word 'relative' is used to point out that the maximal activation observed is relative to a given set of autonomic measurements. Determining the function showing truly maximal activation in a given individual would require simultaneous measurement of all autonomic functions, a task obviously impossible at present.

Procedure

The Subjects

The group chosen was relatively homogeneous with regard to age, sex, and cultural level. Data were secured on 85 male college students, all volunteer subjects; aged 19 to 21 years.

The Stresses

Each subject was exposed to four stresses in sequence.

The first stress was *mental arithmetic*, requiring the multiplication of a two-digit number by a one-digit number and the subsequent addition of a two-digit number ('multiply 4 by 67 and then add 39'). As soon as the subject announced the answer, another problem was given to him. Problems were given orally over an intercommunication system connecting the recording room to the laboratory. This stress was continued at a staccato pace for 2 min.

The second stress was *hyperventilation*. The subject was required to breathe deeply at the rate of one complete respiration per second. He was paced by the experimenter, who called off each second over the intercommunication system. This stress was continued for 45 sec.

The third stress was *letter association*, in which the subject was required to name all the words he could think of that began with the letter 'w'. Each time the subject faltered, he was urged to continue. The stress continued for 2 min.

The fourth stress was a modified *cold pressor test*, in which the left foot was immersed to the level of the internal malleolus for 60 sec in water maintained at 4° C.

The Physiological Measures

Palmar conductance (reflecting sweat gland activity), heart rate, and variability of heart rate were continuously and simultaneously recorded, using Brush electromagnetic recorders.

Palmar conductance was measured with the Fels Dermohmmeter, which passed 4 μA through the subject no matter what the subject's resistance. A zinc plate electrode [5] was used on the right palm, and contact was made with the skin by means of a jelly composed of 1 per cent zinc sulfate in agar-agar. The other lead was connected to the right ear lobe, after puncture with a spring lancet. Under these conditions, only changes in conductance of the right palmar skin surface were registered [13]. The ear lobe electrode consisted of a zinc plate soldered to an earring; connection was made by the zinc sulfate jelly. The use of the extremely low current value of 4 μA permitted large changes in skin conductance to occur but introduced an appreciable error because body polarity effects are marked at low currents. To eliminate this error completely, the current polarity was automatically reversed every 30 sec. Conductance readings were then corrected to the value that would be secured if no body polarity existed by taking the conductance value midway between the 2 values secured with opposite polarities. Conductance was read in micromho units.

Simultaneously with this recording, heart rate and heart rate variability were measured with the Fels Cardiotachometer[2]. This instrument records the duration of individual cardiac cycles (R-R intervals) as a vertical distance. A continuous graph of cardiac rates is thus drawn, permitting the measurement of rate and variability of rate. Electrical connections were made to the skin surfaces overlying the right mastoid and right knee cap, an arrangement which practically eliminates interference from muscular activity. The zinc plate electrodes were fastened with collodion.

The Experimental Routine

All measurements were made in an air-conditioned room maintained at approximately 74°F and 50% relative humidity. The palmar electrode for the measurement of skin conductance was attached to the subject as soon as he reported to the laboratory. In every case the critical physiological measurements were not made until at least 20 min later; sufficient time was thus provided for the subject to become partially acclimatized. More important, this delay allowed the stratum corneum underlying the palmar electrode to become hydrated before skin conductance measurements were taken [2]. The sequence of events was explained in detail to each subject so that he would know what to expect. The following details, however, were not revealed: the time to elapse before the first stress was administered, the actual nature of the mental arithmetic problems, the letter to be used in the letter association stress, and the purpose of the experiment. Each subject was given practice in hyperventilating in rhythm with the experimenter's count until he could perform satisfactorily. The volume displacement of his

left foot was measured so that only enough water would be used in the cold pressor foot bath to guarantee immersion to the level of the internal malleolus. He was seated comfortably in an easy chair; electrical connections were completed; and the experimenter retired to the recording room. All further instructions were given via the intercommunication system.

The subject was asked to close his eyes and relax. This relaxation period was continued for 15 min, a period sufficient for all individuals to show physiologic stability under the conditions of our experiment. The mental arithmetic stress was then administered. At the end of 2 min the subject was told to stop and relax once again. After a variable time permitted for recovery, the hyperventilation stress was administered, and following recovery from this, the letter association stress. Midway through the recovery from letter association, the experimenter entered the laboratory, prepared the cold water bath, and then returned to the recording room. The cold pressor test was administered when recovery was complete.

Each recovery period was continued as long as was necessary for the subject to return to the same physiologic status he was in just before the first stress was administered. This return to the general 'base level' was defined primarily by the return of palmar conductance to its base level. If the heart record approximately back to its base, the next stress was administered. If the heart was not yet back to its base, or was showing momentary acceleration, further recovery time was permitted. Recovery times were extremely variable, ranging from 2 to 30 min. This procedure insured that the physiological background upon which each stress was imposed was approximately the same for a given subject.

The Measure of Autonomic Activity

The degree to which a given physiological function has been activated by stress may be studied in two ways. First we may direct our attention simply to the *level* the function has reached – so many milimeters mercury of blood pressure, so many heart beats per minute. Or we may compute some measure of the *displace-*

[2] Constructed and supplied by the Yellow Springs Instrument Company, Yellow Springs, Ohio.

ment the function has shown under stress by computing percentage change or absolute change from the base level at which the stress was imposed to the level reached during stress. Since no rationale exists as to which computational method is appropriate, both have been used in this study. We call the first approach, the one dealing with level reached during stress, the measurement of *autonomic tension*, the second, dealing with displacement, the measurement of *autonomic lability*. These terms are generalizations of THERON's nomenclature [14].

Since it was necessary in this study to use equivalent units so that the reactivity of different functions within a given individual might be quantitatively compared, all autonomic tension measurements were expressed in T-score form. That is, all measures have a mean of 50 and a standard deviation of 10. The utility of this method can be illustrated by the following example: If a subject reached a maximum heart rate of 93 during the cold pressor test and a maximum palmar conductance of 1.74 log micromhos, the presentation of these figures would not be as informative

as saying that his T score for heart rate was 50, or exactly average, whereas his T score for palmar conductance was 70, or two standard deviations above average. The interpretation of T scores is more precise if the measures are distributed normally. By referring to the table of the normal curve, we can state that his heart rate exceeds 50 % of the population, but his palmar conductance exceeds 97.7 % of the population. This is the basis for the construction of the *reaction profile* for a given individual [8]. McCALL's method [6] was used to normalize and T-score all stress-level measurements.

Stress levels were read as follows: (a) for palmar conductance, the maximum palmar conductance reached during stress; (b) for heart rate, the average of the 6 fastest beats; (c) for heart rate variability, the average of the 6 greatest beat-to-beat variations (that is, the kymograph record was inspected and the greatest difference between two *successive* heart rates was found; then the pair of successive heart rates showing the next greatest difference was found, and so on for six pairs of successive beats).

Table 1. Cases exemplifying each of the degrees of response specificity, as seen in the number of variables in which peak autonomic tension appears

Degree of response specificity	Case No.	Stress No.	Autonomic tension T-scores *		
			Palmar con- ductance	Heart rate	Variability of heart rate
Maximum (maximum reactions in one variable only)	1	1	43	*75*	52
		2	44	*60*	45
		3	46	*71*	34
		4	46	*64*	37
High (maximum reactions in two variables, one variable appearing three times)	18	1	*64*	49	35
		2	*66*	57	41
		3	69	*75*	29
		4	*67*	63	47
Low (maximum reactions in two variables, each appearing twice)	4	1	40	*51*	42
		2	39	44	*53*
		3	34	48	*60*
		4	36	*56*	46
Minimum (maximum reactions in all three variables)	5	1	64	54	*71*
		2	*66*	75	61
		3	*60*	56	43
		4	*64*	59	40

* Peak T scores are set in italics.

Autonomic lability scores were also put in T score form. However, since it is commonly found that both percentage change and absolute change depend upon the base value of the physiological function [9, 15] the measurement of autonomic lability presents a special problem. For example, if a stress is imposed upon an individual whose heart rate is already near his 'ceiling', only a small increase in heart rate can possibly occur; interpretation of absolute and percentage changes are therefore unclear. However, appropriate statistical technics can eliminate this interrelationship. The details and mathematical justification for the statistical procedure used will be presented in a separate report [9].

The essence of the procedure is: From the product-moment correlation coefficient between base level and stress level, and from the distribution statistics (means and standard deviations), a series of normal frequency distributions may be inferred, showing the stress levels that would be secured for an infinite population of individuals *with a given base level*. For example, there is a hypothetical infinite population of individuals with a base heart rate of 79 beats/min. The specific members of this study who actually exhibited a base heart rate of 79 beats/min are a sample of this population. If all individuals in this infinite population were subjected to the cold pressor test, the distribution of stress levels would be normal, with an estimated mean value of 93 and an estimated standard deviation of 8. If a given individual with a base level of 79, then, shows a stress level of 101, he is one standard deviation above expectation (93 plus 8) and is given a T score of 60. If his heart rate under stress were 81, he would be one and one-half standard deviations below normal, and his T score would be 35. Such distributions of stress levels may be inferred for any given base level. These inferences are completely valid, however, only if certain assumptions (linearity of regression, homoscedasticity, and bivariate normality) are shown to hold true. The assumptions are satisfied by the data of this experiment [9].

This statistically derived measure of autonomic lability is highly correlated with both percentage change and absolute change. For the present study, for example, the correlations of the lability scores with absolute change range from 0.74 to 0.93, with a median

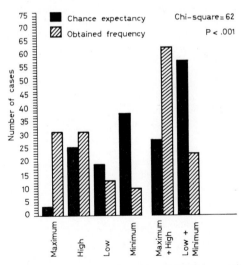

Fig. 1. Degree of specificity: Peak autonomic tension. Maximum specificity: cases showing maximum reactions in one variable only. High specificity: cases showing maximum reactions in two variables, one variable appearing three times. Low specificity: cases showing maximum reactions in two variables, each appearing twice. Minimum specificity: cases showing maximum reactions in all three variables.

value of 0.90; with percentage change they range from 0.76 to 0.92, with a median of 0.83 [9]. They have the important attribute, however, that their correlations with base levels are necessarily zero.

Base levels were read in the same manner as stress levels. The base palmar conductance was the conductance which existed just prior to the administration of stress. Heart rate and heart rate variability were read for the minute just preceding stress. The raw data were again transformed into McCALL's T scores.

Results

Autonomic Tension

Peak Autonomic Tension

The data permit the specification of four degrees of relative response specificity: (1) 'Maximum' response specificity, within the limits of the experiment, is shown by an individual who exhibits his maximum T score in the same physiological variable in all four stresses. (2) 'High' response specificity is shown by one exhibiting peak reactivity in one variable three times, and in another variable the fourth time. (3) 'Low' response specificity is shown by an individual whose peak response is in one physiological variable for two of the four stresses, and in another physiological variable for the other two stresses. (4) 'Minimum' response specificity is shown by one exhibiting peak response in all three variables over the four stresses.

Examples of each of these categories, drawn from actual cases, are presented in table I. The large intra-individual variability in the response of the different physiological functions shown by this tabulation is not unusual [7, 8].

In figure 1 the observed number of cases showing each of the four degrees of response specificity is compared with the frequencies expected on the hypothesis of independent and equally probable events[3]. These chance frequencies are easily calculated, using the probability calculus. On the chance hypothesis, the probability that an individual

will show his peak response in a given function on a given stress is $1/3$. From the multiplicative theorem, the joint probability that he will show his peak response in the same given physiological variable all four times is $1/3^4$, or $1/81$. From the additive theorem (since there are three variables, each of which may appear as the maximum response) the expected frequency of individuals showing maximum response specificity is $3/81$ times 85, or 3.15 cases. The other chance frequencies may be computed similarly, although some combinatorial analysis is required.

It can be seen in figure 1 that there is a marked excess of obtained frequency over expected frequency in the category 'maximum degree of response specificity'. There is a slight excess for the high specificity, a slight deficiency in the low specificity, and a marked deficiency in the minimum specificity category. For purposes of testing the significance of these observed deviations from the theoretical distribution, the data were recombined into two classes. This brings the theoretical frequency in each cell above 10, and a chi-square test may legitimately be employed as follows:

Degree of response specificity	Expected frequency	Obtained frequency	Discrepancy
Maximum and high	28	62	+34
Low and minimum	57	23	−34

[3] That the 'events' (palmar conductance, heart rate, or variability of heart rate appearing as maximum response) were in fact equally probable *in the population* was checked by appropriate chi-square tests. Theoretically, each variable should appear as the maximum reaction for one-third of the cases for each stress. The deviations from the theoretical frequencies were never statistically significant. This empirical check was performed whenever chance frequencies were computed in the study.

Table II. Cases exemplifying varying degrees of response specificity, as seen in the reproducbiliity of the whole pattern of autonomic tension scores

Degree of response specificity	Case No.	Stress No.	Autonomic tension T-scores*		
			Palmar con- ductance	Heart rate	Variability of heart rate
Shows only one pattern in all	12	1	*58*	45	38
four stresses		2	*58*	50	49
		3	*57*	52	38
		4	*55*	49	40
Shows one pattern in three stresses	3	1	31	*56*	50
and another pattern in the fourth stress		2	36	40	*60*
		3	33	55	*56*
		4	36	51	*57*
Shows one pattern in two stresses	16	1	46	56	*60*
and another pattern in the		2	41	44	*48*
other two stresses		3	43	*51*	44
		4	44	65	50
Shows one pattern in one stress,	7	1	*52*	44	39
another pattern in another stress,		2	*54*	41	52
and still another pattern in two stresses		3	55	*57*	43
		4	*56*	54	50
Shows four different patterns	70	1	52	42	*53*
		2	*48*	42	45
		3	*51*	49	47
		4	44	*48*	43

* Peak T scores are set in italics.

The obtained chi-square is 61.566. Since for one degree of freedom a chi-square of 10.827 is required at the 0.001 confidence level, the obtained discrepancies certainly could not have occurred by chance alone. Clearly, the hypothesis that there is independence from stress to stress of the physiological function in which an individual exhibits his maximum reaction must be rejected. Or, put more precisely, it is not true that *each individual* studied is so constituted that the physiological variable in which he exhibits maximum response varies at random from stress to stress, with equal likelihood of any variable showing the peak reaction. The principle of relative response specificity is therefore strongly supported.

Pattern of Autonomic Tension Scores

The previous section dealt only with the physiological function showing maximal activation. We now turn our attention to the whole pattern of activation.

There are 6 possible patterns of response that may appear. If we let PC stand for palmar conductance, HR for heart rate, VHR for variability of heart rate, and use the usual symbol > for 'greater than', then the six patterns are PC > HR > VHR; PC > VHR > HR; HR > PC > VHR; HR > VHR > PC; VHR > PC > HR; and VHR > HR > PC. In the four stresses, a given individual may exhibit only one hierarchy of response, or 2 or 3, or 4. Actual examples are given in table II.

Figure 2 shows the observed number of cases falling in each of the above categories, in comparison with the chance expectancies. There is a marked excess of cases showing 1 or 2 patterns and a marked deficiency of cases showing 3 or 4 patterns. The chi-square for the data regrouped into 2 categories, as shown on the right-hand side of the graph, is 177.349, compared to the 10.827 required at the 0.001 level! Unquestionably the appearance of a given hierarchy of response in a given individual for one stress is not a haphazard event. There is a very strong tendency to reproduce the pattern of response, no matter what the stress.

Pattern Index Scores

So far we have studied only the rank order of the reactivity of the different physiological functions without regard to the size of the differences. The pattern index scores [8] however, permit quantitative study. The pattern index score between 2 variables is defined as the difference between the 2 T scores divided by 10. For example, suppose an individual has a palmar conductance T score of 40, and a heart rate T score of 60. The score for the pattern PC–HR (palmar conductance compared with heart rate) is $\dfrac{40-60}{10} = -2.0$.

This index means that the individual's T score for heart rate places him 2 standard deviations higher in the group than does his palmar conductance. If the index had been + 1.5, this would mean that his T score for palmar conductance placed him one and onehalf standard deviations higher than did his heart rate. Each subject has three pattern index scores for each stress: PC–HR, PC–VHR, and HR–VHR.

Table III shows the reproducibility of the pattern index scores from stress to stress. It can be seen that all but one of the correlations are significant far beyond the 0.001 level, and one is significant between the 0.01 and 0.001 levels. There is no doubt that the pattern index scores have fair consistency from stress to stress. None of the correla-

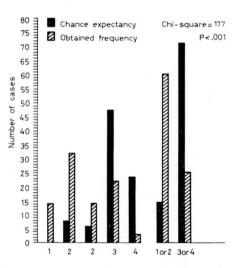

Fig. 2. Number of different autonomic tension patterns. The cases showing two patterns are subdivided into two groups: (a) those showing one pattern in three stresses and another pattern in the fourth stress; (b) those showing one pattern in two stresses and another pattern in two stresses.

Table III. Reproducibility of autonomic tension pattern index scores from stress to stress, shown by means of product-moment correlation coefficients

Pattern index score											
(Palmar conductance T-score minus heart rate T-score) ÷ 10				(Palmar conductance T-score minus heart rate variability T-score) ÷ 10				(Heart rate T-score minus heart rate variability T-score) ÷ 10			
Stress	1	2	3	4	Stress	1	2	3	4	Stress	1	2	3	4

Stress	1	2	3	4	Stress	1	2	3	4	Stress	1	2	3	4
1	X	0.73	0.84	0.75	1	X	0.56	0.72	0.66	1	X	0.32	0.71	0.57
2		X	0.81	0.79	2		X	0.66	0.58	2		X	0.45	0.45
3			X	0.85	3			X	0.79	3			X	0.68
4				X	4				X	4				X

N = 85.
An r of 0.28 is significant at the 0.01 level, and of 0.36 at the 0.001 level.

tions, however, reaches a very high level; they range from 0.32 to 0.85, and almost all are below 0.80. This indicates that the *amount* of differentiation between the reactivity of the different physiological measures is not reproduced in high degree from stress to stress, as can be seen from the T scores given for the 9 representative cases in tables I and II.

Table III also indicates that the reproducibility of the pattern index scores depends upon the physiological variables being considered. Taking the correlations between pattern index scores in stresses 1 and 2, for example, we find that they are 0.73, 0.56, and 0.32 for the patterns PC–HR, PC–VHR, and HR–VHR respectively. The same systematic decline is observable for each combination of stresses.

Autonomic Lability

The analysis of response specificity utilizing autonomic lability scores parallels the analysis of autonomic tension scores. One qualification must be added: Variability of heart rate typically increased in all

stresses except hyperventilation. In this stress, most individuals exhibit a decrease in variability, for reasons unknown to the authors. For the second stress, then, the autonomic lability scores were 'reflected', with high T scores being assigned to those individuals whose beat-to-beat variabilities during stress were much lower than the values expected from their base levels. An important by-product of this directional shift in response is that the demonstration of specificity in these circumstances implies that response specificity is independent of the direction of physiological change called for by different stresses. If over-reaction is evidenced by a physiological increment in one kind of stress and by a physiological decrement in another, then an individual who over-reacts with an increment in the first stress tends to over-react with a decrement in the second.

Peak Autonomic Lability

Figure 3 shows the result of the comparison of obtained frequencies with chance frequencies. Again there is a marked excess in the maximum specificity category, a slight excess in the high specificity category, and

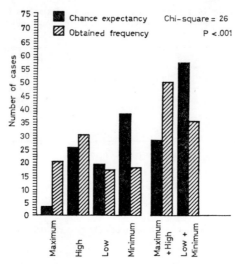

Fig.3. Degree of specificity: Peak autonomic lability. Maximum specificity: cases showing maximum reactions in one variable only. High specificity: cases showing maximum reactions in two variables, one variable appearing three times. Low specificity: cases showing maximum reactions in two variables, each appearing twice. Minimum specificity: cases showing maximum reactions in all three variables.

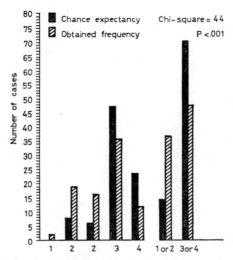

Fig.4. Number of different autonomic lability patterns. The cases showing two patterns are subdivided into two groups: (a) those showing one pattern in three stresses and another pattern in the fourth stress; (b) those showing one pattern in two stresses and another pattern in two stresses.

Table IV. Cases exemplifying each of the degrees of response specificity, as seen in the number of variables in which peak autonomic lability appears

Degree of response specificity	Case No.	Stress No.	Autonomic lability T-scores*		
			Palmar con- ductance	Heart rate	Variability of heart rate
Maximum (maximum reactions in one variable only)	15	1	*57*	54	55
		2	*58*	38	50
		3	*58*	53	52
		4	*70*	32	36
High (maximum reactions in two variables, one variable appearing three times)	6	1	*52*	42	32
		2	54	38	*56*
		3	*50*	39	41
		4	*56*	39	34
Low (maximum reactions in two variables, each appearing twice)	33	1	*85*	54	52
		2	53	51	*56*
		3	*66*	52	56
		4	46	43	*50*
Minimum (maximum reactions in all three variables)	5	1	57	51	*80*
		2	63	*76*	35
		3	46	*50*	43
		4	*58*	44	54

* Peak T scores are set in italics.

deficiencies in the low and minimum categories. The obtained chi-square is 25.777, significant far below the 0.001 level of confidence. Actual representative cases are given in table IV.

Pattern of Autonomic Lability Scores

Figure 4 shows the results of this analysis. Again there is excess in the high specificity groups and deficiency in the low specificity groups with the obtained chi-square far in excess of the value of 10.827 required for significance at the 0.001 level. Representative cases are given in table V.

Pattern Index Scores

Table VI gives the results of this analysis. The results are not as decisive as they were for the pattern index scores of autonomic tension. Three of the correlations fail to be significant even at the 5% level. In every case the relationship between the pattern index scores in 2 stresses is lower for auto-

nomic lability scores than for the parallel autonomic tension scores, as may be seen by comparing corresponding entries in tables III and VI. In particular, the quantitative differentiation between heart rate and variability of heart rate reactivity is seen to be highly unreliable. The reproducibility of pattern index scores for autonomic lability depends upon the physiological variables being compared, just as the pattern index scores for autonomic tension did. PC–HR scores are more reliable than PC–VHR scores, which are in turn more reliable than HR–VHR scores.

Statistical Cross-Validation

Dr. C. J. BURKE, of the Department of Psychology, Indiana University, has pointed out to the authors that the use of chi-squares in this study may be slightly suspect. Proof of this, and a statement of the amount of bias, is an exceedingly difficult task. An empirical study was made, therefore, to determine whether serious error had been introduced by our statistical manipulations.

The possibility of obtaining biased chi-square values is introduced by the use of McCall's method to normalize the distributions. A more direct method would have been to find on an *independent sample* the mathematical transformation that does normalize the data. Then, the means and sigmas of the independent samples should be used to T-score the data of an experimental group. Similarly, the correlations between base levels and stress levels, used in computing autonomic lability scores, should be found for the independent

sample and applied to the experimental sample.

These requirements may be nicely fulfilled by the data of our study. It was first ascertained, using Fisher's g-statistics, that heart rate base levels and stress levels were all distributed normally [6]. The distributions for palmar conductance and heart rate variability, however, were markedly skewed positively, and Fisher's test indicated that the hypothesis of a normal distribution had to be rejected. The use of a logarithmic transformation eliminated the skew, and statistical test indicated the acceptability of normality of distribution.

The 85 cases were then divided into a group of 43 odd-numbered cases, and 42 even-numbered cases. Means, sigmas, and

Table V. Cases exemplifying varying degrees of response specificity, as seen in the reproducibility of the whole pattern of autonomic lability scores

Degree of response specificity	Case No.	Stress No.	Autonomic lability T-scores*		
			Palmar con-ductance	Heart rate	Variability of heart rate
Shows only one pattern in all four stresses	38	1	*65*	46	36
		2	*63*	62	42
		3	*60*	48	38
		4	*61*	53	27
Shows one pattern in three stresses and another pattern in the fourth stress	14	1	47	56	*59*
		2	48	*58*	50
		3	46	*60*	50
		4	51	*55*	53
Shows one pattern in two stresses and another pattern in the other two stresses	23	1	44	45	*58*
		2	45	43	*61*
		3	41	32	*45*
		4	40	49	*54*
Shows one pattern in one stress, another pattern in another stress, and still another pattern in two stresses	9	1	51	*69*	54
		2	*53*	52	40
		3	48	*56*	44
		4	49	*84*	38
Shows four different patterns	13	1	*66*	44	53
		2	*55*	51	41
		3	55	*68*	58
		4	54	45	*66*

* Peak T scores are set in italics.

correlations were then computed for the 'odds' group, which was considered the 'independent sample'. These independently secured statistics were then used for T-scoring the 'evens' group, the 'experimental sample', and for securing autonomic lability scores. The procedure was then reversed; means, sigmas, and correlations were computed for the 'evens' group, and these statistics were used for securing autonomic tension and autonomic lability scores for the 'odds' group. We may call this a method of cross-validation. Corresponding means, sigmas, and correlations for the 'evens' and 'odds' groups were reasonably close to each other, probably because of the fairly large N and the relative homogeneity of the group. To save space, these data are not presented. The relevant conclusions, however, may be drawn from the data presented in tables VII and VIII. Here we see the product moment correlations between the original scores and those secured by this method of cross-validation. All correlations are extremely high, with none falling below 0.91. The conclusions concerning response specificity would not therefore be changed by using the more complex analysis. As a

matter of fact, all the analyses were carried through to completion by this cross-validation method and no discrepancies arose. Since the method employed earlier lends itself more easily to simple report, it was the one chosen for complete presentation.

Discussion and Conclusions

The results of this study clearly support the principle of relative response specificity. For a given set of autonomic functions individuals tend to respond with a pattern of autonomic activation in which maximal activation occurs in the same physiological function whatever the stress. The results further show that there is a strong tendency for the entire pattern of autonomic activation to be reproduced from stress to stress. Of course, these conclusions hold only within the limits of the experiment. Further studies are called for, in which more physiological variables would be measured and a different variety of stresses used.

The evidence for the conclusions may be summarized as follows. First, when the different physiological reactions are expressed

Table VI. Reproducibility of autonomic lability pattern index scores from stress to stress, shown by means of product-moment correlation coefficients

Pattern index score											
(Palmar conductance T-score minus heart rate T-score) ÷ 10				(Palmar conductance T-score minus heart rate variability T-score) ÷ 10				(Heart rate T-score minus heart rate variability T-score) ÷ 10			
Stress	1	2	3	4	Stress	1	2	3	4	Stress	1	2	3	4
1	X	0.39	0.62	0.44	1	X	0.31	0.46	0.39	1	X	0.09	0.42	0.26
2		X	0.48	0.47	2		X	0.22	0.34	2		X	0.12	0.10
3			X	0.53	3			X	0.45	3			X	0.37
4				X	4				X	4				X

N = 85.
An r of 0.21 is significant at the 0.05 level, of 0.25 at the 0.02 level, of 0.28 at the 0.01 level, and of 0.36 at the 0.001 level.

Table VII. Product-moment correlations between autonomic tension scores secured by McCall's method and those secured by method of 'cross-validation'

'Evens' group (N = 42)				'Odds' group (N = 43)			
	Physiological variable				Physiological variable		
Stress	Palmar conduc-tance	Heart rate	Variability of heart rate	Stress	Palmar conduc-tance	Heart rate	Variability of heart rate
1	0.991	0.984	0.990	1	0.993	0.988	0.989
2	0.990	0.991	0.991	2	0.993	0.989	0.996
3	0.995	0.989	0.995	3	0.994	0.991	0.996
4	0.989	0.992	0.994	4	0.993	0.994	0.996

in equivalent units, it is found that each individual shows differential response within himself. For one physiological function he may be markedly over-reactive; for another, average in reactivity; and for still another, markedly under-reactive. This phenomenon of marked quantitative differentiation within the individual has not been formally analyzed in this paper, as it has in previous papers of this series [7, 8] but the 18 representative cases given in tables I, II, IV, and V serve to exemplify it. Secondly, it was demonstrated that the individual does not vary haphazardly in the physiological function showing maximum reactivity, nor does he vary haphazardly in his pattern of reactivity. These findings were true both for autonomic tension scores (maximum levels reached during stress) and autonomic lability scores (maximum displacement during stress). However, the tendency to show response specificity was more marked for autonomic tension than for autonomic lability.

The distribution of cases obtained directly suggests that the group consists of some individuals who have relatively fixed patterning of the physiological variables studied, some who depart occasionally from their modal pattern, and some who vary haphazardly in their pattern of autonomic arousal. Such a postulated quantitative variation among individuals in the degree to which a pattern of response is

stereotyped completely accounts for the observed data.

The study of the reproducibility from stress to stress of the pattern index scores supplements these observations. We find that the *quantitative differential* between physiological functions in their degree of activation is only imperfectly reproduced from stress to stress; that is, while the rank order between two variables may remain the same (palmar conductance activation greater than heart rate activation, for example), there is considerable fluctuation in the amount by which the response of one exceeds the other. The detailed results suggest that reliability of pattern index scores is greater for measures of autonomic tension than for measures of autonomic lability, and that the reliability is a function of the two physiological measures being compared. Comparing pattern index scores for any two stresses, the results invariably show a progressive decline in the reliability coefficients as we go from the pattern index score PC–HR to PC–VHR to HR–VHR. Comparing any two stresses, we also invariably find that the reliability of autonomic tension pattern index scores is higher than the reliability of autonomic lability pattern index scores.

These results, taken together, suggest a revision of the principle of relative response specificity. The revised principle is that for a given set of autonomic functions quantita-

Table VIII. Product-moment correlations between autonomic lability scores secured by McCall's method and those secured by method of 'cross-validation'

'Evens' group (N = 42)				'Odds' group (N = 43)			
	Physiological variable				Physiological variable		
Stress	Palmar conduc- tance	Heart rate	Variability of heart rate	Stress	Palmar conduc- tance	Heart rate	Variability of heart rate
1	0.96	0.97	0.98	1	0.99	0.97	0.98
2	0.94	0.98	0.99	2	0.94	0.94	0.99
3	0.93	0.91	0.96	3	0.96	0.98	0.99
4	0.91	0.97	0.98	4	0.92	0.96	0.99

tive variation among individuals exists in the degree to which a pattern of response is stereotyped. Some individuals are so constituted that they will respond with a given hierarchy of autonomic activation whatever the stress; others will show greater fluctuation from stress to stress, although they will exhibit one pattern more frequently than another; still other individuals will randomly exhibit now one pattern, now another. In addition, although the rank order of reactivity remains the same from stress to stress, the quantitative difference between the degree of activation of the different physiological measures will fluctuate considerably.

It is tempting to speculate that if a different set of physiological measurements had been chosen at least some of the subjects whose patterns of response seem random would show a stereotyped pattern. In other words, we hypothesize that for every individual at least a part of the total response pattern is stereotyped, with other autonomic responses varying at random. Experiments are now under way to test this hypothesis.

The data of this experiment also have some relevance to a doctrine most recently proposed by ALEXANDER [1]. According to the theory of specificity of physiological response to emotional stimuli, 'every emotional state has its own physiological syndrome'. We have previously argued [8]

that our results using a single stress (the cold pressor test) were somewhat in contradiction to this principle. It was impossible to assume that the subjects responded to the cold water stress with as many diverse emotional constellations as the varying patterns of response would suggest. The present experiment lends greater weight to this argument. Each subject was exposed to four stresses, at least three of which differed markedly among themselves. The physiological and psychological demands of the cold pressor test, of hyperventilation, and of the two intellectual stresses appear to be radically different. The emergence of response specificity under these conditions indicates the striking influence that factors other than the nature of the immediate affective response to stress may have.

Summary

Eighty-five male college students were subjected to four stresses in sequence. The stresses were mental arithmetic, hyperventilation, letter association, and the cold pressor test. Palmar conductance, heart rate, and variability of heart rate were simultaneously and continuously recorded. The results were analyzed in terms of autonomic tension and autonomic lability. Autonomic tension was defined as the maximum level a physiological function reaches during stress. Autonomic lability was defined as the maximum displacement a physiological function exhibits during stress.

The experiment was designed to test the hypothesis of relative response specificity, which states that for a given set of autonomic functions individuals tend to respond with a pattern of autonomic activation in which maximal activation occurs in the same physiological function, whatever the stress. This hypothesis was decisively supported.

The detailed results suggested an extension of the principle of relative response specificity. The revised hypothesis is: For a given set of autonomic functions, there exists quantitative variation among individuals in the degree to which a pattern of response is stereotyped. Some individuals are so constituted that they will respond with a given hierarchy of autonomic activation whatever the stress; others will show greater fluctuation from stress to stress, although they will exhibit one pattern more frequently than others; still other individuals randomly exhibit now one pattern, now another. In addition, although the rank order of reactivity remains the same from stress to stress, the quantitative difference between the degree of activation of the different physiological functions will fluctuate markedly.

References

1. ALEXANDER, F.: Psychosomatic Medicine, Its Principles and Applications (Norton and Co., Inc., New York 1950).
2. BLANK, I. H. and FINESINGER, J. E.: Electrical resistance of the skin. Effect of size of electrodes, exercise, and cutaneous hydration. Arch. Neurol., Chicago 56: 544 (1946).
3. CANNON, W. B.: Bodily changes in pain, hunger, fear and rage (Appleton, New York 1929).
4. CANNON, W. B.: The wisdom of the body (Norton and Co., Inc., New York 1939).
5. CLARK, L. C., Jr. and LACEY, J. I.: An improved skin electrode. J. Lab. clin. Med. 35: 786 (1950).
6. JOHNSON, P. O.: Statistical methods in research (Prentice-Hall, Inc., New York 1949).
7. LACEY, J. I.: Individual differences in somatic response patterns. J. comp. physiol. Psychol. 43: 338 (1950).
8. LACEY, J. I.: An experimental study of differential emphasis in somatic response to stress. Psychosom. Med. 14: 71 (1952).
9. LACEY, J. I.: The application of the mathematical model of correlation coefficients to the measurement of autonomic response (in preparation).
10. LACEY, J. I.; BATEMAN, D. E., and VANLEHN, R.: Autonomic response specificity and Rorschach color responses. Psychosom. Med. 14: 256 (1952).
11. MALMO, R. B. and SHAGASS, C.: Physiologic study of symptom mechanisms in psychiatric patients under stress. Psychosom. Med. 11: 25 (1949).
12. MALMO, R. B.; SHAGASS, C., and DAVIS, F. H.: Symptom specificity and bodily reactions during psychiatric interview. Psychosom. Med. 12: 362 (1950).
13. RICHTER, C. P.: Instructions for using the cutaneous resistance recorder, or 'Dermometer', on peripheral nerve injuries, sympathectomies, and paravertebral blocks. J. Neurosurg. 3: 181 (1946).
14. THERON, P. A.: Peripheral vasomotor reactions as indices of basic emotional tension and lability. Psychosom. Med. 10: 335 (1948).
15. WILDER, J.: The law of initial values. Psychosom. Med. 12: 392 (1950).

An Investigation of the Relation Between Life Experience, Personality Characteristics, and General Susceptibility to Illness[1]

L. E. Hinkle, Jr., W. N. Christenson, F. D. Kane, A. Ostfeld, W. N. Thetford and H. G. Wolff

Retrospective comment by Dr. S. Cobb. This is one of a series of similar studies done in Harold Wolff's laboratory at Cornell, which are distinguished for their data gathering and their clinical interpretation, although not yet achieving equivalent sophistication in statistical design and analysis. The importance of this paper lies in the fact that it represents a nodal point in the evolution of the concept of person-environment fit as a predictor of physical and mental health. Earlier psychosomatic studies had tended to focus on the personality of the patient or on the temporal relation of life events to exacerbations and remissions of specific illnesses. Gradually the notion evolved that it is the perceived or subjective social environment that is most closely related to the occurrence of illness. This point is admirably expressed here. Since that time our thinking has become more complex with the recognition that it is the interaction of the personality with the current objective environment that leads to the perceived or subjective environment which in turn leads to behavioral, affective and physiologic responses. An even fuller flowering of this concept came with the presentation of the person-environment fit model to the Stanford Conference on Coping and Adaptation in March of 1969.

This paper is further significant because in it are shown glimmerings of concern over the extent to which findings should be interpreted as disease, as sick role behavior, and/or as reporting artifact. We now know that all three are important and that they are very difficult to separate.

Episodes of illness are not distributed at random among the members of the general population. Even among groups of people of similar ethnic and social background, living in the same general environment, and sharing the same occupation over a period of many years, the likelihood of becoming ill is different from person to person. Differences in age, sex, and opportunities to encounter trauma or infection do not entirely account for this variability. In several groups in which the distribution of illness episodes has been investigated, 25% of the members have experienced approximately 50% of the episodes over a 20-year period of the 'prime of life', and another 25% of the members have experienced fewer than 10% of the episodes [1, 2]. Those experiencing the greater number of episodes were found to have a greater number of disease syndromes, major as well as minor, involving a greater number of organ systems, and falling into a greater number of etiological categories – in short, they appeared to have a greater 'general susceptibility to illness' than other members of the group.

The number of episodes of illness experienced per unit time, therefore, is a rough measure of susceptibility to illness. For people in relatively static life situations it has provided a better basis for predicting future health than has the amount of time a person has been disabled, or, in most instances, the type of illness he has experi-

[1] From The Study Program in Human Health and the Ecology of Man. Departments of Medicine and Psychiatry, New York Hospital-Cornell Medical Center, New York City.

enced in the past. Provided one uses an arbitrary but standardized definition of the term 'episode of illness', it becomes a reproducible measure of 'general health' which, though crude, has advantages over other measures so far tested in studies of this type [3].

Differences in general suceptibility to illness are present early in life, and they appear to be at least in part 'constitutional'. The illness record of an individual, when followed over a period of years, fluctuates around a mean [1]. The various fluctuations are closely related to reactions to the various life situations that are encountered; but the mean level appears to be determined to a large extent by characteristics of the individual himself. Some people exhibit recurrent disturbances of mood, thought, behavior, and bodily function in an environment that the observer evaluates as relatively unchallenging, while others show little or no symptomatic response to major environmental changes. These differences from person to person could arise from differences in the perception and evaluation of the environment, or from innate differences in reactivity, or both.

It is the purpose of this paper to explore some of the characteristics of 10 people who have experienced a large number of illness episodes, and to compare them with 10 similar people who have experienced few illness episodes, in order to illuminate some factors that may be responsible for differences in general susceptibility to illness.

Method

At the time that this report was prepared, the distribution of illness had been studied in five groups of people: 1,527 skilled workmen in New York City [1]; 1,297 semiskilled women workers in the same city [4]; 100 Chinese graduate students, technical, and professional people; 70 refugees from the 1956 revolution in Hungary; and 132 recent graduates of American colleges [5]. The present report is based on the study of the Chinese, a group selected because of the large amount of

dislocation and social change which they had experienced.

The members of the group had these features in common: (1) They were ethnically Chinese. (2) They were reared in China, in the Chinese cultural milieu. (3) During the course of their lives they had been exposed to the effects of the rapid changes in Chinese culture, the social upheavals and the geographic dislocations, which have characterized the last half-century in China; and many of them had had personal experience with wars, revolutions, new customs, and technological changes in their homeland. (4) They had received (or were in the process of receiving) a modern, Western college education, and thus had had to make a personal adaptation to features of two dissimilar cultures. (5) With few exceptions they had come to the United States before 1949, in the pursuit of their education or their professional activities, and had been unable or unwilling to return to China after the Communists seized power. (6) In the United States most of them had been in a situation of uncertainty since that time, without assurance of their future status, their occupation, their careers, or the fate of their families, friends, and possessions in China. They were, therefore, a group who had experienced many major changes in their life situations, and who had had to make many major adaptations during their lives.

When this study was initiated in the fall of 1954, there were several thousand such Chinese in the United States. The 100 selected for study were obtained largely through the mediation of a Chinese educator on the staff of the project, who undertook to obtain a representative group covering the various professions, and the technical and the administrative fields. Altogether, his selections covered some 25 fields, ranging from medicine and art to engineering and business administration, and including a few housewives and some undergraduate students. In age, the informants ranged from 19 to 72, but the bulk of them were in their 30s or late 20s. Thirty-one were women, and 69 were men. Health was not a consideration in their selection. The project was presented to them as an attempt to understand the personality features and the problems of adjustment of their group of Chinese. Informants were selected for participation and then were asked to volunteer. Most of those approached agreed to be seen, and it is likely that the majority of those who refused did so because they were employed full time, and could not spare the two days necessary to complete the investigation of each person. Those who volunteered were motivated primarily by a desire to contribute to the study, which covered points of great concern to all of them; their participation was also a personal favor to the highly respected staff member who obtained them for the project. Each informant received the sum of $ 25 to help cover the expense and effort expended.

Sixteen hours were spent in the study of each informant. Four hours were spent with an internist, who obtained a factual biography, a comprehensive review of all illnesses past and present, a physical examination, and any laboratory tests necessary to clarify diagnostic questions. Four hours were spent with a psychiatrist, partly in directed and partly in undirected interviewing aimed at obtaining an assessment of his personality features and some idea of the dynamics of the development of his personality. Four hours were spent with a clinical psychologist, who administered a series of tests, including the Rorschach, the Wechsler-Bellevue form 1, the Sachs Sentence Completion, the Thurstone Temperament Scale, a projective questionnaire, the Lowenfeld Mosaic, and the Human Figure Drawing Test. Four hours were spent with a cultural anthropologist. In the latter part of the project two hours were spent with a sociologist. One of the goals of the anthropologist and sociologist was to place the informant in the context of his culture and his society, and to obtain an understanding of his culturally determined reactions to his various life situations.

The present report is primarily concerned with some of the medical and psychological observations. When the medical data had been obtained, illness episodes were tabulated by name, classified, and counted, using a prearranged, standardized, written procedure prepared for use in all of these studies. For the purposes of this report, only those illnesses which occurred during the twenty-year period from age 12 through age 31 were considered. Each individual was ranked according to the rate of episodes of illness *per annum* over this 20-year period, and individuals were selected for comparison on the basis of their rank. The men and the women were treated as separate groups.

The psychiatrist and the cultural anthropologist could not escape learning about the health history of each informant during the course of their interviews, although they developed only a general idea of how each would rank on the final analysis of the medical data. Thus it cannot be stated that they evaluated the information in the total absence of knowledge of the health history of the informants: but they did attempt to exclude considerations of health from their evaluations. They made their decisions from analyses of their own data without knowledge of the results of the statistical analyses of the medical data.

Results

Distribution of Illness Episodes

Of the 69 men in the group, 60 were 32 years old or older, and had, therefore, health histories obtainable over a full 20-year period from age 12 through age 31. These 60 were a group large enough to be treated statistically. When the individuals within it were distributed according to the number of episodes experienced over the 20-year period, and the results were plotted by cumulative percentages of individuals, the resulting plot closely approximated the curve of a calculated negative binomial distribution. Such a distribution is in accordance with the assumption that some factor (or factors) in addition to chance operated in determining the distribution of episodes of illness or, in other words, that the likelihood of becoming ill varied from person to person (fig. 1) [1].

When the men were divided into quartiles based on episodes of illness *per annum*, the quartile whose members had the highest frequency of illness had 49.5% of the episodes experienced by the entire group, and the quartile with the lowest frequency rate experienced only 8.5% of the episodes (fig. 2).

When the number of episodes of illness experienced by each man was plotted against the number of organ systems primarily involved in these illnesses, the general upward trend of the data was apparent (fig. 3). The plot closely approximated that obtained from similar data from the American groups [3]. Considering that these data were obtained from memory, and that the recall of minor episodes of illness is relatively inaccurate even under the most careful questioning, there is a noteworthy similarity between these data and those obtained from the detailed and continuous health records of the American working groups.

The various illness syndromes were placed in 'etiological categories' as defined by the *Standard Nomenclature of Diseases and Operations* [6], and the number of episodes experienced by each man was plotted against the number of 'etiological categories' into which they fell. This plot also resembled that obtained from the data from the American groups, trending upward as the number of episodes increased (fig. 4).

Among the 31 women there were 18 who were 32 years old or older, and who therefore provided data over the time span from

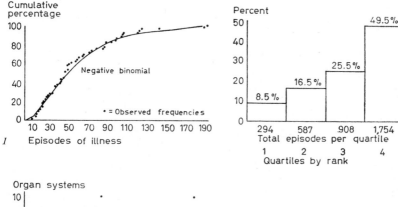

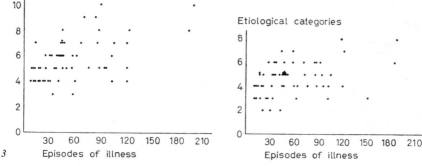

Fig. 1. Distribution of 60 Chinese men (age 12–32) by total number of episodes of illness.

Fig. 2. Distribution of 60 Chinese men (age 12–32) by number of episodes of illness *per annum*.

Fig. 3. Episodes of illness in 60 Chinese men (age 12–32) plotted against the number of organ systems primarily involved.

Fig. 4. Episodes of illness in 60 Chinese men (age 12–32) plotted against the etiological categories in which the illness fell.

Table I. Lowest and highest frequency of illness episodes per annum

Inf.	Age	Illness episodes rate *per annum*	Occupation
		Low-frequency	
L 1	37	0.5	Insurance broker
L 2	72	0.6	Widowed executive
L 3	37	0.65	Chemical engineer
L 4	34	0.7	Graduate student
L 5	37	0.75	Graduate student
L 6	32	0.75	Housewife, mother
L 7	32	0.8	White collar worker
L 8	44	0.85	College instructor
L 9	33	0.85	Department store manager
L 10	27	1.3	Recent bride
		High-frequency	
H 10	31	5.3	Chemical engineer
H 9	31	6.0	Certified public accountant
H 8	33	6.1	Graduate student
H 7	32	6.2	Graduate student
H 6	52	7.1	Philosophy lecturer
H 5	36	9.5	Surgical resident
H 4	33	9.6	Graduate student
H 3	33	13.6	Secretary
H 2	37	15.0	College instructor
H 1	30	20.2	Housewife, mother

age 12 through age 31. The number was too small to be treated statistically as a separate group. When the data from the women were combined with those from the men, and the grouped data were treated as a whole, the results previously described were not significantly altered; but such a procedure creates a mixed sample, which is not desirable, and for this reason, data from the women were excluded from the plots.

Among the 60 men, the number of sickness episodes *per annum* ranged from 0.5 to 9.6. Among the 18 women, they ranged from 0.6 to 20.2. The 7 men and the 3 women having the lowest rates were selected for comparison with the 7 men and 3 women having the highest rates. These 2 groups of informants are listed in table I. The rates *per annum* in the lowest frequency group ranged from 0.5 to 1.3; that in the highest group ranged from 5.3 to 20.2.

Thus, the members of the high-frequency group had experienced approximately ten times as many episodes of symptomatic illness during adolescence and young adulthood as had the members of the low-frequency group.

Comment

Although it is recognized that data obtained from memory are not precise, it is reasonable to conclude that the difference between the 2 groups in respect to number of illness episodes per unit time was real, and of the order of magnitude stated. Their members were comparable in age, sex, and education; the interviews provided no evidence that they differed in their capacity to recall, in their willingness to talk, or in their use of repressive mechanisms, in a manner that would account for this difference in distribution of illness episodes. Their syndromes described were clearly recognizable and their signs and symptoms often detectable by examination; and neither group had more reason to conceal its illness than the other. In the American groups, where records were available for comparison with medical histories, it was found that the recall of major episodes of illness is generally good, and that the recall of minor episodes is generally inaccurate in detail, but accurate in order of magnitude. For example, people who say that they had a severe headache about once a month for 20 years may have had many more or many fewer headaches than they actually describe, but they almost always have had a great many more headaches than have people who maintain that they have never had a headache at all.

The illness episode rates calculated for these Chinese are only an approximation of the facts and should be so regarded. Rankings, and the rates for individual cases, are relative. However, there is no reason to doubt that there is a difference in the number of symptomatic episodes of illness experienced by the two groups as such, and the comparison between them is justifiable on this basis.

Family Histories

A review of the family histories of the members of the two groups revealed no striking differences in the general health or longevity of their kin, or in the incidence of familial diseases among them. In both groups there were some whose parents were healthy and long-lived, and others whose parents were chronically ill and died young.

Childhood Health

Eight members of the low-frequency group reported that they had been robust and healthy in infancy and childhood, and two said that they were thin and sickly during this time. One of the low-frequency group was enuretic to age 10. Seven of the high-frequency group reported that they had been healthy infants and children, and one of the seven said that he had been the healthiest child in his family; three reported that they had been sickly. Two of this group were enuretic to age 10.

Illness Experienced During the Period of Observation

The high-frequency group, during the 20-year-period from age 12 through age 31, experienced 14 major illnesses (mean per person 1.4, range 0–4), 20 disorders of mood, thought, and behavior (mean per person 2.0, range 0–6), and 1,989 minor episodes of illness (mean per person 199, range 108–342). The number of organ systems primarily involved in illness averaged 7.7 per person (range 5–9). Their health histories may be briefly characterized in the following summaries:

H 1. A woman with recurrent attacks of migraine and severe dysmenorrhea, who also had malaria, preeclampsia, and a major depressive illness, as well as recurrent upper and lower gastrointestinal disturbances, anemia, hemorrhoids, and moderately frequent upper respiratory infections.

H 2. A woman with recurrent bouts of low-grade arthritis, who also had malaria, dysmenorrhea, recurring lower-bowel symptoms, and intermittent respiratory infections, as well as myopia, exfoliative dermatitis, hemorrhoids, and extensive dental caries.

H 3. A woman with recurring episodes of gastric hyperfunction, but without a demonstrable ulcer; she also had hyperthyroidism, acute appendicitis, the Stevens-Johnson syndrome, a spontaneous abortion, many vascular headaches, and recurrent symptoms of tension and anxiety, plus fairly frequent upper respiratory infections.

H 4. A man highly susceptible to respiratory infections, who also had chronic bronchitis, allergic rhinitis, and sinusitis, as well as recurrent vascular headaches, constipation, fissure in ano, myopia, a chalazion, and symptoms of muscle tension and anxiety.

H 5. A man with the 'irritable colon syndrome' and migraine, who also had malaria, typhoid, dengue, and appendicitis, as well as trachoma, frequent respiratory infections, severe dental caries, myopia, hemorrhoids, acne, acute epididymitis, and a number of accidents.

H 6. A man with severe migraine, who also had malaria, and a depressive illness.

H 7. A man highly suceptible to respiratory infections, who also had vasomotor rhinitis, recurrent otitis media, malaria, and episodes of anxiety and depression, as well as myopia and severe dental caries.

H 8. A man with recurrent respiratory infections, who also had vascular headaches and gastric hyperfunction, as well as vasomotor rhinitis, malaria, depressive and neurasthenic symptoms, and nonspecific arthritis.

H 9. A man susceptible to respiratory infections and sore throat, who also had typhoid, gastric hyperfunction, and a great deal of dental caries, as well as myopia, allergic rhinitis, chronic sinusitis, and an accident.

H 10. A man with gastric hyperfunction, tension headaches, and fairly frequent respiratory infections, who also had infectious hepatitis, mumps, dental caries, and a few anxiety symptoms.

The low-frequency group, from age 12 through age 31, experienced 11 major illnesses (mean per person 1.1, range 0–2), 11 disorders of mood, thought, and behavior (mean per person 1.1, range 0–2), and 123 minor episodes of illness (mean per person 12.3, range 3–21). The number of organ systems primarily involved in illness averaged 4.3 per person (range 3–7). Their health histories are briefly characterized:

L 1. A man who on most careful questioning could recall only two symptomatic illnesses during the 20-year-period: a brief febrile illness, probably infectious, at age 22, and a sprained wrist at age 15. He denied all other symptoms during this time, and stated that he had always felt healthy. The only finding on examination was myopia.

L 2. A woman who had a behavior disturbance at age 12, in a setting of family conflict, and whose only other illnesses were mild respiratory infections occurring approximately every 2 years.

L 3. A man whose recalled illnesses were four episodes of dental caries, two respiratory infections, cholera, a contusion of the arm, and a two-day febrile illness of unknown etiology.

L 4. A man whose recalled illnesses were appendicitis, the fracture of two teeth, ten upper respiratory infections (estimated), and a few days of anxiety and depression when his wife obtained a legal separation.

L 5. A man who during the war had beriberi and two severe bouts of malaria, but, except for these, denied all illnesses and symptoms other than a few respiratory infections, a dog bite, and a few days of impotence and premature ejaculation shortly after his wedding.

L 6. A woman who had a tonsillectomy at age 12 at her parents' insistence, had had a few respiratory infections thereafter, and had been well otherwise, except for one episode of fainting, one of bleeding, and two of anorexia and nausea during her four pregnancies.

L 7. A man who had acne, two bouts of malaria, a mild episode of bacillary dysentery, a short period of dejection after the death of a sister, and who insisted that he had had only two upper respiratory infections during this period.

L 8. A man who stated that he had been well except for two brief periods of loneliness and slight depression, about ten respiratory infections, malaria, staphylococcal septicemia, and a pilonidal cyst.

L 9. A man who was well except for malaria, a minor patch of psoriasis, and about ten respiratory infections, despite the fact that he had a noticeable congenital deformity, and said that he had been shy, discouraged, and resentful about this all of his life.

L 10. A woman who was ill for six months because of minimal tuberculosis, which did not recur; but who otherwise had only about 15 respiratory infections, mumps, myopia, and two short periods of moderate anxiety and tension.

Life Experiences

During their lives, the members of both groups had faced many difficulties including problems of interpersonal relations, the attainment of a modern education, geographic changes, shifts in their social and cultural milieu, the hazards of war and similar threats and deprivations, and a variety of individual responsibilities and frustrations. There is no adequate way of counting or measuring these, but they can be epitomized briefly for each informant, beginning with the high-frequency group:

H 1. The child of a concubine of a high government official, she was given away at birth to be reared by a foster mother until age three. Returned to her family, she had a barren existence until her invalid mother died when she was nine. After three more years with the foster mother, she was sent to a village at age 12, to escape the Japanese war. She had six months of hardship there, and then went to Chungking and Chengtu, obtaining a modern college education under difficulties in the midst of war. At 22, she married a religious scholar and businessman, went to an East Asian country with him, and taught school there until his business collapsed. She then came to the United States, where she worked variously in grocery stores and laundries in order to support her husband, parents, and two children. Recently she had been living precariously on her husband's small fellowship while he resumed his studies of Oriental religion.

H 2. The first of seven children of the sickly wife of a Chinese who had become a poor Protestant parson. She was sent to mission schools in Treaty Ports. At the onset of the Japanese war, she was separated from her family and evacuated with other adolescents to rural China, then went across country to southwest China, enduring many privations and bombings while obtaining a modern education. After her graduation she became a teacher by necessity. She came to the United States for advanced training in the late 1940s, and was unable to return. She had held various mediocre teaching jobs in small colleges in the United States since that time, and was still unmarried.

H 3. The only child of a self-made Army officer who married a scholar's daughter and became an important military leader. Her parents took her all over China in the 1920s, with many nurses and servants and no playmates. Her mother was a chronically depressed woman. At the age of 10 she was sent to mission school, and attended six different schools in as many years, accompanied by her ill mother: she finally graduated from college at age 23. A year later a marriage was 'arranged', and at a large and fashionable wedding she was married to a Chinese businessman, who was unfaithful and squandered her money. After having one child she divorced him at age 26 and went to Taiwan, where she got a government job. Transferred to the United States several years ago, she brought with her her mother and her daughter, whom she supports.

H 4. Born in Canton, the son of an American-born Chinese businessman who went to China to have a family. The father returned to the United States when H 4 was several months old, and did not come back. H 4 was reared happily up to age 13 in a large family compound with many children, and attended Chinese schools. At 13 he went to a modern middle school. During the war he escaped across country to Chungking and went to college there, with some difficulty and privation. At age 26 he went to Singapore to learn English, and a year later he became a journalist. In the late 1940s he came to the United States to study and was supported on a grant, when his funds were cut off. He later married a Chinese girl with a good job, who helped to support their mutual household.

H 5. Born in Hong Kong, the son of a Chinese educator. He attended a Chinese school to age 10; then, after some rebellion, he went to modern Roman Catholic mission schools. During the war he was sent to a Catholic college in a coastal city, and after one year there he was persuaded to shift from engineering to medicine. He graduated at 26, and had an internship and residency in Chinese hospitals. In the late 1940s he came to the United States for further training, and he had remained here since in the status of a 'permanent surgical resident', being unwilling to return to China, and unable to practice here because he is an alien.

H 6. The eldest son of a Chinese scholar, he was reared in comfort and with solicitude in a traditional, well-to-do, large family compound. Educated by tutors, and then sent to a modern university, from which he graduated at age 22. His parents having died, he took over the leadership of the large family, marrying a 'cousin' by arrangement. Friction soon developed between them and the marriage was never satisfactory. He held a number of teaching positions in China until he came to the United States before the war for further study, leaving his family behind. Moving in a leisurely fashion from university to university, he finally obtained his degree eight years later. In the 11 years since, he had lived on lecture fees and meager grants from foundations, occasionally teaching. He had not attempted to return to China, and had found no solution to his marital situation.

H 7. The eldest son of a rural landowner

who became a politician. His parents were solicitous and affectionate, but his family moved around a great deal during the political upheavals of the 1920s. He was separated from them and sent to boarding school at age 13, and was evacuated to southwest China with other students at age 15. He was leader of his student group, and, in Chungking, while obtaining an education under difficulties, he remained a leader and became active in politics. He completed his studies after the war in a large Chinese university, standing first in his class. He then went to Europe to study political science, coming to the United States the next year. He completed his doctorate three years later. Since then he has worked at various incidental jobs in order to support himself, and has done some teaching. He has been unwilling to return to China, and has not established a career or marriage here.

H 8. The third son of an uneducated but well-to-do restaurant owner in Canton, he was raised by a nursemaid while his parents traveled. They were away from home most of the time until he was seven, when he was sent to a mission school. He attended this and another school until age 14, when his father took him to another area in China to escape the war. There he attended an English religious school for two years, until he was expelled for taking part in a riot. He traveled overland to west China, where he continued his education, while suffering serious privations. He was briefly in the Chinese Army. After the war he continued his studies, graduating at 26. Forced to flee from the Communists, he came to the United States and studied for a higher degree at several midwestern universities until his funds were cut off. After that he worked at various incidental jobs to support himself.

H 9. The youngest son of a well-to-do publisher, his childhood was spent in a comfortable home, with affectionate parents, good sibling relations, and solicitous servants. He went to a Chinese private school to age 12, when his family fled to the French Concession in Shanghai to escape the Japanese. He was sent to a British-type middle school and college, remaining in the same city throughout the war. After his graduation, he took a job in a bank. Shortly after the war he came to the United States, and in 2 years obtained a Master's degree from an important university. Finding that this did not help him to obtain a job, he took a second Master's degree in another field and since then has worked successfully for an important corporation. A few years ago he married a Chinese girl of similar background. They have one child, are satisfied with the marriage, and have a comfortable home.

H 10. The thirteenth child of a well-to-do bank manager who had a modern education, but ran his household as an old-fashioned large family. The home was stable, and interpersonal relations were good. He was cared for by an amah to age 10. His mother was kidnapped that year, but returned unharmed. From age 11 to 13, he was taught at home by tutors; thereafter, he attended a modern middle school, and later went to college, remaining in Shanghai during the war. In the mid-1940s he came to the United States to join an older brother and obtain further education. He tried several schools and considered several courses of study before deciding to become an engineer. Cut off from funds a few years later, he soon obtained a well-paid job as an engineer in the United States, and shortly thereafter married a Chinese girl of similar background. He lives in a comfortable apartment with his wife and mother-in-law.

The same information for the low-frequency group may be epitomized thus:

L 1. The second son of a wealthy businessman, he grew up in a large, semimodern household, with many children, who were cared for much of the time by servants because the parents were away from the home. He had private tutors in childhood, and was then sent away to a Protestant boarding school. During the war his father sent him in comfort and with ample funds to join his brother in Chungking, where he obtained a college education while carrying out successful business ventures on the side. Graduating in political science at age 24, he obtained a job in a government agency, and the next year married a well-to-do girl of his own choice. After the war he obtained a post with the government, and in the next 2 years he and his wife had two children. He was sent overseas, and shortly thereafter was left without a job or funds when the government was defeated. Moving to the United States on his own resources, he took a course in business, established his own firm, and has prospered. He has a substantial house with servants in a suburb of a large city.

L 2. Born before the fall of the Empire, the bound-foot daughter of an old Chinese family, she was reared in the Confucian tradition until she rebelled at age 13 and demanded a modern education. With great effort she learned English at a mission school, soon excelling in this and other studies. Gradually she broke away entirely from the traditional restrictions upon women, becoming a Christian, participating in political activity, becoming a respected executive, and ultimately marrying a man of her own choice, while overcoming the vigorous opposition of her family and the strong sanctions of her friends in order to do so. When her husband died tragically shortly after the marriage, she resumed her career and raised and educated her children through the difficult period of the Japanese occupation. She left China with great reluctance in the late 1940s and has established a comfortable home for herself and her two daughters in the United States.

L 3. The third son of a banker, he was reared in a harmonious large family setting, with many children and servants, who continued with him through the private school and the private middle school which he attended. His family remained in Shanghai during the Japanese war, in comfort, and he went to college there, studying engineering. Upon his graduation at 22, he worked for six months in a factory, and then went to Hong Kong. He went through the siege of Hong Kong in 1941, escaped across country to Chungking with some hardship and privation, and lived and worked there throughout the war. Shortly after the war he came to the United States to complete his studies. Entering a top-grade engineering school, he obtained a creditable record. At 30 he married a Chinese girl of similar background. After their funds were cut off in 1949, he obtained a job as an engineer with a Chinese concern, and did well financially. His wife continued her education intermittently, while rearing their two children. He bought a home in the suburbs of a large American city, and continued to prosper, as did the members of his family.

L 4. The son of a village landowner who became a Christian because his opium-smoking uncles were squandering the family inheritance. There was some conflict in the family because of this. L 4 was the first child in the village to go to a modern school, to high school, and then to college. For four months, early in the war, he fought against the

Japanese as a soldier; then he walked on foot over a thousand miles to Chungking, where he attended school, took part in student activities, and partly supported himself. At age 24 he became the principal of a Christian high school, and rose rapidly in the field of education. At 27 he became dean of students at a large university, and made a marriage of choice to a girl of similar background, with whom he was very happy. Coming to the United States to continue his studies, he was forced to leave his wife behind. Shortly thereafter the Communists took over the government and his funds were cut off. Soon he lost contact with his family: a few years later he was notified by mail that his wife had received a 'political divorce'. During the course of these events he continued his studies, obtained his degree, and found a job in the United States in his chosen field, where he continued to work steadily and productively thereafter.

L 5. The fifth child of a wealthy rural landowner. His father died when he was two years old, and his mother took the large family to a nearby town, where the children could get a modern education. He attended various Chinese schools near his home. During the war he went to western China to a displaced university, where he completed his education with a good deal of hardship and privation. After a brief period of postgraduate work, he volunteered for youth work with the Army, which he continued until the end of the war, when he returned to his native village and married a girl chosen by his family. The girl wanted the marriage, but he was unenthusiastic about it. It has worked out very satisfactorily. He became the protégé and assistant of a prominent Nationalist general, and accompanied this general to Taiwan, taking his family with him. He had moved steadily ahead as an administrator there. He came to the United States to do postgraduate work, and was seen during his brief visit here.

L 6. The ninth of ten children of a wealthy politician. She grew up in a large, old-fashioned family with an uneducated mother and many servants, having no very close associations in childhood. At age 9 she was sent to boarding school with a maid. Thereafter she was in a succession of schools, being at home only on vacations. She was sent to Chungking when the Sino-Japanese war broke out, and completed her education there in semicomfort, with the maid still in attendance.

At age 19 she made a marriage of choice to a wealthy 'playboy', and lived with him and his parents until the end of the war. She then accompanied him to the United States, where he soon established himself as an able and responsible businessman, and prospered. He has taken over the support of those members of both families who lost their income after the Communist revolution. She had four children, a comfortable home, and was pursuing the career of housewife.

L 7. The only son of a self-made military man who became a successful Nationalist officer. He was sent with his mother to live with the grandparents in a rural village at age 3, and from then to age 10 he was reared in a traditional setting. He then rejoined his father, and was sent to modern schools and middle school; during the war he continued his education at Chungking with great difficulty, suffering many bombings and much privation. Later in the war he accompanied his father to Europe and attended a European medical school for three and a half years. In the late 1940s his father returned to China, leaving him in the United States. Failing to get into an American medical school, he made no further attempt to obtain an education, but settled down and lived on his remaining money until this gave out, making only nominal attempts to continue his medical education. After his last few thousand dollars had been stolen, he moved to another city and obtained a full-time job in another field, which he found dull, but which he continued out of necessity.

L 8. The seventh of eight children of a convert to Protestantism, who worked for the church. His father had tuberculosis, and turned him over to a stern, cold, rejecting uncle and aunt for adoption. He had a barren, deprived, and restricted childhood. He was sent to mission schools, where he did poorly, and to a Christian college, which he left two years later after failing two subjects. Marrying a wife of his choice, whom he found compatible, he became a technician, and moved west to work in a large industrial plant when the Sino-Japanese war began. A sister, married to a wealthy and influential man, made it possible for him to come to the United States after the war. Here he enjoyed going to a number of colleges over the course of a decade, starting as a premedical student, shifting to physics, and finally to engineering, in which he ultimately received a degree. Thereafter he

obtained a job as a teacher of engineering, bought a house, and lived comfortably with his wife. He had no children.

L 9. The third son of a well-to-do judge, he had a prominent congenital deformity. His early years were spent in a large and quarrelsome family; then he was sent to Chinese public schools, where he was a poor student, and was teased and ridiculed. During the war he went to school in Shanghai and later in Chungking, but did little and followed no regular academic course. His marriage was arranged by his mother, and after it, he lived with his wife's parents. With money supplied by his father-in-law, he and his wife came to the United States after the war, leaving their two children behind. He briefly attended a junior college on the West Coast, intermittently studied art, then worked in a factory and a retail store. A third child was born before his wife left him. Thereafter he moved to a new city, taking this child with him, and obtained a job as a stockboy in a department store, which he has held since.

L 10. The only daughter of a government official, she was a thin, sickly child and a feeding problem during the first 18 months of her life. Thereafter her childhood was healthy. She went to various mission schools, and traveled about to various cities with her parents. She stayed with them in Hong Kong until the Japanese occupation of that city, then escaped to Chungking, where she went to boarding school and her family soon joined her. Still with her family, she returned to Shanghai after the war and resumed her college career. Her first separation from them occurred when she was sent to the United States in the late 1940s for further schooling, but they came over and rejoined her after her graduation. Thereafter she worked for a while in a department store, while continuing to live with her parents. Her father died, and her brother caused some difficulties during this time. She was engaged to a young Chinese when she was seen.

The Realization of Potentialities

There appeared to be a difference, but not a great difference, between the members of the two groups in the degree to which they had realized their apparent potentialities, and had fulfilled the responsibilities of their position in life, as these were estimated by the project staff.

In these respects the high-frequency group were characterized thus by the staff:

H 1 was a woman who had striven conscientiously to fulfill the role of a faithful daughter and wife, as she understood it.

H 2 was an inflexible old maid, rigidly pursuing a career in which she could expect neither success nor reward.

H 3 was a woman whose family had made poor choices for her, but who tried conscientiously to fulfill her responsibilities nevertheless.

H 4 was a striving, ambitious man, who had got ahead partly by his own effort, but had not succeeded as much as he wished.

H 5 had acquired good surgical training in spite of many difficulties; but he had not solved many other problems in his life.

H 6 was a passive man who had not discharged his family responsibilities, solved his marital problems, or worked out a career suitable to his present life situation.

H 7 was a striving and ambitious man, with a record of leadership and achievement, who was caught in a situation for which he could find no solution.

H 8 was a man whose early life experiences had not prepared him for a life of hardship and decision, and who had had difficulty in dealing with these.

H 9 was a striving, ambitious, and able man, who had made a good adaptation to his present situation.

H 10 was a likable and conscientious man, who had had more responsibility thrust upon him than he would have sought of his own accord, and had tried to meet it adequately.

The members of the low-frequency group were epitomized thus by the staff:

L 1 was a likable man, generally looked upon as resourceful and successful, but primarily interested in taking care of himself.

L 2 was a woman deeply convinced that her course in life was proper and justifiable, quite adept at attaining her goals, and highly respected.

L 3 was an able man, who became a good engineer, and made a good adaptation to American life.

L 4 was a man deeply convinced that his course in life was proper and justifiable, and successful in following his own career in the United States.

L 5 was a man without fixed goals, who had taken advantage of his opportunities, and had done well for himself.

L 6 was a girl who had faced rather few responsibilities, had made few decisions, and was fortunate to have had an easy life.

L 7 was a man who had moved ahead as long as opportunities were present, but had made no serious effort to solve the first major problem in his life.

L 8 was a man who had rejected his first opportunities and, more by luck than by design, had ultimately found a life situation that was satisfactory for him.

L 9 was a man with a modest intelligence, who had not made very much of his life, and had not attempted to do so. His family and his friends regarded him as a conspicuous failure.

L 10 was an immature young woman who had had a relatively easy life under the protection of her family, and was only beginning to encounter the problems of adult independence.

Perceptions of Life Experiences

On the other hand, there was a notable difference in the way that the members of the two groups had viewed their own lives.

The perceptions of the high-frequency group may be epitomized thus:

H 1 saw herself as an unloved and unwanted child, who had had a lonely and difficult life, and now had a husband and children who were a burden to her.

H 2 saw herself as a restricted and deprived child, who had had a lifetime of hardship and responsibility, and a career that was not really satisfying. She would have liked to be married, but she could not find a man who came up to her standards, and in any case, she found it difficult to let herself go emotionally.

H 3 saw herself as a lonely child, with an ill and unhappy mother who had always been a burden to her; she regarded her marriage as a tragic mistake, and her present lot in life as extremely difficult.

H 4 was a suspicious and resentful man, who saw his life as full of obstacles, many of which were created by other people.

H 5 saw himself as the child of an unhappy mother and a demanding father, who had been persuaded to go into a profession that was extremely difficult, and now found himself in a demanding, unsatisfactory, and insolubly difficult life situation.

H 6 saw himself as a man who had been trained as a scholar, but who had not received from his parents, his wife, or his associates the affection, the support, or the status, which a Chinese scholar should receive.

H 7 saw himself as a man of special abilities, with a promising future in Chinese politics, who had accepted unusual responsibilities and challenges, and had been repeatedly frustrated by misfortune.

H 8 saw himself as having been reared by a very strict father, and a demanding older brother. He had wanted to be a musician, but felt it to be his duty to work at an uninteresting career, and to take on many onerous responsibilities.

H 9 saw himself as a serious, responsible person, whose early life had been easy, but who had had to struggle hard ever since then in order to attain his present position.

H 10 saw himself as a person without any special demands or ambitions, who had had a happy childhood, and had tried to do whatever was necessary thereafter, even though some of it had been hard.

The perceptions of the low-frequency group may be epitomized thus:

L 1 saw himself as a man who had had an easy life, involving a number of changes, none of which had been as great as he had thought they might be, and each of which had led to a new and interesting experience.

L 2 did not question the correctness of any of the major decisions she had made and saw herself as destined to overcome any obstacle she might encounter; she took it for granted that she would hold positions of leadership and responsibility. She looked back upon her life with satisfaction.

L 3 saw his childhood as happy and secure, his schooling as enjoyable, and his life as full of interesting experiences and unexpected opportunities.

L 4 saw himself as a man who had had a fortunate childhood, and whose father had provided him with a reliable guide to the course of conduct that he should follow under any circumstances; his life had been full of change and adventure, and some hardship, but he had no doubts and no conflict about any of his decisions.

L 5 saw his childhood as secure, and his later life as interesting and full of opportunity; he regarded his wartime experiences as interesting, though hard, and looked upon his marriage as a move which had turned out well.

L 6 saw herself as a 'lucky person'; she regarded herself as a good mother and a good wife, who was happily married, had had a 'nice time' in childhood, and had never experienced any real hardship.

L 7 saw himself as a person who had had a rather secure and pleasant childhood, who had studied medicine because he had liked it, and who had had to quit through no fault of his own: he regarded his wartime experiences as physically hard, but not otherwise difficult, and saw his present situation as not of his own making; he expected that something would turn up after a while.

L 8 saw himself as a man who had been treated unfairly and deprived of his just due in childhood, who had had to fight for his rights, and had gradually begun to attain them.

L 9 has always been angry, ashamed, and somewhat discouraged about his deformity; he saw himself as a man who wanted to be jolly and well-liked, and become an artist: he had no interest in higher education, regarded his wife with indifference, rather enjoyed his work as a salesman, and enjoyed the companionship of his young son. He looked upon his experiences in the United States as the best part of his life.

L 10 saw herself as a person who was very close to her family, and had spent her life in the midst of them; life had been pleasant and not at all difficult until she came to the United States and went to school and was separated from them. Recently her father's death and the difficulties with her brother had upset her, but she expected that things would be better as soon as she was married.

Summary of Data

The observations and conclusions drawn from the study of the life histories of these two groups of people, described in the foregoing paragraphs, may be summarized thus:

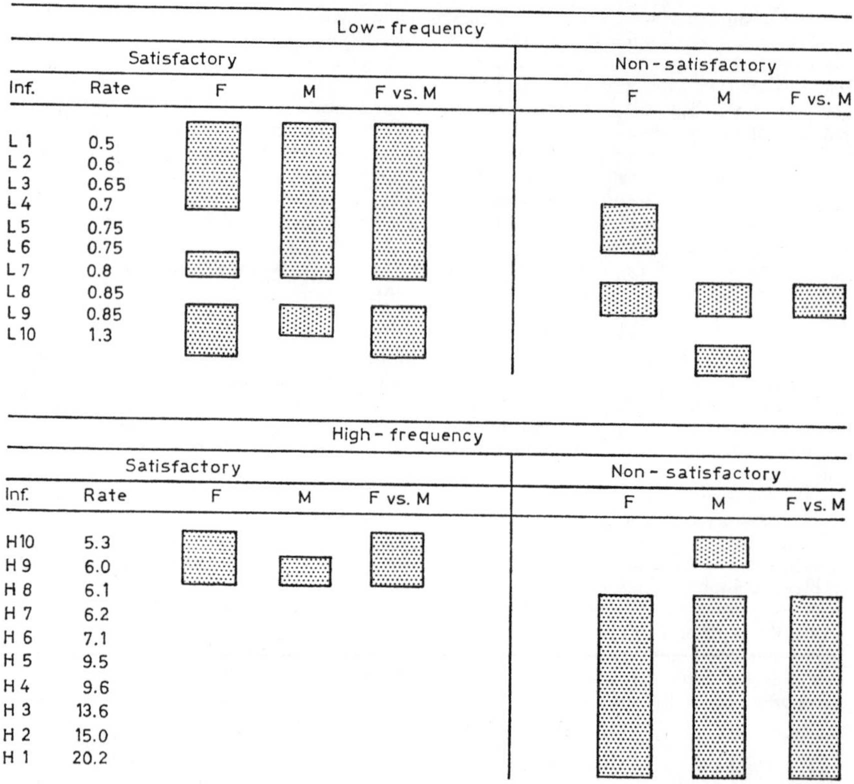

Fig. 5 and 6. Psychiatrist's independent evaluation of each informant's perception of his relation with both parents and the relationship of the parents between themselves. F = father; M = mother; F vs. M = relationship between father and mother.

1. The lifetime environments and the various life experiences of the members of the two groups did not appear to be significantly different, as viewed by an outside observer.

2. On the basis of estimates of trained observers one could not establish a significant difference between the 2 groups with regard to the degree to which members had realized their potentialities and had fulfilled the responsibilities of their positions in life. If anything, the data suggested that some of the more frequently ill were superior in these respects.

3. The members of the 2 groups were notably different in the way in which they had perceived their lives and the various situations that they had encountered.

It was the judgment of the staff that the members of the high-episode group were more predictably oriented toward an identification with goals in which their own self interest was not of paramount importance, and with duties, responsibilities, and ideologies; and they showed more concern about, and reaction to, the events and situations which they encountered than did the members of the 'low frequency' group. It was generally agreed that some of the low-frequency group had shown an unusual lack of concern when confronted by situations which the external observer would have expected to cause them the greatest

Low - frequency				High - frequency			
Inf.	Rate	Emotionally insulated	Emotionally vulnerable	Inf.	Rate	Emotionally insulated	Emotionally vulnerable
L 1	0.5			H 10	5.3		
L 2	0.6			H 9	6.0		
L 3	0.65			H 8	6.1		
L 4	0.7			H 7	6.2		
L 5	0.75			H 6	7.1		
L 6	0.75			H 5	9.5		
L 7	0.8			H 4	9.6		
L 8	0.85			H 3	13.6		
L 9	0.85			H 2	15.0		
L 10	1.3			H 1	20.2		

Fig. 7. Summary of the independent integration of data from all psychological tests for both low-frequency and high-frequency groups. Crosshatching indicates overall patterns. See text for explanation of these categories. The open boxes under the low-frequency group indicate test results not falling clearly into either of these two categories.

concern. They were more concerned with fulfilling those social expectations which advanced their own interests.

When those who make such judgments have prior knowledge of the classification of those judged, their own bias is liable to enter into their decisions. An attempt was made to escape this by submitting the 20 cases to the psychiatrist, without informing him of their ranking and without indicating their grouping. He was asked only whether he could divide these informants into two groups of ten upon any basis, using the psychiatric data alone. In his opinion they were so divisible. 10 of them having perceived their childhood environment, their relationships with their parents, and the relationship between their parents as generally satisfactory, and 10 having perceived these relationships as generally unsatisfactory. When the groupings of the psychiatrist were compared with the ranking of the informants made on the basis of episodes of illness, it was found that 8 of the 10 who saw their childhood environment as 'satisfactory' fell into the low-frequency group, and that 8 of the 10 who saw their childhood environment as 'un-

satisfactory' fell into the high-frequency group. It is improbable that this is a coincidence due to chance alone ($\chi^2 = 7.2$, $p = <0.01$) (fig. 5 and 6).

The independent analysis of the psychological tests indicated personality differences between the two groups [13] (fig. 7). Seven members of the low-frequency group were described as people who 'experienced little conflict or anxiety arising out of interpersonal relations. They showed little insight into themselves, or awareness of emotional problems. In general, they appeared self-centered, morally righteous, insensitive to the needs of others, and rigidly insulated from close interpersonal involvements. However, they were skillful as role players in highly structured situations where demands and expectations were clearly understood and ritualized. Their defense pattern emphasized the use of denial, reaction formation, intellectualization and rationalization.'

All of the informants in the high-frequency group presented psychological test patterns interpreted as showing 'anxiety, tenuous contact with reality, and a pattern of restriction in many important areas of functioning. This pattern of restriction was not a successfully integrated one, and these informants experienced a great deal of tension as a result of their inability to gratify many of their most pressing needs.' They readily discussed emotional and interpersonal problems, partly because of the intensity with which they experienced such problems and their awareness of them. They were more inner-directed, more self-absorbed, and more preoccupied with their difficulties in dealing with other people.

One of the low-frequency group was said to show a pattern similar to those evidenced by the members of the high-frequency group. Two others fell into neither of these categories.

Assessment of the social data allowed less clear-cut conclusions, but directions were apparent. The members of the low-frequency group in general came from more stable families, that were capable of lending more support to their members and had a far lower proportion of polygamous marriages – which had become a source of difficulty among the segment of society from which these Chinese originated. There were more complete families in the group also. More of the members of the low-frequency group also had occupied a preferred sibling position, and had had a positive experience in their schooling, marriages, and careers.

Discussion

Like their American counterparts, these Chinese exhibited differences in susceptibility to illness, which were general as well as specific. Those who had experienced the greater number of sickness episodes per unit time had had more syndromes, involving more organ systems, and falling into a greater number of etiological categories. Biologically they behaved as if they were more easily displaced from an ideal state of 'health' by a variety of means, and in a variety of directions.

The family histories of the members of

the two groups were not notably different with regard to the illness or longevity of the family members. This fact is not of great help in deciding the part that genetic factors may play in such differences in susceptibility, because from a genetic point of view these family histories are very limited and of poor reliability. This is not to say that the informants were themselves unreliable, but simply that they did not possess the pertinent information. That genetic determinants may be of great importance, however, is strongly suggested by the known familial occurrence of many of the syndromes experienced by the members of the high frequency group, such as migraine [7], myopia [8], allergic rhinitis [9] and recurrent depressive illnesses [10].

It is hard to find convincing evidence that the external aspects of the lifetime experiences of the members of the 2 groups were significantly different. Physical hardship, geographic dislocation, social change, and interpersonal difficulties occurred with approximately equal frequency in both groups. Many of those who had few episodes of illness had had an abundant exposure to demanding life experiences. One can only conclude that physical hardship, geographic dislocation, social change, and interpersonal difficulties, even when experienced in large amounts and over long periods of time, did not inevitably cause these Chinese to become ill. The same thing can be said of the members of the 2 American groups that were studied; difficult and demanding life situations not inevitably associated with the occurrence of illness among members of these groups also.

Yet, on the other hand, there can be no doubt that there is some relationship between difficult and demanding life situations and the occurrence of illness. A great majority of these Chinese (as well as a majority of the membres of the American and Hungarian groups who were studied at other times) described many of their periods of illness as being associated with periods of hardship and difficulty [11]. The clue to the relationship appears to lie not so much in the nature of the life situations themselves as in the way that these situations are perceived by those who experience them. This was illustrated by some contrasts between the Chinese in the high- and low-frequency groups. Those who had had a great many illness episodes commonly had viewed their lives (or portions of them) as difficult, demanding, and unsatisfactory, whereas those who had had few illness episodes generally had viewed their lives as interesting, varied, and relatively satisfying. It seems evident that the occurrence of illness is less closely associated with situations which are 'objectively' difficult to the external observer than it is with those situations which are perceived as difficult by the person who experiences the illness.

It is possible that this relationship between the occurrence of illness and the perception of the life situation may be one of parallelism. In other words, viewing life as threatening and unsatisfying may simply be a personality feature associated with whatever constitutional limitations of adaptive capacity lead to an increased susceptibility to illness. However, such a hypothesis does not provide a total explanation of the relationship between illness and the perception of the life situation. The relationship between a man and his social environment is such that he can react only to his evaluation of the configurations which he perceives within it, rather than to the 'actual' life situation itself, as it might be perceived by independent observers [2]. Laboratory experiments have demonstrated the widespread physiological changes that may take place as a part of the reaction to perceived situations, and have also demonstrated the frequency with which such physiological changes are evoked as a part of defensive reaction patterns when a situation is perceived as threatening [12]. Hence, it seems more likely that those who perceive their life situations as threatening, demanding, and unsatisfactory may become more susceptible to illness because of the physio-

logical changes evoked during attempts to adapt to the threats which they perceive.

The observations of the present study lead one to prefer this hypothesis. The intellectual and social accomplishments of the frequently ill Chinese were at least the equals of those of the rarely ill Chinese, some of whom were 'conspicuous failures'. In terms of their responsibility to others, their dedication to principles, and the tenacity with which they pursued goals, the frequently ill Chinese sometimes exceeded the rarely ill, many of whom were self-centered, opportunistic, and without direction or purpose in life. In short, it appeared that some of the frequently ill Chinese viewed their lives as challenging, demanding, and full of conflict because, regardless of the situations in which they found themselves, they tried to abide by principles, to attain goals, or to pursue courses of behavior which might be unrealistic but which they regarded as praiseworthy and socially desirable. On the other hand, some of the rarely ill Chinese viewed their lives as easy, interesting, and varied, because they had not attempted to pursue any particular course in life. They were less bound by abstract principles, and they were more free in pursuing whatever line of behavior rebounded to their own benefit at any given time. Thus, even though the externally observable facts of the lives of these 2 groups of Chinese were similar, it appeared that the frequently ill people were more often challenged and threatened by their life situations, and experienced more physiological and psychological disturbances as a result.

Conclusions

1. The members of this group of Chinese exhibited differences in their general susceptibility to illness such that 25% of the individuals experienced approximately 50% of all episodes of illness over a standard period of young adult life. Those having the greater number of episodes per unit time displayed a greater variety of syndromes, in-

volving a greater number of organ systems, and falling into a greater number of etiological categories.

2. From the total sample, two groups of 10 were selected upon the basis of the number of episodes of illness experienced, the members of one group being frequently ill, and the members of the other rarely so. When the two groups were compared, the following observations were made: a) Family histories revealed no striking differences in the health or longevity of the kin: but many of the syndromes exhibited by the frequently ill are known to be familial in their occurrence. b) The lifetime experiences of the members of both groups were similar in most respects; members of both had faced many difficult life situations. c) In general, the frequently ill appeared to be more predictably oriented toward goals, duties, and responsibilities, and showed more concern about, and reaction to, the events and situations which they encountered. d) The more frequently ill commonly viewed their lives as difficult, demanding, and unsatisfactory, whereas the less frequently ill commonly viewed their lives as interesting, varied, and relatively satisfying. e) Eight of the ten who were frequently ill viewed their relationships with their parents as having been unsatisfactory; a similar proportion of the less frequently ill viewed their relationships with their parents as having been satisfactory. f) The frequently ill were more innerdirected, more self-absorbed, and more highly aware of emotional and interpersonal problems; whereas the less frequently ill had experienced little conflict or anxiety in their interpersonal relations, and showed little awareness of having emotional problems.

3. The findings suggest that the determinants of general susceptibility to illness are both genetic and environmental, but that the actual life situations encountered are less important in this respect than the way in which these situations are perceived. The differences in the number of illness episodes experienced by the members of these groups appear to be related in part to the fact that the more frequently ill people perceived their life experiences as more challenging, more demanding, and more conflict-laden, and experienced more disturbances of bodily processes and of mood, thought, and behavior as a result of their efforts to adapt to a greater number of perceived challenges.

References

1. HINKLE, L. E. Jr., et al.: The distribution of sickness disability in a homogeneous group of healthy adult men. Amer. J. Hyg. 64: 220 (1956).
2. HINKLE, L. E., Jr. and WOLFF, H. G.: The nature of man's adaptation to his total environment and the relation of this to illness. Arch. intern. Med. 99: 442 (1957).
3. HINKLE, L. E., Jr. et al.: Differences in general susceptibility to illness occurring among the members of a group of adult men over a twenty-year period.
4. HINKLE, L. E., Jr. and PLUMMER, N.: Life stress and industrial absenteeism: The concentration of illness and absenteeism in one segment of a working population. Industr. Med. Surg. 21: 363 (1952).
5. HINKLE, L. E., Jr. et al.: Reports in preparation.
6. Standard Nomenclature of Diseases and Operations (ed. 4) (McGraw-Hill, New York 1952).
7. GOODELL, H.; LEWONTIN, R., and WOLFF, H. G.: The familial occurrence of migraine headache: A study of heredity; in Genetics and the inheritance of integrated neurological and psychiatric patterns. Res. Publ. Ass. nerv. ment. Dis. 33 (1954).
8. GATES, R. R.: Human genetics, vol. 1, p. 192 (Macmillan, New York 1946).
9. NEEL, J. V. and SCHULL, W. J.: Human heredity, pp. 20, 81 (Univ. Chicago, Chicago Press, 1954).
10. KALLMANN, F. J.: The genetics of psychotic behavior patterns; in: Genetics and the inheritance of integrated neurological and psychiatric patterns. Res. Publ. Ass. nerv. ment. Dis. 33 (1954).
11. HINKLE, L. E., Jr. et al.: Studies in human ecology: Factors governing the adaptation of Chinese unable to return to China; in Experimental psychopathology, pp. 170–186 (Grune & Stratton, New York 1957).
12. WOLFF, H. G.: Stress and disease. Publication No. 166, American Lecture Series, Monograph in Bannerstone Division of American Lectures on Physiology, R. F. PITTS (ed.) (Thomas, Springfield 1953).
13. THETFORD, W. N.: A cross-cultural approach to the study of personality and illness.

Relationship of Specific Attitudes and Emotions to Certain Bodily Diseases[1]

W. J. GRACE and D. T. GRAHAM

Retrospective comment by Dr. P. Knapp. GRACE and GRAHAM introduce in the following paper their concept of *specific attitudes* in psychosomatic illnesses. This notion represents a way station in the continued effort by psychosomatic research workers to deal with the tantalizing problem of specificity, so easy to inspire a subjective sense of conviction, so difficult of objective demonstration. Coming on the heels of earlier propositions about specific personalities and specific unconscious emotional conflict, and growing out of the 'life stress' studies by HAROLD WOLFF and his group, the attitude hypothesis had simple and appealing features. It circumscribed the areas which individuals, who obviously differ, might necessarily share in sharing the same syndrome; and it suggested that manifest, verbalizable, and observable features might be as important, or more so, than deeper, inferential, and less accessible factors. Of still greater value, their view of attitude broke down the complex range of phenomena subsumed under the term 'emotion'. It focussed particularly on the relatively persistent, expressive aspects of emotional behavior. In suggesting that 'attitude' might be crucial to bodily symptom formation the authors thus formed a sort of bridge, running between one view, that of ALEXANDER, that psychosomatic symptoms were an obligatory consequence of stereotyped autonomic nervous and glandular mobilization, and another view, that of early psychodynamic investigators like FELIX DEUTSCH, who saw such symptoms as a form of primitive 'pregenital' conversion.

New scientific ideas appear in various guises, sometimes as the culmination of a series of long and elegantly executed steps, sometimes as part of a more preliminary phase of investigation. The latter is the case here. After a decade and a half, when one reviews the actual evidence contained in this single paper by GRACE and GRAHAM, one is left with gaps. Many of these were filled out in subsequent publications, particularly those by GRAHAM and his group. Their original report, and its ideas, have heuristic, and enduring importance.

There is now evidence that many symptoms and diseases occur in settings of difficult life situations [1, 6, 14]. In spite of this, however, the reason why some individuals suffer from one disease or symptom and others from another continues to arouse considerable discussion.

Previous attempts to find something in common among persons with any given disease, other than the disease itself, fall into several loosely defined and not mutually exclusive categories. In the first place, there have been attempts to demonstrate a particular kind of personality pattern in all patients with the same disease. Migrainous individuals, for example, have been described as having 'feelings of insecurity with tension, manifested as inflexibility, conscientiousness, meticulousness, perfectionism, and resentment' [22]. A modification of this has consisted of the identification of a single personality trait or characteristic, defined in terms of overt behavior in association with a particular disease, as for

[1] From the Department of Medicine, of the New York Hospital-Cornell Medical Center.

instance, 'obsessive-compulsive behavior' and 'subnormal assertiveness' with arterial hypertension [9] or 'non-participation' with rhinitis [12]. A prominent psychoanalytic point of view, which could in some instances be combined with the preceding, is that the common denominator in individuals with the same disease is a 'nuclear conflict' or 'dynamic configuration' unique to the disease in question, the significant factors being largely unconscious [1]. An older formulation is the notion of 'organ inferiority', the assumption that certain individuals have particular organs predisposed to disturbance, so that in some persons any kind of life stress will result in gastric dysfunction, for example.

A somewhat different approach to the problem has revolved around an investigation of what has happened to the patient previously, especially in childhood, with relatively little attention paid to the aspects of the present situation which are important to his disease. An example of this is the search for toilet-training conflicts in the histories of patients with constipation and diarrhea [11].

Finally, there have been efforts to correlate the occurrence of particular symptoms with particular situations, as, for instance, asthmatic attacks with withdrawal of a mother's love. These have usually not been rigidly restricted to an objective description of the situation, however, since some qualification in terms of the patient's perception of it is ordinarily introduced. Perhaps the closest approach to the views expressed in the present paper is GROEN's [10] statement that the onset of ulcerative colitis occurred at times of 'acute love-loss and painful humiliation'.

These formulations contain considerable truth and have contributed significantly to our understanding and knowledge of human behavior, but they have been unsatisfactory in some respects. There are, for example, some persons with migraine who do not show the personality features described to an outstanding degree, just as there are individuals who show these features and do not have migraine. Also, many patients manifest a great variety of symptoms during their lives, often with fairly rapid changes; this phenomenon is difficult to reconcile with the notion of fixed personality patterns belonging to different diseases. The same objection can be raised against the idea of 'organ inferiority'. (In addition, an organ such as the colon cannot be considered 'weak' if it is working all the time [21].) We have seen one patient who had at different times angina pectoris, eczema, vasospastic retinopathy, diarrhea, vomiting, and backache; and there are many persons who show at least 2 diseases, such as vasomotor rhinitis and ulcerative colitis, or peptic ulcer and migraine. It seems, in fact, that the majority of patients if followed for an extended period will show more than one symptom, although of course one may predominate over the others.

The concept of the single, significant personality trait has not been much explored. It is an attractive notion, since a single individual may have many traits. It does appear, however, that traits will be found in many persons free of the corresponding diseases and that some with a disease may not have the trait in question. The correlations of 'obsessive-compulsive behavior' and 'subnormal assertiveness' with arterial hypertension, for example, although significant statistically, were far from perfect [9]. Obvious difficulties arise also in connection with the definition of traits and in their measurement. Similar considerations apply to the 'specific dynamic configuration' theory, and it has been explicitly stated [1] that there are persons who have the configuration without having the disease in question. In both of these approaches there is a relative lack of emphasis on correlating definite events in the individual's life with exacerbations of symptoms.

Attempts to find common factors in early life experiences of individuals with the same disease have not met with uniform success. For instance, difficulty in early toilet training seemed to play no part in ulcerative colitis [15]. There may well be such factors, however, which have been missed because the relevant variables have not been isolated.

Finally, there is not necessarily any striking external similarity among the situations which provoke exacerbations of any one disease in the same patient or in different patients; nor is the same situation always associated with attacks. The greater the extent to which the patient's way of looking at the situation is introduced into this formulation, the more closely it approaches the thesis of the present paper. No one, however, has given clear-cut statements of the patients' attitudes.

In the course of attempting to resolve these difficulties it became apparent that there was associated with each symptom a definite attitude which was peculiar to it, and without which it did not occur. In order to explore this approach further, a systematic method of questioning patients was employed.

Method

One hundred and twenty-eight patients, who had one or more of the 12 symptoms or diseases studied, were followed in treatment in the outpatient department. Interviews with the patients by one or the other of the authors were the only method of obtaining the information used in this paper. Interviews usually lasted about 1 h, and took place as often as twice a week and as infrequently as once in 3 months. Most of the patients made a total of 10 or more visits to the clinic.

In the interviews, emphasis was first placed on defining the situations temporally associated with attacks of the patient's symptoms. After such a situation had been identified, the next step was to obtain from him a description of his *attitude, by which is meant a clear and unambiguous statement of what he felt was happening to him, and what he wanted to do about it, at the time of the occurrence of the symptom.* This last point is of major importance, as it was found that often an individual felt in one way about the precipitating event during an interview, but in another way at the

time symptoms were developing. Conventional names of 'emotions', such as 'anger', 'resentment', 'sadness', etc., were not accepted without further definition.

It was noted, in the first place, that many of the patients with the same symptom-complex spontaneously referred to their life-situations and their own reactions in the same way. Those who did not were asked to describe the situation in the terms outlined above. Patients who were still unable to grasp the task were given a set of possibilities from among which they were told to select those most applicable to themselves.

No attempt was made to utilize dream or associative material in collecting the data used in this study. All of the conclusions are based entirely on direct statements by the patients.

Surprisingly little difficulty was encountered with most patients in obtaining unequivocal answers to the questions asked. Obstacles arose chiefly with reticent or bland individuals in trying to discover exactly what the stressful situation was. Without this information the method described of eliciting the patient's attitude cannot be employed. There was an occasional patient who, although willing to say that he was 'upset' by some event, refused to go any further without strong urging.

Results

All patients with the same symptom-complex described their attitudes toward the situation which precipitated it in essentially the same way.

The following attitudes and physiological disturbances were found to be associated:

1. Urticaria (31 patients) occurred when an individual saw himself as being mistreated. This mistreatment might take the form of something said to him or something done to him. He was preoccupied entirely with what was happening to him, and was not thinking of retaliation or of any solution of his problem. Typical statements were: 'They did a lot of things to me and I couldn't do anything about it.' 'I was taking a beating.' 'My mother was hammering

on me.' 'The boss cracked a whip on me.' 'My fiancée knocked me down and walked all over me but what could I do?'

2. Eczema (27 patients) occurred when an individual felt that he was being interfered with or prevented from doing something, and could think of no way to deal with the frustration. His preoccupation was with the interference and the persons or things thwarting him, rather than with the goals or aims which concerned migraine patients. Typical statements were: 'I want to make my mother understand, but I can't.' 'I couldn't do what I wanted but there wasn't anything I could do about it.' 'It upset me because it interfered with what I wanted to do.' 'I felt terribly frustrated.'

In addition, however, minor attacks of urticaria or exacerbations of eczema occurred when the individual felt that he was being looked at and had no response to make – the feeling commonly called 'embarrassment'. An additional feature in many instances of eczema was the aggression directed toward the self, expressed in the statement, 'I take it out on myself'.

3. Cold and moist hands (10 patients) occurred when an individual felt that he should undertake some kind of activity, even though he might not know precisely what to do. Typical statements were: 'I wanted to hit him.' 'I just had to be doing something.' 'Something ought to be done.' 'I wanted to do something.' In Raynaud's disease (4 patients) the coldness of the hands is carried to the extreme. The action contemplated by those with Raynaud's disease was characteristically a hostile one. Typical statements were 'I wanted to hit him.' 'I wanted to put a knife through him.' 'I wanted to strangle him.'

4. Vasomotor rhinitis (12 patients) occurred when an individual was facing a situation with the wish that he didn't have to do anything about it, or that it would go away, or that somebody else would take over the responsibility. The essential feature was the desire to have nothing to do with the situation at all, to deal with it by excluding it. Typical statements were: 'I wanted them to go away.' 'I didn't want to have anything to do with it.' 'I wanted to blot it all out, I wanted to build a wall between me and him.' 'I wanted to hole up for the winter.' 'I wanted to go to bed and pull the sheets over my head.'

5. Asthma (7 patients) occurred in association with attitudes exactly like those associated with vasomotor rhinitis. Presumably in asthma the feelings are more intense, but since no measure of strength of attitude was employed, this cannot be categorically stated. It is consistent with this formulation that attacks of asthma are almost invariably accompanied by vasomotor rhinitis, although the reverse is not true. In short, the two seem to be essentially the same disease, the difference between them being one of severity. Typical statements were: 'I wanted them to go away.' 'I didn't want to have anything to do with it.' 'I just couldn't face it.'

6. Diarrhea (27 patients) occurred when an individual wanted to be done with a situation or to have it over with, or to get rid of something or somebody. One man who developed severe diarrhea after he had purchased a defective automobile said: 'If I could only get rid of it!' 'I want to dispose it.' Typical statements of others were: 'If the war was only over with.' 'I wanted to get done with it.' 'I wanted to get it finished with.'

7. Constipation (17 patients) occurred when an individual was grimly determined to carry on even though faced with a problem he could not solve. Typical statements were: 'I have to keep on with this, but I know I'm not going to like it.' 'It's a lousy job but it's the best I can do.' 'This marriage is never going to be any better but I won't quit.' 'I have to keep on with this but I don't like it.' 'I'll stick with it even though nothing good will come of it.'

8. Nausea and vomiting (11 patients) occurred when an individual was thinking of something which he wished had never happened. He was preoccupied with the mistake he had made, rather than with what he should have done instead. Usually he felt responsible for what had happened. Typical statements: 'I wish it hadn't happened.' 'I was sorry I did it.' 'I wish things were the way they were before.' 'I made a mistake.' 'I shouldn't have listened to him.'

9. Duodenal ulcer (9 patients) occurred when an individual was seeking revenge. He wished to injure the person or thing that had injured him. Typical statements were: 'I wanted to get even.' 'I wanted to get back at him.' 'I wanted revenge.' 'He hurt me so I wanted to hurt him.' 'I did it for spite.'

10. Migraine headache (14 patients) occurred when an individual had been making an intense effort to carry out a definite planned program, or to achieve some definite objective. The headache occurred when the effort had ceased, no matter whether the activity had been associated with success or failure. The essential features were striving and subsequent relaxation. Typical statements were: 'I had to get it done.' 'I had to meet a deadline.' 'I had a million things to do before lunch.' 'I was trying to get all these things accomplished.'

11. Arterial hypertension (7 patients) occurred when an individual felt that he must be constantly prepared to meet all possible threats. Typical statements were: 'I had to be ready for anything.' 'It was up to me to take care of all the worries.' 'Nobody is ever going to beat me, I'm ready for everything.'

12. Low back pain (11 patients) occurred when an individual wanted to carry out some action involving movement of the entire body. The activity which such patients were most commonly thinking about was walking or running away. One 16-year-old girl spent most of her waking hours contemplating various schemes for running away from home. Typical statements were: 'I just wanted to walk out of the house.' 'I wanted to run away.' 'I wanted to get out of there.' 'I felt like taking a flying leap off that island.'

Comment

It is interesting to inquire whether a generalization concerning these observed relations can be found. It appears that in many cases the attitude can be considered as a description of the function of the physiological process with which it is associated. This is an extension of the formulation previously made particularly by CANNON [5] and WOLFF [21].

1. Vasodilatation is the reaction of the skin to trauma. Whealing occurs when vasodilatation is intense. The patient with urticaria feels that he is receiving a blow, and that there is nothing he can do about it [8].

3. Cold skin is the result of cutaneous vasoconstriction [3]. Its occurrence in the individual who is contemplating some kind of action probably represents the functioning of a mechanism to raise body temperature by reducing heat loss. That an elevated body temperature is desirable for the active organism is suggested by the fact that the elevation occurs to the same extent with a standard amount of exercise whether heat loss is experimentally facilitated or interfered with [17].

4 and 5. The reaction of the respiratory mucous membrane to a noxious agent is to exclude it by swelling of the membrane with consequent narrowing of the passageway, and to dilute it and wash it out by hypersecretion [12]. When these changes are limited to the nose, the reaction is called vasomotor rhinitis; when they are sufficiently intense to include the bronchi, so

that wheezing occurs, the name 'asthma' is applied.

6. Defecation is a way of ridding the body of substances which have been taken in but are no longer useful. Diarrhea, or frequent defecation, occurs in the setting of an intense desire to get something over with or to dispose of something.

7. Constipation is a phenomenon of holding on without change. This corresponds to the patients' attitudes of trying to continue with things as they are, without hope of immediate improvement, or definite desire to do anything different [2, 7].

8. Vomiting is a way of undoing something which has been done. It thus corresponds to the patient's wishes to restore things to their original situation, as if nothing had ever happened.

9. Duodenal ulcer is probably the end-result of protracted gastric hyperfunction. It has been suggested that such hyperfunction is part of the preparation for eating [20]. Directing aggression into the particular channel of eating seems to make sense biologically, for the only way an injured animal can use the animal which injured him as a source of materials for tissue repair is to devour him. An individual with duodenal ulcer desires revenge – that is, he wishes to hurt the person who hurt him.

12. The backache which accompanies the desire of the individual to walk out of his situation is probably consequent to the tension of the lumbar muscles. The latter fix the spinal column in preparation for locomotion [19]. It has been shown that thinking about lifting a weight is associated with increased electrical activity in the appropriate muscles [13]. It has also been demonstrated that sustained contraction of skeletal muscles can be painful [18].

The biological function of the bodily changes underlying others of the symptoms

is obscure. The value of elevation of the diastolic blood pressure is not clear at present, although it seems probable that there are circumstances under which it is a useful response. The vasodilatation of frustration, seen in eczema, may possibly represent a method of heat loss by an organism which has abandoned its readiness for action. The occurrence in the head of vasoconstriction followed by vasodilatation, which underlies migraine, has no useful function which is obvious at present.

Discussion

The present approach differs from those discussed in its emphasis on the nature of the patient's reaction to the situations which precipitate attacks of his illness. The reaction of an adult human being consists of an *attitude*, which can be expressed verbally, and accompanying *bodily changes*. By 'attitude' is meant the way in which he perceives his own position in the situation, and the action, if any, which he wishes to take to deal with it. The bodily changes, if sufficiently intense and prolonged, give rise to experiences which have names and are called 'symptoms', such as palpitations or diarrhea. If the phenomena recur or persist, and especially if they lead to structural changes, they are said to represent a 'disease'. Most of the common diseases can be viewed as the outcome of physiological adjustments which, although perfectly appropriate in some circumstances, may eventually entail discomfort, disability and danger to the organism.

It will be noted that, although the above definition of attitude has two aspects, in many of the specific attitudes discussed – for example that accompanying diarrhea – there is no mention of the first component. The reason for this is that no consistencies were discovered in the statements of patients in question about what they felt was happening to them, although they all wished to deal with the traumatic situation in the same way. It is possible that further investigation in certain of the syndromes will reveal common denominators in the first component of the attitude as well as the second, and to this extent the attitude statements given may be incomplete. It may be, for instance, that persons with duodenal ulcer always regard the situations responsible for their symptoms as injuries of a particular kind.

The results of this study suggest that each attitude is associated with its own unique set of bodily changes. The possibility of the existence of such a relationship has been suggested by BULL [4]. Nothing is implied in this connection about a cause-and-effect relation between 'mental' and 'physical' events, and, indeed, it seems unprofitable to look at the matter in this light.

This conclusion is in opposition to the widely-held view [16] that there is no predictable relation between the 'emotion' felt and the physiological changes which accompany it. There seem to have been at least three reasons for the adoption of this position. The first was the attemps to work with an inadequate vocabulary, so that the range of possible attitudes was not sufficiently explored. Second, questioning was not conducted in such a way that precise attitudes were ascertained, the experimenter or therapist remaining content with the 'name' of the emotion supplied by the subject or patient, or suggested by his own appraisal of the situation. This introduces the difficulty that not all individuals attach the same meanings to the common words denoting feelingstates. Third, only a very few of the large number of possible physiological variables were measured, for example cardiovascular changes and the galvanic skin responses.

These considerations suggest the advisability of defining the word emotion[2], so that it means *an attitude and the associated bodily changes*. This implies that there are a very large number of possible emotions, probably many more than are conventionally considered, since there are a large number of possible attitudes toward situations. It also implies that there is no such thing as 'non-emotional' behavior, since it is presumably impossible to do anything or think about anything without adopting some attitude. In ordinary speech, however, emotions are not recognized until they reach a certain intensity.

Looked at in this way, it becomes apparent that most emotions have no specific or appropriate name. There are, however, suitable words in the English language to describe some of them, with at least some degree of exactness. According to Webster's Collegiate Dictionary (1939), for instance, *resentment* is a 'feeling of indignant displeasure because of something regarded as a wrong, insult, etc.'. This is a good description of the attitude of patients who have urticaria. *Hostility* is 'antagonism, especially as manifested in action'. Wishes to take hostile action are associated with Raynaud's disease. *Regret* is 'a wishing that something had not happened'. (Funk and Wagnalls College Standard Dictionary, 1933.) This is the attitude associated with vomiting.

'Anxiety' is a term which is widely used in psychiatry, but one for which there is no generally accepted precise definition. If one considered those individuals who have the symptoms ordinarily considered those of 'anxiety', it is fairly evident that their attitude consists of two major components. The first is *apprehension*, the feeling that something bad is about to happen, and the second is an urge to action of some kind, a feeling that something must be done (even though there is no clear idea of what to do) which may be named *tension*. The names are not important, but it is important that there are such feelings, and that they can be clearly expressed by patients. The complete anxiety syndrome, then, consists of a feel-

[2] There is considerable dissatisfaction with present definitions of emotion especially with respect to the distinction between 'emotional' and 'non-emotional' behavior. See, for example, the series of papers on emotion in Psychological Review during 1948 and 1949.

ing that something bad will happen, together with an urge to do something. The physiological correlates of these attitudes, however, have not been clarified. It is suggested that the term 'anxiety' be reserved for the co-existence of these two attitudes with their accompanying physiological changes.

It may be well to emphasize again that the correlation of attitudes with bodily changes given above is based entirely on the patient's statements about their feelings, and not on interpretation of dream or fantasy material with inferences concerning the content of the unconscious. In other words, a clear-cut statement of any attitude was accepted at its face value. It is, in fact, surprising how aware patients are of their attitudes toward particular circumstances, and how readily they can verbalize them. The reasons, on the other hand, which determine the way a situation is viewed are very likely to be unconscious.

It is commonly held that patients' declarations about their feelings are of little significance. Some individuals, for example, may say of a situation which is repeatedly associated with attacks of their symptoms, 'It doesn't bother me'. It is however, highly significant that if a patient admitted to an awareness of any emotional disturbance at all, and could be made to describe his attitude toward the precipitating event in the terms outlined above, he always did so in the same way as all the other patients with the same syndrome. The importance of such statements is supported by the correlations between them and the observed physiological changes. If what the patients said was really completely 'unreliable', no consistent relation between verbalizations and bodily changes would be possible.

It sometimes happened that a patient expressed about some situation one of the attitudes listed, without developing the corresponding symptoms. This is presumably because the feeling was not sufficiently intense or long-lasting, so that only transitory and minor physiological changes occurred.

Such findings are therefore not evidence against the thesis of this paper. What is crucial, however, is that no attack of any of the symptoms mentioned occurred in the absence of the appropriate attitude. It is probable that all human beings develop at one time or another the attitudes and associated somatic changes described. The person who gets symptoms severe enough to make him a patient simply feels a particular way very intensely and for a long time.

Most persons show some consistency in the attitudes they have. A single individual, in other words, 'selects' from the wide range of possible attitudes one or a few which he develops often and intensely, to the relative exclusion of others. Since different attitudes lead to different kinds of overt behavior, one would predict some correlation between personality traits and diseases. This individual consistency in attitude seems also to be of importance in keeping disease processes active. Asthmatics, for instance, often state that they wish not to have to think about or deal with their asthma, and persons with diarrhea say that they wish to be rid of their symptoms.

It is important to know what it is in the life history of a patient which predisposed him to adopt the response (attitude and bodily change) which eventually culminated in disease. Are there common factors in the lives of persons with asthma, for instance, which have made them especially prone to wish to shut unpleasant things away from them? It seems probably that there are certain experiences, particularly exposure to attitudes and behavior of parents, which result in the development of predictable attitudes in any individual exposed to them, and that all patients with the same disease have had lives with these experiences in common. Their reactions to their present situations are, of course, in large part determined by their previous learning. There is, however, reason to think that certain situations encountered for the first time in adult life may have intrinsically a high potentiality for evoking particular attitudes and bodily changes, just as they would in a child.

It is probably also true that some persons have been exposed to environments producting more than one kind of traumatic situation, repeated often enough to be significant. These individuals are presumably those who react as adults with many different symptoms, the nature of which is determined by the situation.

With a few of the common syndromes it has been possible to identify experiences of early life which seem highly relevant to adult attitudes and diseases, and which are found in the background of many of the patients with the syndrome. One girl whose chief complaint was backache, for instance, had a mother who constantly threatened to pack her bags and walk out of the home. Another woman, who developed severe vomiting as a reaction to her life situation, had been thoroughly indoctrinated with the idea of the impossibility of atonement for sin, so that having once done something which she felt was wrong she was completely preoccupied with wishing it hadn't happened.

This is a first report, and greater objectivity in the evaluation of attitudes is desirable in order to obviate the criticism that patients' statements are so loose as to be open to any number of interpretations, or that suggestion by the therapist may have played a part. The method of questioning was designed to avoid these difficulties, but, in addition, a questionnaire has been made up to be presented to patients after the event responsible for an attack of their symptoms has been clearly defined. It consists of about fifty questions representing a variety of possible attitudes toward life situations, the patient answering 'yes' to those he thinks best represent his attitudes at the time the symptoms developed. For example, questions pertinent to diarrhea are, 'Did you feel that you wanted to get rid of someone or something?', and 'Did you feel that there was something you wanted to get over with or done with?'.

Summary and Conclusions

1. One hundred and twenty-eight patients who had one or more of the following symptoms or diseases as responses to life situations, were studied: urticaria, eczema, cold hands, vasomotor rhinitis and asthma, diarrhea, constipation, nausea and vomiting, duodenal ulcer, migraine, arterial hypertension, low back pain.

2. It was found that each of these conditions was associated with a particular, completely conscious, attitude toward the precipitating situation. There were, in other words, physiological changes specific to each attitude.

3. These changes are biologically appropriate to the attitudes they accompany.

4. It is proposed that 'emotion' be defined to mean 'an attitude with its associated physiological changes'.

References

1. ALEXANDER, F. G.: Psychosomatic medicine, its principles and applications (Norton & Co., New York 1950).
2. ALMY, T. P.; KERN, F., and ABBOT, F.: Constipation and diarrhea. Ass. Res. nerv. ment. Dis., Proc. 29: 724 (1950).
3. BROBECK, J. R.: Regulation of energy exchange; in FULTON A textbook of Physiology, ed. 16 (Saunders Co., Philadelphia 1949).
4. BULL, N.: Toward a clarification of the concept of emotion. Psychosom. Med. 7: 210 (1945).
5. CANNON, W. B.: Bodily changes in pain, hunger, fear and rage (Appleton and Co., New York 1929).
6. DUNBAR, F.: Emotions and bodily changes, ed. 3 (Columbia University Press, New York 1947).
7. GRACE, W. J.; WOLF, S., and WOLFF, H. G.: The human colon (Hoeber, Inc., New York 1951).
8. GRAHAM, D. T.: The pathogenesis of hives. Ass. Res. nerv. ment. Dis., Proc. 29: 987 (1950).
9. GRESSEL, G. C.; SHOBE, F. O.; SASLOW, G.; DuBois, P. H., and SCHROEDER, H. A.: Personality factors in arterial hypertension. J. amer. med. Ass. 140: 265 (1949).
10. GROEN, J.: Psychogenesis and psychotherapy of ulcerative colitis. Psychosom. Med. 9: 151 (1947).

11. HALLIDAY, J. L.: Psychological medicine (Norton & Co., New York 1948).

12. HOLMES, T. H.; GOODELL, H.; WOLF, S., and WOLFF, H. G.: The nose (Thomas, Springfield 1950).

13. JACOBSON, E.: Electrophysiology of mental activities. Amer. J. Psychol. *44:* 677 (1932).

14. Life stress and bodily disease: Proceedings of the association for research in nervous and mental. Disease, December 2 and 3, 1949 (Williams & Wilkins Co., Baltimore 1950).

15. MAHONEY, V. P.; BOCKUS, H. L.; INGRAM, M.; HUNDLEY, J. W., and YASKIN, J. C.: Studies on ulcerative colitis. Gastroenterology *13:* 547 (1950).

16. MUNN, N. L.: Psychology: The fundamentals of human adjustment (Houghton Mifflin Co., Boston 1946).

17. NIELSEN, M.: Die Regulation der Körpertemperatur bei Muskelarbeit. Skand. Arch. Physiol. *79:* 193 (1948).

18. SIMONS, D. J.; DAY, E.; GOODELL, H., and WOLFF, H. G.: Experimental studies on headache; muscles of the scalp and neck as sources of pain. Ass. Res. nerv. ment. Dis., Proc. *23:* 228 (1943).

19. STEINDLER, A.: Mechanics of normal and pathological locomotion (Thomas, Springfield 1935).

20. WOLF, S. and WOLFF, H. G.: Human gastric function, ed. 2 (Oxford University Press, New York 1947).

21. WOLFF, H. G.: Protective reaction patterns and disease. Ann. Intern. Med. *27:* 944 (1947).

22. WOLFF, H. G.: Headache and other head pain (Oxford University Press, New York 1948).